Practical Guide to Psychiatric Medications

Practical Guide to Psychiatric Medications

Simple, Concise, & Up-to-date

Tanveer A. Padder, MD

Published by MTP Publishing, LLC. Maryland, USA
Feedback: mypsychiatryguide@gmail.com
ISBN-13: 9781514374023
ISBN-10: 1514374021
Printed in the United States of America
Library of Congress Control Number: 2014904606
CreateSpace Independent Publishing Platform
North Charleston, South Carolina
First Edition

Acknowledgements

First and foremost, this guide is dedicated to all of my patients and their family members who made the very idea of this book conceivable through their continued trust and contributions. Thank you for enabling me to enhance and develop my expertise in psychiatry and share this resource with the medical and psychiatric community.

I would like to offer special gratitude to the pioneers in the field of psychopharmacology whose work has been a beacon of light for me in completing this guide. Thank you, Dr. Alan Schatzberg, Dr. Charles Nemeroff, Dr. Jonathan Cole, Dr. Charles Debattista, Dr. Glen Gabbard, and Dr. Stephen Stahl, among others, for your expertise and contributions to the field.

To my editor Amanda, I want to express my sincere appreciation for your expertise and suggestions that have helped form this guide to convey the most relevant clinical material in an accessible, professional, and pertinent manner.

To my research assistants Prakash and Sarah, I offer my gratitude for your hard work in researching, compiling data, and editing as well as condensing various resources.

To my parents and siblings, I offer grateful recognition of your love and support. You have helped shape my passion for psychiatry and have encouraged me to persevere in my clinical efforts.

Above all, I want to express my deepest thanks to my wife and children. Thank you for respecting my busy schedule and for constantly supporting me in my endeavor. This guide would not have been possible without your encouragement and sacrifice.

Finally, I extend my appreciation to the many other extraordinary individuals who assisted me throughout the composition of this guide. Thank you to everyone who discussed data, offered suggestions, granted permission to reference work, and collaborated with me to bring this guide to life.

Disclaimer

The entirety of this guide is provided for informational and educational purposes only and is not intended under any circumstances to replace or be used to disregard professional medical or psychiatric advice. This guide does not propose to treat any medical or psychiatric condition apart from the direction of a qualified, licensed medical and/or psychiatric professional and should not substitute or supersede their professional recommendations. Reliance on this guide is to be practiced solely at the reader's risk.

The author, editors, and publisher have sought to ensure that all information is consistent with the current standards defined by the US Food and Drug Administration (FDA) and by the general medical/psychiatric community. While great care has been taken to ensure accurate drug or supplement dosages, indications, warnings/precautions, adverse effects, contraindications, and other important information, this guide does not exhaustively or definitively represent all of the information that may be necessary for the proper prescription or use of the drugs and supplements listed herein. All readers should consult the drug package insert provided by the manufacturer, the current *Physician's Desk Reference* (PDR), and any latest communications from the FDA to become aware of any changes in the proper administration of a drug.

References to other potential uses of medications are not FDA approved, are considered off-label, and are purely based on standards of care, clinical evidence, and practical experience. These off-label uses are sometimes acceptable, although not recommended, standards within the psychiatric and medical communities. Off-label use of medications should only be considered based on the latest clinical evidence, and this guide should only serve as a reference and is not an endorsement of these uses. Informed consent should always be obtained to apprise patients of any related or anticipated risks, benefits, and treatment alternatives.

Every effort was made to ensure that the information contained herein accurately reflects the presently accepted medical and psychiatric standards at the time of publication. Future research or changes in regulatory procedures may alter clinical standards and practices. Consequently, the author, editors, and publisher make no warranty that this guide is free of human error, omissions, or other perceived inaccuracy. Readers should confirm the information contained in this guide with other current peer-reviewed sources.

The author, editors, and the publisher disclaim any and all liability in any manner for any direct, indirect, incidental, consequential, or punitive damages that may arise from the interpretation of the information presented in this guide, especially any reference to other potential uses of medications.

The content of this guide is not designed to promote or endorse any medical procedures or products. The author has no conflicts of interest to disclose—professional, financial, or otherwise. No part of this guide has been influenced by sponsors. Neither financial support nor any other contributions were received from any of the manufacturers or stakeholders of the products discussed in this guide.

Table of Contents

Preface

For many years now, medical and mental health professionals have desired a straightforward, portable reference guide offering a comprehensive but concise resource on psychiatric medications—myself included. As the medical director of multiple mental health clinics, I have witnessed firsthand the obstacles faced by my colleagues in the day-to-day practice of prescribing and monitoring these medications. The lack of such a guide has condemned mental health clinicians to spend an exhaustive portion of their time and energy digging through the literature to review the nuances of medications—time that could be better spent with patients. Although there is an enormous range of resources on psychiatric medications available online and in print, to date no definitive guide has offered essential information in a unified, portable, reliable, user-friendly, and elegant way.

I began constructing this guide by reflecting upon the past 12 years of my career, asking myself fundamental questions about the type of information clinicians need in everyday practice and seeking to distill the information down to its purest form. I then reached out for guidance from the best resources, reading hundreds of books and articles, reviewing lectures, speaking with fellow clinicians, and reviewing patient treatments in various settings. Compiling all of the material was simple; condensing it down to the most pertinent information was laborious, to say the least. The result is a guide that not only covers the major facts about the most commonly used psychiatric drugs but also provides clinically actionable information such as the latest FDA-approved indications, dosing protocols, warnings, drug interactions, common side effects, contraindications, use in special populations, and more. All of these components are incorporated in this guide through evidence-based clinical recommendations presented in an accessible manner, without superfluous intricacy.

Of all the challenges encountered in the creation of this guide, the biggest one was balancing a copious amount of information with what was practically important. I chose to base many content decisions on my own clinical and educational experiences. Many psychopharmacological manuals often present an overwhelming amount of information, reviewing every known possibility. Such breadth of knowledge is a double-edged sword, often leading busy clinicians and their patients astray. In contrast, I have intentionally structured this book for ease of use, categorizing and explaining various drugs in their specific pharmacological classes and only offering the most clinically-relevant information. Further, this book's compact format is priced affordably and is designed for the busy clinician in practice, the young medical professional in training, and all others responsible for prescribing and monitoring the use of psychiatric medications.

I trust that this guide will enable clinicians to quickly and effectively glean current, comprehensive information about psychiatric drugs, both to strengthen performance in daily practice and to broaden knowledge. Ultimately, I see this guide as a tool that will positively impact how clinicians work by equipping them with all of the information they need to provide the best possible care to their patients.

Tanveer A. Padder, MD
June 27, 2015

Introduction

Despite decades of research and medical advancements, the epidemic of mental illness continues to plague the world's population with no relief in sight. The World Health Organization (WHO) predicts that mental illness will become the leading contributor to the global burden of disease by the year 2020. According to the National Institute of Mental Health (NIMH), about one in four Americans (approximately 61.5 million people) have been diagnosed with some form of mental illness.[1] With a significant part of the population at risk and the burden of illness contributing to over $317 billion per year in costs, it has become more important than ever to develop better medications and to improve our understanding of the psychopathology of mental illness.[1]

Efforts to combat this growing problem have resulted in the creation of new drugs, replacing many of the older drugs which are now obsolete due to either poor efficacy or harmful adverse effects. Currently, more than 119 medications with novel mechanisms of action are being developed to treat an array of mental health conditions.[1] Some of these innovative and fascinating approaches include an intranasal medication for treatment-resistant depression, an anti-cocaine vaccine, and a rapidly dissolving tablet for autism.[2] Additionally, the discovery of the glutamate system marks a major breakthrough in treatment for many psychiatric conditions, including depression and suicide.[2] Triple reuptake inhibitors, brain-derived neurotrophic factor (BDNF), corticotropin-releasing hormone (CRH), and melatonin are just a few of the substances currently receiving significant attention from researchers. Similarly, the NMDA-receptor antagonist ketamine has shown promising results for the rapid treatment of severe depression and acutely suicidal patients. The field of pharmacogenetics is receiving a great deal of attention from both public organizations and drug companies, and it may not be too long before physicians could be developing personalized treatment plans via gene scanning, RNA fingerprinting, brain mapping, and brain imaging.[2] In light of these breakthroughs and developments, prescribers have an added responsibility to their patients to stay abreast of the latest psychopharmacological advancements.[1]

The interplay of evolving treatment options, new diagnoses, redefined disorders, and changing treatment recommendations from various professional and regulatory organizations places a tremendous burden on prescribers who need to keep their knowledge current. Maintaining such a robust scientific literacy can be overwhelming and, in many ways, is as daunting as the problem of mental illness itself. In an era where quick access to information is essential for the effective treatment of patients, it is evident that a comprehensive and up-to-date guide for psychiatric medications is needed.

Over the last decade, I have served as the medical director for multiple high-volume mental health clinics, working with thousands of patients amidst a diverse assortment of difficult circumstances. Throughout my career, I have witnessed the challenges faced by clinicians in day-to-day practice, struggling to recall minute details across a wide range of psychiatric medications. An inordinate amount of valuable time and energy is spent combing through the literature for information on medications needed for accurate prescribing, such as dosing, side effects, interactions, precautions, withdrawal symptoms, and use in special populations. This book condenses all of this information into a practical guide that is immensely useful to busy clinicians.

This guide contains a wealth of knowledge in a readily digestible form that retains scientific detail, displacing texts that focus solely on basic overviews or specific classes of drugs. Rigorously composed and current, this essential resource covers the most clinically relevant psychiatric medications and their latest indications, dosing protocols, warnings, interactions, common side effects, and other important prescribing information. Further, this guide examines the most prevalent psychiatric disorders seen in clinical practice, including major depression, anxiety, substance abuse, bipolar disorder, ADHD, and schizophrenia. In addition, it contains dedicated sections for must-know DSM-5 changes and the treatment of sleep disorders, eating disorders, dementia or cognitive disorders, and personality disorders. Other current mental health issues explored in detail include psychiatric emergencies (e.g., suicide and violence), PTSD, and future advances in mental health. This guide also discusses medication use in special populations in-depth, addressing areas such as use in pregnancy, lactation, elderly, children, and comorbid illnesses (e.g., renal/hepatic impairment and HIV). Moreover, due to growing interest related to the use of alternative medications in the treatment of psychiatric ailments, a separate chapter is devoted to the most commonly used dietary, herbal, and over-the-counter medications currently available on the market. In addition to psychiatric medications, this guide also expands upon the emerging non-pharmacological psychiatric interventions that are currently utilized in practice. Electroconvulsive therapy (ECT), vagus nerve stimulation (VNS), deep brain stimulation (DBS), transcranial direct current stimulation (tDCS) and other brain stimulation therapies are covered thoroughly, enabling clinicians to sharpen their interventional knowledge and related skills.

The contents of this guide form an exceptionally beneficial tool for clinicians, allowing them to economize their valuable time and succeed in the modern era of medicine through its straightforward and to-the-point presentation, portability, and reliability. In essence, this book bridges the gap between bulky, intricate textbooks and brief, minimal booklets. As a result, it will be of tremendous help to any medical or mental health clinician who requires a short, clearly-presented account of the latest medications used in psychiatry. As a manual that intersects clinical psychiatry with psychopharmacology, this guide is intentionally accessible to students, residents, counselors, therapists, psychologists, family physicians, pediatricians, and psychiatrists alike. Evidence-based and written from clinical expertise, this book is an indispensable resource for those responsible for prescribing, dispensing, or administering drugs to patients with mental health disorders.

References:

1. Goff, D.C. and J.T. Coyle. 2001. "The Emerging Role of Glutamate in the Pathophysiology and Treatment of Schizophrenia." *Am. J. Psych.* 158:1366–1377. Accessed January 1, 2015. http://www.ncbi.nlm.nih.gov/pubmed/11532718.
2. Pharmaceutical Research and Manufacturers of America (PhRMA). 2014. "Mental Health Medicines in Development Report, 2014." Accessed January 12, 2015. http://www.phrma.org/mental-health-medicines-in-development-report-2014.

How To Use This Guide

This guide covers both general information about psychiatric disorders and specific information about the drugs used to treat these disorders. Chapters 1–3 and 13–22 contain clinically significant information about important psychiatric topics, including a basic overview of psychopharmacology, notable trends in the field, and medication use in special populations. Chapters 4–12 examine the most prevalent disorders encountered in day-to-day psychiatric practice (depression, bipolar disorder, anxiety, ADHD, psychosis/schizophrenia, disorders caused/exacerbated by psychiatric medication, sleep disorders, substance abuse, and cognitive disorders) and provide comprehensive prescribing information on the medications used to treat those disorders. Essential information is presented in a detailed profile covering the most critical and relevant aspects of a medication including:

- Generic and brand names
- FDA-approved indications
- Other potential uses (off-label)
- Medication forms
- Dosage
- Mechanism of action (MOA)
- Pharmacokinetics
- Warnings
- Drug interactions
- Common side effects

- Contraindications
- Lab tests recommended
- Overdose information
- Tapering/withdrawal
- Special populations: use in pregnancy, lactation, elderly, hepatic and renal impairment
- Important notes: evidence-based clinical context and recommendations

Full profiles are provided for the most clinically-relevant medications, and less frequently used medications may have abbreviated profiles. For medications that apply to more than one chapter, an abbreviated profile will direct you to the chapter containing the medication's full profile. For ease of use, medications are presented in alphabetical order within their class.

The following classes of medications also contain general profiles which are placed before the profiles of the individual medications within that class: SSRIs, SNRIs, SARIs, MAOIs, TCAs, benzodiazepines (benzos), CNS stimulants, atypical (second generation) antipsychotics, and typical (first generation) antipsychotics. These class profiles contain an overview of the characteristics shared by medications in these groups, including mechanism of action, warnings, drug interactions, contraindications, side effects, and withdrawal symptoms. When researching a medication in one of these classes, both the *class profile* and the *individual medication profile* need to be consulted together to obtain all relevant and available information for that particular medication. The presence of the phrase "Similar to *Class Profile*" in an individual medication profile signifies that you should refer to the class profile for that particular information. In many cases, individual medication profiles will contain information in addition to the phrase "Similar to *Class Profile*," which indicates that the medication has unique characteristics for that particular topic beyond what is contained in the class profile.

A detailed table of contents has been provided to allow you to quickly hone in on the location of the medications or sub-topics that you desire to access.

Please refer to Appendix A for a list of helpful references and to Appendix B for a list of medical/psychiatric abbreviations.

Chapter 1
The Role of Psychopharmacology

Psychopharmacology is the study of the interactions between medications and receptors in the central nervous system resulting in the alteration of brain function. This discipline dictates the prescription and appropriate use of medications for psychiatric and neuropsychiatric conditions.[12,13] Psychopharmacological agents, especially antidepressant, anxiolytic, and antipsychotic medications, are among the most commonly prescribed drugs throughout the world.[2]

Psychopharmacology encompasses the following classes of medication[4,15]:

- Antipsychotics
- Anxiolytics
- Antidepressants
- Mood stabilizers
- Sedatives/Hypnotics

- Stimulants
- Hallucinogens
- Opiates
- Cannabinoids
- Others

classes of meds

Research and practice guidelines demonstrate that psychotropic medications are effective and safe when used prudently to control psychiatric symptoms.[12] Due to the complex and expanding nature of psychopharmacology, comprehensive knowledge of each drug's mechanism of action, pharmacokinetics, dosage, side effects, and drug interactions is crucial for safe prescribing.

The Key to Successful Psychopharmacological Practice

The last 30–35 years saw a tremendous shift towards the increased use of psychiatric medications in the practice of clinical psychiatry. The development of progressively newer psychiatric medications moved the focus away from psychotherapeutic techniques towards the prescription of psychopharmacological agents.[12] Adjusting to this newer model was a difficult challenge for mental health professionals, especially psychologists and therapists. However, after a few years of novelty, the preferred treatment model has now evolved into a biopsychosocial model which utilizes all three modalities: medication, therapy, and psychosocial intervention.[12]

Although psychiatric medications can be very effective for a variety of conditions, they do not chan.ogy of a mental health disorder is highly sensitive to intrapsychic, interpersonal, and psychosocial stressors.[12] As a result, the key to successful psychopharmacological practice involves the combination of psychopharmacology, psychotherapy, and psychosocial intervention in a holistic approach.[12]

Practice Guidelines

A multidisciplinary approach with evidence-based practices and protocols should be utilized to provide safe, high-quality continuing care.[12] Successful practice guidelines include the following principles:

- Effective treatment should be based on an empathic, integrated, and collaborative mental health program.[10]
- Treatment should be based on a holistic approach.[10]
- Clinical experience and knowledge of the latest treatment modalities should always determine treatment guidelines.[12]
- Mental health professionals should become well-versed with medications and their dosages, side effects, and interactions.[10,15]
- Physicians should work with patients in the decision-making process of choosing a medication. [10,12, 15]
- Informed consent is mandatory and should always be obtained from the patient.[12]
- Both patients and their families should be educated about any possible side effects before starting any medications.[10,15]
- Unless otherwise stated, medications should always be prescribed at a low dosage and increased gradually.[12]
- FDA approval is critical to prescribing appropriate medications and dosages.[12]
- Off-label treatment should be based on a high standard of care, clinical evidence, and medical experience. [12]
- Cost being a factor, generic medications may be preferable to brand name medications.[12,15]

Improving Compliance

Noncompliance includes poor adherence to treatment, such as not using medications as prescribed, stopping medications without informing the physician, and/or not following the correct directions regarding medication usage.[15] It is the leading cause of treatment failure, relapse, and disease recurrence.[10] To improve patient compliance, it is essential to pinpoint the causes of noncompliance and to formulate strategies to prevent them from occurring.[12,14] Some of the most common causes of noncompliance and the best practices for preventing them include the following:

- Psychiatric medications are still associated with significant stigma.[10] Educating patients and their families can promote compliance.
- Medication affordability can also lead to noncompliance, as most brand name medications are expensive; this can especially affect lower income and elderly patients. Prescribing less expensive brands or generic drugs, suggesting nonprofit assistance programs, and refering to discount programs like *goodrx.com* can help patients adhere to their medication regimens.[12,15]

- Unpleasant side effects are a major cause of noncompliance.[10] To improve adherence, clinicians should explain potential side effects and suggest ways of dealing with them. This can boost the confidence of patients and improve their compliance.[12,15]
- Some patients do not remember to take medications on time. Suggestion tools such as pillboxes, medication apps, calendars, post-it notes, timers, and cell phone alarms can promote better patient compliance.[5,15]
- Increasing medication frequency often leads to a higher chance of missed doses. Offering a once-daily formulation or a longer-lasting option can help clients adhere to their medication programs.[5,15] Once-monthly depot medications can be useful for noncompliant patients.[12]
- Many psychiatric medications, especially antidepressants, take four to six weeks before there are any signs of improvement in symptoms. Patients should be informed of this before the start of any medications so that there are no unrealistic expectations.[10]

The Integrated Biopsychosocial Model of Treatment

As discussed earlier, the biopsychosocial model considers the complex interaction of biological, psychological, and social factors when understanding disease etiology and treatment.[1,3,9] This model offers an evidence-based approach for integrating physical and mental health services into a single primary setting. It also aids community outreach as well as the long-term monitoring and management of patients. Furthermore, this integrated model is cost-effective and is therefore embraced by healthcare professionals as "the best practice of care."[3]

An integrated model of treatment, especially with the advent of medical homes, is becoming increasingly popular. Rather than treating just one component of a patient's condition, research shows that treating all components under one roof can provide safe, quality care to patients in some populations.[11]

Pharmacogenetics

Pharmacogenetics studies the genetic variations associated with the body's response to pharmacological compounds. This discipline encompasses both the pharmacokinetics and pharmacodynamics of medications.[7] With the rapid expansion of this field, the use of a patient's genetic profile is expected to revolutionize clinical practice in the near future, resulting in the ability to predict a patient's response to a particular psychotropic agent.[7] Consequently, a prescriber will be able to employ a more individualized approach when recommending the most appropriate medication for a patient based on the assessment of biomarkers that will interact with the medication.[7] Pharmacogenetics can offer the opportunity to identify the safest drug and the most effective dosage for an individual.

Pharmacogenetic analyses focus on single-nucleotide polymorphisms (SNPs) in a candidate gene associated with a drug's action.[6] These SNPs are subsequently tested for any connection with the clinical response to the drug. Microarrays are now able to screen as many as 100,000 SNPs in a patient's genome within a few hours. With advancements in DNA microarray technology, SNP screening in the clinic to determine a patient's response to a particular medication prior to prescribing is soon expected to become commonplace.[6]

Currently, the FDA has approved only one commercial pharmacogenetics test for use in psychiatry. This specific test can identify the genotypes for two CYP450 genes: CYP2D6 and CYP2C19.[7] Utilizing this technology, a clinician could predict a patient's metabolic capacity for drugs associated with these enzymatic pathways, influencing the choice of medication and dosing.

References:

1. Borrell-Carrio, F., A. L. Suchman, and R. M. Epstein. 2004. "The biopsychosocial model 25 years later: principles, practice, and scientific inquiry." *Ann Fam Med* 2(6):576–582. doi: 10.1370/afm.245.

2. Brooks, M. 2014. "Top 100 Most Prescribed, Top Selling Drugs." *Medscape*. Accessed January 21, 2015. http://www.medscape.com/viewarticle/825053.

3. Engel, G.L. 1980. "The clinical application of the biopsychosocial model." *Am J Psychiatry* 137:535–544.

4. Hilal-Dandan, Randa, and Laurence Brunton. 2013. "General Principles." *In Goodman & Gilman's: The Pharmacological Basis of Therapeutics*. 2nd ed.1–98. New York: Pergamon Press.

5. Julius R.J., M.A. Novitsky Jr., and W.R. Dubin. 2009. "Medication adherence: a review of the literature and implications for clinical practice." J Psychiatr Pract 15:34–44.

6. McCarthy, Jeanette J., and Rolf Hilfiker. 2000. "The use of single-nucleotide polymorphism maps in pharmacogenomics." *Nat Biotech* 18(5):505–508.

7. Narasimhan, S., and F.W. Lohoff. 2012. "Pharmacogenetics of antidepressant drugs: current clinical practice and future directions." *Pharmacogenomics* 13(4):441–464. Accessed January 13, 2015. http://www.ncbi.nlm.nih.gov/pubmed/22380000.

8. National Institute of Mental Health. 2015. "Statistics." Accessed February 3, 2015. http://www.nimh.nih.gov/health/statistics/index.shtml#Refs.

9. Pilgrim, David. 2002. "The Biopsychosocial Model in Anglo-American Psychiatry: Past, Present and Future?" *Journal of Mental Health* 11(6):585–594.

10. Preston, John D., and Johnson, J. 2011. *Clinical Psychopharmacology Made Ridiculously Simple*. 7th ed. 61–65. Miami: MedMaster Inc.

11. Sandmaier, M., Bell, A., Fox, H., McManus, M., and Wilson, J. 2007. "Under one roof: Primary care models that work for adolescents." *The National Alliance to Advance Adolescent Health*. http://www.thenationalalliance.org/pdfs/Report1.%20Under%20One%20Roof%20-%20Primary%20Care%20Models.pdf.

12. Schatzberg, Alan F., Jonathan O. Cole, and Charles DeBattista. 2010. *Manual of Clinical Psychopharmacology*. 7th ed. 1–4. Washington, DC: American Psychiatric Publishing.

13. Schatzberg, Alan F., and Charles B. Nemeroff, eds. 2009. *The American Psychiatric Publishing Textbook of Psychopharmacology*. 4th ed. 261–530. Washington, DC: American Psychiatric Publishing.

14. Shea, S.C. 2006. *Improving Medication Adherence: How to Talk with Patients About Their Medications*. Philadelphia: Lippincott, Williams and Wilkins.

15. Wegmann, J. 2008. *Psychopharmacology: Straight Talk on Mental Health Medications*. 169–172. Eau Claire: Pesi.

Chapter 2
Black Box Warnings

A black box warning is the strongest caution designated by the FDA for medications. Named after the black border surrounding the text of the warning, the FDA requires pharmaceutical companies to include a black box warning on the labels of particular prescription medications to alert patients and healthcare providers about significant safety concerns associated with their use.[8,12]

Black Box Warning Regarding Antidepressant Use in Children

In 2004, the FDA issued a black box warning for all antidepressants concerning an increased risk of suicidality in children and adolescents.[3,8,12,16] In 2007, the warning was updated to include young adults aged 18 to 24 during the first one to two months of treatment.[8,11,12] According to the FDA, a pooled analysis of credible studies in this area indicated a 4% risk of suicidal thinking or behavior amongst the patients receiving an active drug compared to a 2% risk in those receiving a placebo.[9,19]

The black box warning includes the following statement:

Antidepressants increased the risk of suicidal thinking and behavior in children, adolescents, and young adults in short-term studies with major depressive disorder (MDD) and other psychiatric disorders. This risk must be balanced with the clinical need. Monitor patients closely for clinical worsening, suicidality, or unusual changes in behavior. Families and caregivers should be advised of the need for close observation and communication with the prescriber.[6,8,19]

The warning applies to any and all use of antidepressant drugs in children, adolescents, and young adults. Any clinician prescribing antidepressants must caution patients and their families about the potential risks associated with these medications.[14] In addition, the FDA has determined that all patients receiving these medications should be given a patient medication guide explaining any associated risks and precautionary measures.[6,12]

Clinicians and family members must monitor pediatric patients with depressive disorders on antidepressants for the following adverse responses, particularly during the initial months of therapy and when the dosage is adjusted[6,19]:

- Worsening depressive symptoms
- Suicidality
- Unusual changes in behavior
- Agitation

- Irritability or hostility
- Impulsivity
- Akathisia
- Hypomania or mania

children, Teens, young adults

The recommended management program includes periodic in-person checkups for children and adolescents who have been prescribed antidepressants. These checkups should occur every week for weeks 1–4, every other week for weeks 5–8, during week 12, and whenever clinically prudent from week 13 onward.[16,19] The patient's family must be educated about these potentially serious indications of clinical worsening and should notify the clinicians immediately if these symptoms occur.[14]

Possible Causes of Increased Suicidality in Children Taking Antidepressants

Researchers speculate that increased suicidality in children using antidepressants may be due to the following factors[8]:

- Most MDD episodes are not diagnosed/treated by psychiatrists
- Incorrect diagnosis
- Inadequate treatment
- Ineffective treatment
- Immature brain development of the children
- Altered response to antidepressants
- Behavioral activation from antidepressants
- Pediatric-onset bipolar disorder: The use of antidepressants in these patients may induce hypomania or mania

SSRIs and Children

The NIMH estimates that 11% of American adolescents suffer from a depressive disorder.[13] SSRIs are an effective form of treatment for major depressive disorder (MDD) and are preferred over other classes of antidepressants, as they have fewer side effects and are rarely lethal in cases of overdose. However, SSRIs may trigger agitation and suicidal thinking in some individuals.[11] Although fluoxetine (Prozac) and escitalopram (Lexapro) are the only FDA-approved medications for treating depression in children and adolescents, some other SSRIs (e.g., citalopram, sertraline) are often used off-label. In June 2003, the FDA advised against the use of paroxetine (Paxil) for treatment of MDD in children and adolescents.[13] The FDA also recommended that children who are using SSRIs should be monitored closely and that children who are benefiting from SSRIs continue the medication with the understanding that parents should promptly seek medical help if any suicidal thinking or behavior arises.[19]

The Link between Depression and Suicide

Depression and suicide are strongly linked, as depression is one of the strongest risk factors for suicide.[1,2] Multiple studies have demonstrated that about 65–70% of people who commit suicide were depressed at the time of their death. In one analysis, approximately 90% of people who committed suicide were found to have been suffering from depression, bipolar disorder, or some other psychiatric disorder according to a "psychological autopsy."[9] Adolescents suffering from MDD are much more likely to attempt suicide compared to adolescents who are not depressed,[9] and individuals with recurrent depression and substance abuse are at a much higher risk for suicide.[15] The summation of this evidence clearly demonstrates a strong connection between clinical depression and suicide, which has led some researchers to question the black box warning.

Controversy and Consequences of the FDA Warning

Since the implementation of the black box warning for antidepressant use in children and adolescents, the question has been raised as to whether it is necessary.[20] A 2012 study of the antidepressant fluoxetine failed to show any evidence that the drug increases the risk of suicide in youth.[10] Furthermore, evidence of serious design flaws was documented in the study that resulted in the FDA warning initially, as the trials were not originally designed to measure suicidal tendencies but were, in fact, intended to assess the efficacy of antidepressants.[7,9] Lack of any evidence of increased suicides in children and adolescents has also been reported by earlier studies.[17] Some people question whether the black box warning has done more harm than good.[10] Moreover, practitioners are concerned that the current controversy has lowered the use of effective antidepressants and has caused some successfully treated patients to stop taking SSRIs needlessly.[8,14]

Potential consequences of the FDA black box warning include:

- Many physicians are now hesitant to prescribe SSRIs to depressed children and adolescents, even when the use of these medications is clinically warranted.[14]
- Though the FDA recommends frequent vists with the prescriber after starting antidepressants in youth, a high percentage of parents are unwilling or unable to bring their children for follow-ups on such a frequent basis.[9]
- One study concluded that suicide rates have tripled among children and adolescents since the warning's initiation,[14] as prescribers have been hesitant to start SSRIs in this population.
- Another study found that 91% of practitioners misunderstood the FDA warning of increased suicidality by wrongly interpreting it as an increased risk of death.[14]

It is important to note that a recent study funded by the NIMH suggests that the benefits of antidepressant medications likely outweigh their risks to children and adolescents with major depression and anxiety disorders.[13]

Black Box Warning Regarding Antipsychotic Use in the Elderly

Behavioral disturbances such as agitation and aggression are common in people suffering from dementia, creating a major challenge for medical professionals and families. In the absence of other approved agents, many physicians have turned to the off-label use of antipsychotics to manage their patients.[4] Due to the increased mortality risk in elderly patients with dementia-related psychosis taking these medications, the FDA initially warned prescribers in 2003 against prescribing risperidone and later in 2005 against using any atypical antipsychotics in this population.[18] Based on observational studies, a black box warning was applied to atypical antipsychotics as a class and was further revised in 2008 to include conventional or typical antipsychotics.[18]

The black box warning includes the following statement:

Elderly patients with dementia-related psychosis treated with atypical antipsychotic drugs are at an increased risk of death compared with placebo. Although the causes of death in clinical trials were varied, most of the deaths appeared to be either cardiovascular (e.g., heart failure, sudden death) or infectious (e.g., pneumonia) in nature. Observational studies suggest that antipsychotic drugs may increase mortality. It is unclear from the observational studies to what extent these mortality findings may be attributed to the antipsychotic drug as opposed to patient characteristics.[18]

Although the practice of FDA-approved and off-label use of antipsychotics in elderly patients decreased after the black box warning was instituted, atypical antipsychotics still comprise 9% of the prescription drugs used to treat dementia.[5] This ongoing use despite the FDA warning can pose a significant mortality risk.

Medications Receiving a Black Box Warning in the Elderly

Atypical antipsychotics

- Abilify (aripiprazole)
- Clozaril (clozapine)
- Geodon (ziprasidone)
- Invega (paliperidone)
- Risperdal (risperidone)

- Seroquel (quetiapine)
- Symbyax (Zyprexa/Prozac [olanzapine/fluoxetine])*
- Zyprexa (olanzapine)

Symbyax also contains a black box warning for antidepressant use in children because it contains the SSRI fluoxetine

Typical antipsychotics

All medications in this class carry the black box warning.[5]

References:

1. Barlow, D.H., and V.M. Durand. 2011. *Abnormal Psychology: An Integrated Approach*. 212. New York: Wadsworth Cengage Learning.
2. Bridge, Jeffrey A., S. Iyengar, C. Salary, R. Barbe, B. Birmaher, H.A. Pincus, L. Ren, and D. Brent. 2007. "Clinical Response and Risk for Reported Suicidal Ideation and Suicide Attempts in Pediatric Antidepressant Treatment: A Meta-Analysis of Randomized Controlled Trials." *JAMA* 297(15):1683–1696.
3. Center for Drug Evaluation and Research (CDER). 2004. "FDA Public Health Advisory: Suicidality in Children and Adolescents Being Treated With Antidepressant Medications." Accessed February 3, 2015. http://www.cchrint.org/pdfs/2004-10-15-FDA-warning-SSRIs.pdf.
4. Cassels, Caroline. 2010. "Inappropriate Use of Antipsychotics in the Elderly Continues Despite FDA Warnings. *Medscape Medical News*. Accessed February 18, 2015. http://www.medscape.com/viewarticle/715257.
5. Dorsey, E.R., Atonu Rabbani, Sarah A. Gallagher, Rena M. Conti, and G. Caleb Alexander. 2010. "Impact of FDA Black Box Advisory on Antipsychotic Medication Use." *Arch Intern Med*. 170(1):96–103. doi:10.1001/archinternmed.2009.456.
6. Gartlehner, Gerald, Richard Hansen, Ursula Reichenpfader, Angela Kaminski, Christina Kien, Michaela Strobelberger, Megan Van Noord, Patricia Thieda, Kylie Thaler, and Bradley Gaynes. 2011. Drug Class Review: Second-Generation Antidepressants: Final Update 5 Report [Internet]. In *Appendix F, Black box warnings of drugs approved by the US Food and Drug Administration*. Portland: Oregon Health & Science University.
7. Gibbons, R.D., C. Brown, K. Hur, J. M. Davis, and J. Mann. 2012. "Suicidal thoughts and behavior with antidepressant treatment: Reanalysis of the randomized placebo-controlled studies of fluoxetine and venlafaxine." *Archives of General Psychiatry* 69(6):580–587. doi: 10.1001/archgenpsychiatry.2011.2048.
8. Gutierrez, M. 2007. "Antidepressants Black Box Warnings." NAMI Annual National Convention. Brentwood, California. Accessed February 18, 2015.
9. Kennedy, Lucas. 2008. "SSRI's and the Black Box Warning: Patient Advocacy or Alarmist Propaganda?" Master's Project Presentation, University of Kentucky. Accessed February 19, 2015. http://www.uky.edu/~hadleyr/PA2009/Kennedy.ppt.
10. Lowry, Fran. 2012. "No Link Between Antidepressant and Suicide in Kids Study Calls FDA Black Box Warning Into Question." *Medscape Medical News*. Accessed February 18, 2015. http://www.medscape.com/viewarticle/758917.
11. McCain, Jack A. 2009. "Antidepressants and Suicide in Adolescents and Adults: A Public Health Experiment with Unintended Consequences?" P&T 34(7):355–367, 378.
12. National Alliance on Mental Illness (NAMI). 2004. "FDA Advisory Committee Recommends 'Black Box Warnings' for Anti-depression Medications." Accessed February 18, 2015. http://www2.nami.org/Template.cfm?Section=Child_and_Adolescent_Action_Center&template=/ContentManagement/ContentDisplay.cfm&ContentID=17662.

13. National Institute of Mental Health (NIMH). 2015. "Antidepressant Medications for Children and Adolescents: Information for Parents and Caregivers." Accessed February 5, 2015. http://www.nimh. nih.gov/health/topics/child-and-adolescent-mental-health/antidepressant-medications-for-children-and-adolescents-information-for-parents-and-caregivers.shtml.

14. Rudd, David M., Liliana Cordero, and Craig J. Bryan. 2009. "What Every Psychologist Should Know About the Food and Drug Administration's Black Box Warning Label for Antidepressants." *Professional Psychology: Research and Practice* 40(4):321–326.

15. Shaffer, D., M.S. Gould, P. Fisher, and et al. 1996. "Psychiatric diagnosis in child and adolescent suicide." *Archives of General Psychiatry* 53(4):339–348. doi: 10.1001/ archpsyc.1996.01830040075012.U.

16. Simon, G.E., J. Savarino, B. Operskalski, and P.S. Wang. 2006. "Suicide risk during antidepressant treatment." Am J Psychiatry 163(1):41–47.

17. Sondergard L., K. Kvist, P.K. Andersen, and L.V. Kessing. 2006. "Do antidepressants prevent suicide?" *Int Clin Psychopharmacol* 21:211–218.

18. US Food and Drug Administration (FDA). 2008. "Information for Healthcare Professionals: Conventional Antipsychotics." Accessed April 18, 2015. http://www.fda.gov/Drugs/DrugSafety/ PostmarketDrugSafetyInformationforPatientsandProviders/ucm124830.htm.

19. US Food and Drug Administration (FDA). 2009. "Labeling Change Request Letter for Antidepressant Medications." Center for Drug Evaluation and Research. Accessed March 24, 2015. http://www.fda. gov/Drugs/DrugSafety/InformationbyDrugClass/ucm096352.htm.

20. Valuck, Robert J., A.M. Libby, M.R. Sills, A.A. Giese, and R.R. Allen. 2004. "Antidepressant Treatment and Risk of Suicide Attempt by Adolescents with Major Depressive Disorder: A Propensity-Adjusted Retrospective Cohort Study." *CNS Drugs* 18(15):1119–1132.

Chapter 3
Important DSM-5 Changes

The final diagnostic criteria for DSM-5 were approved on December 1, 2012 after the extensive collaborative work of over 1500 experts from 39 countries. This fifth edition of the DSM was officially released on May 18, 2013 at an annual meeting of the American Psychiatric Association (APA) in San Francisco, CA. The DSM-5 saw the addition of 15 diagnoses, the elimination of two, the combination of 28, and the amendment of many others.[5] These changes resulted in a net reduction of diagnoses from 172 in DSM-IV to 157 in DSM-5.[5] Other modifications from DSM-IV to DSM-5 involved adjustments to structure, developmental approach, severity measures, biological markers and an increased focus on culture and gender.[5] This edition was named DSM-5 and not DSM-V as future updates will be done "software style" with decimal points (e.g., DSM-5.1).[1]

General Updates in DSM-5
Organization of DSM-5[1]
- Section 1: Introduction to DSM-5
- Section 2: Outline of categorical diagnoses according to revised chapter organization
- Section 3: Conditions requiring further research, cultural formulations and glossary, and a listing of all individuals involved in the development of DSM-5

Major Changes in DSM-5[1,2]
- Removal of the multi-axial system
- Non-axial documentation of diagnoses: combining axes I, II, and III
- Separate notations for psychosocial and contextual factors (formerly Axis IV) and disability (formerly Axis V)
- Axis V eliminated
- Severity scales added to diagnostic categories (mild, moderate, severe)
- Chapters restructured based on several disorders' apparent relatedness, as reflected by similarities, vulnerabilities, and symptom characteristics
- Certain "not otherwise specified (NOS)" diagnoses were removed, such as mood disorder NOS and pervasive developmental disorder NOS
- "Unspecified" and "other specified" replaced "not otherwise specified"

Coding and Reporting Procedures
In DSM-5, each disorder has an identifying diagnostic and statistical code that is used for billing purposes. The official coding system in the US as of the publication of

DSM-5 was ICD-9-CM. However, DSM-5 reflects changes aligned with the newer system, ICD-10-CM. Official adoption of ICD-10-CM is scheduled to take place on October 1, 2015.[4]

New Disorders in DSM-5[1,2,3,5]

- Binge eating disorder
- Caffeine withdrawal
- Cannabis withdrawal
- Central sleep apnea
- Disinhibited social engagement disorder
- Disruptive mood dysregulation disorder
- Excoriation disorder
- Hoarding disorder
- Major neurocognitive disorder (NCD) with Lewy body disease and mild NCD
- Premenstrual dysphoric disorder (PMDD)
- REM sleep behavior disorder
- Restless leg syndrome (RLS)
- Sleep-related hypoventilation
- Social communication disorder

Disorder Specific Changes in DSM-5[1,2,3,4,5]

Neurodevelopmental Disorders:

- *Intellectual Developmental Disorder:* "Mental retardation" has been replaced by "intellectual disability."
- *Autism Spectrum Disorder:* Incorporates autistic disorder, Asperger's syndrome, childhood disintegrative disorder, and pervasive developmental disorder NOS.
- *Attention-Deficit/Hyperactivity Disorder:* Onset criterion has changed from age 7 to age 12. A co-morbid diagnosis with autism spectrum disorder is now allowed.
- *Specific Learning Disorder:* Incorporates reading disorder, mathematics disorder, disorder of written expression, and learning disorder NOS.
- *Motor Disorder:* Includes developmental coordination disorder, stereotypic movement disorder, Tourette's disorder, persistent/chronic motor or vocal tic disorder, and provisional tic disorder.
- *Communication Disorder:* Includes language disorder, mixed receptive-expressive language disorder, speech and sound disorder, social (pragmatic) communication disorder, and childhood-onset fluency disorder.

Schizophrenia Spectrum and Other Psychotic Disorders:

- *Schizophrenia:* DSM-IV subtypes (paranoid, bizarre, catatonic, undifferentiated, and residual) have been eliminated.

- *Schizoaffective Disorder:* Major mood episode must be present for majority of the duration.
- *Delusional Disorder:* No longer requires that delusions must be "non-bizarre."
- *Catatonia:* Now diagnosed as a specifier for depressive, bipolar, and psychotic disorders and as a separate diagnosis in the context of another medical condition.

Bipolar and Related Disorders: Criterion A for manic and hypomanic episodes now includes an emphasis on changes in activity and energy as well as mood. Two new specifiers, with mixed features and with anxious distress, have been added.

Depressive Disorders: Now contains several new disorders, including disruptive mood dysregulation disorder, PMDD, and persistent depressive disorder. Anxious distress specifier has been added, and bereavement exclusion has been removed.

Anxiety Disorders: No longer includes OCD, PTSD, or acute stress disorder. Agoraphobia is now distinct from panic disorder. Social phobia has been renamed as social anxiety disorder. Panic disorder can now be used as a specifier. Separation anxiety may have "adult onset." Selective mutism is now classified as an anxiety disorder.

Obsessive-Compulsive Disorder and Related Disorders: Have been removed from anxiety disorders. Now includes hoarding disorder, excoriation disorder, trichotillomania, and others.

Trauma-and-Stressor-Related Disorders: PTSD has moved from anxiety disorders to this new class. Class includes acute stress disorder, PTSD, adjustment disorder, and reactive attachment disorder.

Disruptive, Impulsive-Control, and Conduct Disorders:

- *Oppositional Defiant Disorder:* Symptoms are grouped into three types including angry/irritable mood, argumentative/defiant behavior, and vindictiveness.
- *Conduct Disorder:* A descriptive feature has been added for individuals who not only meet full criteria but also present limited pro-social emotions.
- *Intermittent Explosive Disorder:* The type of aggressive outburst has changed. Verbal aggression and non-destructive/non-injurious physical aggression also meet criteria.

Dissociative Disorders: Dissociative fugue is now a specifier for dissociative amnesia rather than a separate diagnosis. Depersonalization disorder has been renamed as "depersonalization/de-realization disorder."

Somatic Symptom and Related Disorders: Somatoform disorders have been renamed as "somatic symptom and related disorders." Diagnoses of somatization disorder, hypochondriasis, pain disorder, and undifferentiated somatoform disorder have been removed. A new diagnosis of "psychological factors affecting other medical conditions" has been added.

Feeding and Eating Disorders: "Feeding and eating disorders" now contains several disorders previously included in "feeding and eating disorders of infancy or early childhood" (which is renamed "avoidant/restrictive food intake disorder"). The criteria have been expanded significantly. Criteria for pica and rumination disorder are modified for clarity and now refer to people of any age. Diagnosis of anorexia nervosa no longer requires amenorrhea to be present. Elimination disorders previously classified under "disorders usually first diagnosed in infancy, childhood, or adolescence" now form an independent classification.

Sleep-Wake Disorders: "Sleep disorders related to another mental disorder" and "sleep disorders related to a general medical condition" have been removed. Primary insomnia has been renamed "insomnia disorder." Breathing-related sleep disorders are now divided into three relatively distinct disorders: obstructive sleep apnea (OSA)/hypopnea, central sleep apnea, and sleep-related hypoventilation.

Sexual Dysfunctions: For females, sexual desire and arousal disorders have been combined into "female sexual interest/arousal disorder." "Genito-pelvic pain/penetration disorder" has been added and combines vaginismus and dyspareunia from the DSM-IV. Sexual aversion disorder has been excluded. The DSM-5 has removed two subtypes: sexual dysfunction due to a general medical condition and sexual dysfunction due to psychological versus combined factors.

Gender Dysphoria: A new diagnostic class, "gender dysphoria," has been added, highlighting the phenomenon of "gender incongruence."

Substance-Related and Addictive Disorders: Substance abuse and dependence are combined into "substance use disorder." Criteria for cannabis and caffeine withdrawal have also been added. Gambling disorder and tobacco use disorder have been added.

Neurocognitive Disorders (NCD): "Dementia and amnestic disorders" has been incorporated under "major or mild NCDs." For personality disorders, personality traits and functioning can be assessed to find those who do not meet the criteria for personality disorder. Personality disorder is now under one axis.

Paraphilic Disorders: Distinguishes between paraphilic behaviors (paraphilias) and paraphilic disorders. Pedophilia has been revised to pedophilic disorder, but the criteria remain unchanged.

Sample DSM-5 Diagnostic Documentation[1,5,6]

Behavioral Diagnosis:

- Diagnosis Category 1 Diagnosis Code 1 Description
- Diagnosis Category 2 Diagnosis Code 2 Description
- Diagnosis Category 3 Diagnosis Code 3 Description
- Diagnosis Category 4 Diagnosis Code 4 Description
- Diagnosis Category 5 Diagnosis Code 5 Description

Primary Medical Diagnosis:

- Diagnosis Category 1 Diagnosis Code 1 Description
- Diagnosis Category 2 Diagnosis Code 2 Description
- Diagnosis Category 3 Diagnosis Code 3 Description

Social Elements Impacting Diagnosis:
(Check all that apply)

- ☐ None
- ☐ Housing problems
- ☐ Educational problems
- ☐ Occupational problems
- ☐ Financial problems
- ☐ Homelessness
- ☐ Abuse: physical, emotional, sexual
- ☐ Substance abuse
- ☐ Recent life stressors
- ☐ Family history of mental illness
- ☐ Personal history of mental illness

- ☐ Problems related to access to healthcare
- ☐ Problems related to social environment
- ☐ Problems related to crime/legal system
- ☐ Problems related to primary support group
- ☐ Other psychosocial/environmental factors
- ☐ History of violence
- ☐ Dysfunctional family
- ☐ Difficult childhood
- ☐ Sexual identity
- ☐ Unknown

Functional Assessment (If Applicable)

References:

1. American Psychiatric Association (APA). 2013a. *Diagnostic and Statistical Manual of Mental Disorders*. 5th ed. (DSM-5®). Washington, DC: American Psychiatric Publishing.

2. American Psychiatric Association (APA). 2013b. "Highlights of Changes from DSM-IV-TR to DSM-5." Last accessed January 13, 2015. http://www.dsm5.org/Documents/changes%20from%20dsm-iv-tr%20to%20dsm-5.pdf.

3. American Psychiatric Association (APA). 2013c. "Recent Updates to Proposed Revisions for DSM-5." Last accessed Jan 13, 2015. http://www.dsm5.org/Pages/RecentUpdates.aspx.

4. American Psychiatric Association (APA). 2014. "The DSM-5® Coding Update. Supplement to Diagnostic and Statistical Manual of Mental Disorders, Fifth Edition." Last accessed March 25, 2015. http://dsm.psychiatryonline.org/pb/assets/raw/dsm/pdf/DSM-5%20Coding%20Update_Final.pdf.

5. Regier, Darrel A., Emily A. Kuhl, and David J. Kupfer. 2013. "The DSM-5: Classification and criteria changes." *World Psychiatry* 12 (2):92–98. doi: 10.1002/wps.20050.

6. ValueOptions. 2014. "ProviderConnect®DSM-5 Screen Modifications Effective June 28, 2014." Accessed April 17, 2015. http://maryland.valueoptions.com/provider/clin_ut/ProviderConnect-DSM-5-Powerpoint-Review-6-28-14.pdf.

Chapter 4
Depressive Disorders And Antidepressants

Major depressive disorder (MDD) is the leading cause of disability worldwide as well as for people in the US between the ages of 15 and 44.[36] According to the NIMH, more than 15 million American adults are affected by MDD. Only one third of people with depression are ever diagnosed, only half of those are treated, and only 6% of those are treated sufficiently.[36] MDD can affect anyone regardless of age, gender, ethnic background, or socioeconomic status.[59] While MDD can develop at any age, the median age of onset is 32, and the condition is more prevalent in women than in men.[36] More importantly, MDD is associated with over half of all suicide attempts.[23,28] The incremental economic burden of individuals with MDD has increased by 21.5% (from $173.2 billion to $210.5 billion) between 2000 and 2015.[22] According to the WHO, depression will become the second leading cause of "lost years of healthy life" worldwide by 2020.[36] The specific cause of depression is still unknown, but genetics and environmental factors are thought to play a pivotal role in the etiology of MDD, in addition to stress and neuroendocrine abnormalities.[23,24]

With appropriate treatment, about 70–80% of individuals with MDD achieve a significant reduction in symptoms.[44] While all antidepressant medications approved by the FDA for MDD have comparable ability, it is difficult to predict which specific agent will be the most effective for each patient.[59] Medication selection depends on the patient's family history, drug tolerability, and treatment history.[44] Educating the patient and his or her family members about the risk factors of depression, side effects of medication, importance of compliance, and the recommendation of a healthy diet and exercise is essential for better prognosis.

DSM-5 Types[5]
Depression can be categorized into mild, moderate, and severe, and it includes the following categories and subtypes:
- Major Depressive Disorder
    - Specifier:
        - With anxious distress
        - With mixed features
        - With melancholic features
        - With atypical features
        - With mood-congruent psychotic features
        - With mood-incongruent psychotic features

- • With catatonia
- • With peripartum onset
- • With seasonal pattern
- Disruptive Mood Dysregulation Disorder
- Persistent Depressive Disorder
- Premenstrual Dysphoric Disorder (PMDD)
- Substance/Medication-Induced Depressive Disorder
- Depressive Disorder Due to Another Medical Condition

Black Box Warning Regarding Antidepressant Use in Children[35,55]

This warning applies to any and all use of antidepressant drugs in children and adolescents. The black box warning includes the following statement:

Antidepressants increased the risk of suicidal thinking and behavior in children, adolescents, and young adults in short-term studies with major depressive disorder (MDD) and other psychiatric disorders. This risk must be balanced with the clinical need. Monitor patients closely for clinical worsening, suicidality, or unusual changes in behavior. Families and caregivers should be advised of the need for close observation and communication with the prescriber.[55]

Antidepressants

Selective Serotonin Reuptake Inhibitors (SSRIs)[19,23,28,39,44,45,46,59]

Class Profile

Overview: SSRIs are used to treat a wide spectrum of psychiatric disorders and are first-line treatment for depression and anxiety.[45] Although they have comparable efficacy to TCAs, SSRIs have a faster onset of action, better response, fewer side effects, improved tolerance, and a higher safety margin. Common SSRIs include citalopram, escitalopram, fluoxetine, fluvoxamine, paroxetine, and sertraline.[4]

MOA: SSRIs increase the level of extracellular serotonin in the synaptic cleft by inhibiting the reuptake of serotonin by the serotonin transporter protein, thereby increasing the amount available for binding with the postsynaptic receptor. SSRIs also enhance the transcription of neurotrophic factors, including brain-derived neurotrophic factor (BDNF), which is associated with an increase in synaptogenesis, neurogenesis, and neuronal resilience.[19]

Efficacy: All SSRIs have a similar spectrum of efficacy and comparable side-effect profiles but have distinct pharmacokinetic properties, including differences in half-life and drug-drug interaction potential.[46]

Warnings:
- **Black box warning:** All antidepressants carry a black box warning for increased risk of suicidal thinking and behavior in children, adolescents, and young adults

- May result in clinical worsening and increased risk of suicide
- Risk of PPHN and feeding difficulties in neonates if used during pregnancy
- May lower seizure threshold, trigger angle-closure glaucoma, and interfere with cognitive/motor performance
- Risk of abnormal bleeding, hyponatremia (due to SIADH), serotonin syndrome, and QTC prolongation
- Can activate mania/hypomania; screen for bipolar disorder

Drug interactions:

- Risk of serotonin syndrome when combined with SSRIs, SNRIs, TCAs, MAOIs, or other serotonergic agents, such as buspirone, triptans, fentanyl, lithium, tryptophan, St. John's wort, linezolid, or IV methylene blue; do not use for at least 2 weeks after stopping MAOIs
- Can cause increased bleeding when combined with medications such as NSAIDs, aspirin, warfarin, or other drugs that affect hemostasis
- Can alter the concentration of plasma-protein-bound drugs, such as digoxin and warfarin, which can increase the levels of these drugs
- Many SSRIs—especially fluoxetine, paroxetine, and fluvoxamine—are potent inhibitors of the cytochrome P450 system; use caution when combining any SSRI with drugs whose metabolism is predominantly dependent upon this enzymatic pathway
- Not recommended for concurrent use with drugs that prolong the QT interval (including pimozide and thioridazine)
- Can increase levels of various medications when used together including TCAs, carbamazepine, phenobarbital, haloperidol, clozapine, theophylline, encainide, and flecainide
- Use caution when combined with alcohol or other CNS acting drugs

Class side effects: Usually mild and dose-related, and most of them abate over time—anorexia, asthenia, diarrhea, dizziness, drowsiness, dry mouth, fatigue, headache, sweating, insomnia, nausea, nervousness, sexual dysfunction, somnolence, sweating, tremors, weight gain.

Contraindications: Patients with hypersensitivity or taking MAOIs, pimozide, IV methylene blue, or linezolid.

Discontinuation syndrome: Abrupt cessation of SSRIs may lead to discontinuation syndrome characterized by a wide variety of symptoms such as psychiatric, neurological, and sleep disturbances, transient electric shocks, and flu-like symptoms.[19,58] Symptoms usually resolve within three weeks. Discontinuation symptoms may lead to misdiagnosis and inappropriate treatment, particularly in patients with another active medical illness. It may also deter future compliance. Discontinuation problems often occur when using SSRIs with a short duration of action, such as paroxetine.[44]

Individual Drug Profiles

Citalopram[4,8,12,13,14,19,29,43,44,45,47,52,53,56]

Brand name: Celexa

FDA approved for: MDD

Other potential uses (off-label): Alcoholism, eating disorder, fibromyalgia, GAD, OCD, panic disorder, pathological gambling, premature ejaculation, PTSD

Medication forms: *Tab* (10, 20, 40 mg); *oral sol* (10 mg/5ml)

Dosage:
- Depression: 20 mg qd initially, can be increased based on tolerance/response to max 40 mg/day

MOA: Similar to *SSRI Class Profile*

Pharmacokinetics: t_{max}=4 hrs, $t_{1/2}$=35 hrs

Warnings:
- Similar to *SSRI Class Profile*
- **Black box warning**: Increased risk of suicidal thinking and behavior in children, adolescents, and young adults; not approved for use in pediatric patients
- Can cause dose-dependent QTc prolongation in susceptible individuals

Drug interactions:
- Similar to *SSRI Class Profile*
- Do not exceed 20 mg/day if prescribed with cimetidine, fluconazole, or omeprazole

Common side effects: Asthenia, diarrhea, drowsiness, dry mouth, ejaculation disorder, increased sweating, insomnia, nausea, palpitations, somnolence, tremor

Contraindications: Similar to *SSRI Class Profile*

Recommended lab tests: None

Overdose: Seizure, rigidity, hyperthermia, hypertension or hypotension, QRS and QTc interval prolongation, coma, and death (rare)

Tapering/withdrawal: Slow taper recommended

Special populations:

Pregnancy: Risk Category C

Lactation: Use caution

Elderly: 10–20 mg/day recommended due to increased exposure and risk of QT prolongation

Hepatic impairment: 20 mg/day max

Renal impairment: No dose adjustment in mild to moderate, use caution in severe

Cardiac impairment: Risk of QT prolongation in susceptible individuals; dose <20 mg recommended

Important notes:
- Doses above 40 mg/day not recommended due to risk of QT prolongation
- Among least expensive SSRIs available

Escitalopram[4,8,12,13,16,23,29,43,44,45,47,52,53,56]

Brand name: Lexapro

FDA approved for: MDD and GAD in adults, MDD in adolescents (ages 12–17 yrs)

Other potential uses (off-label): Alcoholism, autism, eating disorders, fibromyalgia, hot flashes, migraines, premature ejaculation, PTSD, social anxiety disorder

Medication forms: *Tab* (5, 10, 20 mg); *cap* (5, 10, 20 mg); *oral sol* (5mg/5ml)

Dosage:
- MDD: 10 mg qd initially, can be increased based on tolerance/response to max 20 mg/day
- GAD: 10 mg qd initial/max

MOA: Similar to *SSRI Class Profile*

Pharmacokinetics: t_{max}=5 hrs, $t_{1/2}$=27–32 hrs

Warnings:
- Similar to *SSRI Class Profile*
- **Black box warning:** Increased risk of suicidal thinking and behavior in children, adolescents, and young adults; not approved for use in pediatric patients <12 yrs

Drug interactions:
- Similar to *SSRI Class Profile*
- Can increase metoprolol levels, which can decrease cardioselectivity

Common side effects: Dry mouth, ejaculation disorder, headache, increased sweating, insomnia, nausea, somnolence

Contraindications: Similar to *SSRI Class Profile*

Recommended lab tests: None

Overdose: Agitation, confusion, tremor, nausea, vomiting, hyperreflexia, seizure, rigidity and hyperthermia; OD is rare

Tapering/withdrawal: Tapering generally not required

Special populations:

Pregnancy: Risk Category C

Lactation: Safer/preferred option

Elderly: 10 mg/day max

Hepatic impairment: 10 mg/day max

Renal impairment: 10 mg/day max, use caution in patients with severe impairment

Important notes:
- Among best-tolerated antidepressants and is considered a "clean" SSRI
- Can be combined with other medications for augmentation

Fluoxetine[4,8,10,12,13,19,29,43,44,45,47,52,53,56]

Brand name: Prozac, Prozac Weekly, Rapiflux, Selfemra, Sarafem

FDA approved for: MDD in adults and children/adolescents (ages 8–17 yrs), bulimia nervosa, panic disorder, PMDD, depressed bipolar I disorder (in combination with olanzapine), treatment-resistant MDD (in combination with olanzapine), OCD in adults and children/adolescents (ages 7–17 yrs)

Other potential uses (off-label): Body dysmorphic disorder, BPD, dysthymia, fibromyalgia, IBS, Raynaud's phenomenon, premature ejaculation, PTSD, selective mutism, social anxiety disorder

Medication forms: *Tab* (10, 20, 60 mg); *cap* (10, 20, 40 mg); *DR cap* (90 mg); *oral sol* (20 mg/5 ml)

Dosage:
- MDD:
  - *Prozac:* 20–40 mg/day, can be increased based on tolerance/response to max 80 mg/day
  - *Prozac Weekly:* 90 mg/week
- OCD:
  - *Prozac:* 20–60 mg/day
  - *Prozac Weekly:* 90 mg/week
- Bulimia nervosa: 20 mg/day initially, can be increased based on tolerance/response to max 60 mg/day
- Panic disorder: 10 mg/day initially, can be increased based on tolerance/response to max 20 mg/day
- PMDD:
  - *Continuous (Sarafem):* 20 mg/day
  - *Intermittent:* 20 mg/day starting 14 days before menstruation
- Treatment-resistant depression: olanzapine 5 mg and fluoxetine 20 mg qd

MOA: Similar to *SSRI Class Profile*

Pharmacokinetics: t_{max}=6–8 hrs, $t_{1/2}$=4–6 days

Warnings:
- Similar to *SSRI Class Profile*
- **Black box warning:** Increased risk of suicidal thinking and behavior in children, adolescents, and young adults
- When using fluoxetine and olanzapine in combination, also refer to the Boxed Warning section of package insert for Symbyax
- May cause serious allergic reactions (e.g., rash, vasculitis), anxiety, and insomnia

Drug interactions:
- Similar to *SSRI Class Profile*
- Can alter lithium concentration; monitor lithium levels regularly
- Potent inhibitor of CYP2D6 enzyme; use caution when combining with drugs metabolized by this pathway

Common side effects: Anorexia, anxiety, diarrhea, dizziness, dry mouth, fatigue, headache, indigestion, insomnia, nausea, nervousness, pharyngitis, rash, sinusitis, somnolence, tremor, yawning

Contraindications:

- Similar to *SSRI Class Profile*
- Agitated insomnia

Recommended lab tests: LFTs

Overdose: Seizures, QTc prolongation, and serotonin toxicity; OD rare

Tapering/withdrawal: Tapering not required

Special populations:

Pregnancy: Risk Category C

Lactation: Avoid

Elderly: Lower dose recommended

Hepatic impairment: Lower dose recommended

Renal impairment: No dose adjustment necessary

Important notes:

- May cause emotional flattening, especially at higher doses
- May cause activation and appetite suppression in some patients
- Use once-weekly form for maintenance phase of treatment only
- Wait for 5 weeks when changing from fluoxetine to an MAOI

Fluvoxamine[4,8,12,13,19,20,29,43,44,45,47,52,53,56]

Brand name: Luvox, Luvox CR

FDA approved for: OCD in adults and children/adolescents (ages 8–17 yrs), social anxiety disorder

Other potential uses (off-label): Depression, alcoholism, autism, diabetic neuropathy, eating disorders, gambling addiction, PMDD, PTSD

Medication forms: *Tab* (25, 50, 100 mg); *ER cap* (100, 150 mg)

Dosage:

- OCD: 50 mg qhs (**or** 100 mg *ER cap* qhs) initially, can be increased based on tolerance/response to max 300 mg/day
- Social anxiety disorder: 100 mg *ER cap* qhs, can be increased based on tolerance/response to max 300 mg/day
- Depression: 100–200 mg/day

MOA: Similar to *SSRI Class Profile*

Pharmacokinetics: t_{max} =3–8 hrs, $t_{1/2}$ =16–20 hrs

Warnings:

- Similar to SSRI Class Profile

- **Black box warning:** Increased risk of suicidal thinking and behavior in children, adolescents and young adults; not approved for use in pediatric patients except for patients with OCD
- May cause allergic reaction and rash

Drug interactions: Similar to *SSRI Class Profile*

Common side effects: Anorexia, diarrhea, dizziness, ejaculation disorder, headache, insomnia, nausea, nervousness, somnolence, weakness

Contraindications: Similar to *SSRI Class Profile*

Recommended lab tests: None

Overdose: Seizures, serotonin syndrome; OD rare

Tapering/withdrawal: Slow taper recommended

Special populations:

Pregnancy: Risk Category C

Lactation: Safe/preferred option

Elderly: Lower dose recommended

Hepatic impairment: Lower dose recommended

Renal impairment: No dose adjustment necessary

Important notes:

- Appears more effective than other SSRIs for obsessive-compulsive symptoms
- Advise patient to consult a healthcare professional before using any new drugs or OTC supplements

Paroxetine[4,7,8,12,13,19,29,43,44,45,47,52,53,56]

Brand name: Paxil, Paxil CR, Pexeva, Brisdelle

FDA approved for: MDD, OCD, panic disorder, social anxiety disorder, PTSD, GAD, PMDD, vasomotor symptoms of menopause (Brisdelle only)

Other potential uses (off-label): Alcoholism, eating disorders, IBS, premature ejaculation

Medication forms: *Tab* (10, 20, 30, 40 mg); *ER tab* (12.5 mg, 25 mg, 37.5 mg); *cap* (7.5 mg); *oral suspension* (10 mg/5 ml)

Dosage:

- Depression:
  - *IR:* 20 mg/day initially, can be increased based on tolerance/response to max 50 mg/day
    or
  - *Paxil CR:* 25 mg/day initially, can be increased based on tolerance/response to max 62.5 mg/day
- OCD: 20 mg/day initially, can be increased based on tolerance/response to max 60 mg/day

- Panic disorder:
  - *IR:* 10 mg/day initially, can be increased based on tolerance/response to max 60 mg/day
    or
  - *Paxil CR:* 12.5 mg/day initially, can be increased based on tolerance/response to max 75 mg/day
- Social anxiety disorder:
  - *IR:* 20 mg/day
    or
  - *Paxil CR:* 12.5 mg/day initially, can be increased based on tolerance/response to max 37.5 mg/day
- GAD: 20 mg/day initially, can be increased based on tolerance/response to max 50 mg/day
- PTSD: 20 mg/day initially, can be increased based on tolerance/response to max 50 mg/day
- PMDD: 12.5 mg/day (*Paxil CR*), can be increased based on tolerance/response to max 25 mg/day
- Menopausal vasomotor symptoms:
  - *Brisdelle:* 7.5 mg qhs
    or
  - *Paxil CR*: 12.5–25 mg/day

MOA: Similar to *SSRI Class Profile*

Pharmacokinetics: t_{max}=5.2–10 hrs, $t_{1/2}$=approx 15–21 hrs

Warnings:
- Similar to *SSRI Class Profile*
- **Black box warning:** Increased risk of suicidal thinking and behavior in children, adolescents, and young adults; not approved for use in pediatric patients
- Greater risk of discontinuation syndrome due to short half-life

Drug interactions:
- Similar to *SSRI Class Profile*
- Fosamprenavir/ritonavir may decrease levels of paroxetine
- Use with cimetidine increases levels; phenytoin and phenobarbital reduce levels
- May inhibit TCA metabolism; use caution if combined
- Use caution if used with other drugs metabolized by CYP2D6

Common side effects: Constipation, diarrhea, dizziness, dry mouth, ejaculation disorder, headache, insomnia, nausea, somnolence, sweating, tremors, withdrawal syndrome

Contraindications:
- Similar to *SSRI Class Profile*
- Patients taking thioridazine or tamoxifen

Recommended lab tests: None

Overdose: May cause ataxia, emesis, lethargy, tachycardia, seizures; OD rare

Tapering/withdrawal: Very slow taper recommended (25% dose decrease per week), can be cross-tapered with longer acting agent like fluoxetine

Special populations:

Pregnancy: Risk Category D

Lactation: Safe/preferred option

Elderly: 10 mg/day initially, max 40 mg

Hepatic impairment: 10 mg/day initially, max 40 mg

Renal impairment: No dose adjustment necessary in mild to moderate, reduce dose 50% in severe

Important notes:

* Preferred treatment for MDD with severe anxiety symptoms and loss of appetite

Sertraline[4, 8,12,13,19,29,41,43,44,45,47,52,53,56]

Brand name: Zoloft

FDA approved for: MDD, OCD in adults and children/adolescents (ages 6–17 yrs), panic disorder, PMDD, PTSD, social anxiety disorder

Other potential uses (off-label): Eating disorders, fibromyalgia, GAD, hot flashes, migraines, post-MI depression

Medication forms: *Tab* (25, 50, 100 mg); *oral conc* (20 mg/ml)

Dosage:

* Depression: 50 mg qam initially, can be increased based on tolerance/response to max 200 mg/day
* OCD: 50 mg qam initially, can be increased based on tolerance/response to max 200–300 mg/day
* Panic disorders/PTSD/social anxiety disorder: 25 mg qam initially, can be increased based on tolerance/response to max 200 mg/day
* PMDD: 50 mg/day throughout the menstrual cycle or limited to the luteal phase, can be increased based on tolerance/response to max 150 mg/day

MOA: Similar to *SSRI Class Profile* but also has very weak effects on norepinephrine and dopamine neuronal reuptake

Pharmacokinetics: t_{max}=4.5–8.4 hrs, $t_{1/2}$=26 hrs

Warnings:

* Similar to *SSRI Class Profile*
* **Black box warning:** Increased risk of suicidal thinking and behavior in children, adolescents and young adults; not approved for use in pediatric patients except for patients with OCD
* Can cause weak uricosuric effect and weight loss

- Use caution in patients with latex allergy due to rubber solution dropper

Drug interactions:

- Similar to *SSRI Class Profile*
- Can alter metabolism of cisapride and levels of lithium and risperidone
- Do not use concomitantly with disulfiram due to ETOH in solution

Common side effects: Diarrhea, dizziness, drowsiness, dry mouth, ejaculation disorder, fatigue, GI problems, headache, insomnia, nausea, somnolence, tremor

Contraindications:

- Similar to *SSRI Class Profile*
- Patients taking disulfiram or procarbazine

Recommended lab tests: None

Overdose: Serotonin syndrome, seizures, hyponatremia; OD rare

Tapering/withdrawal: Slow tapering recommended

Special populations:

Pregnancy: Risk Category C

Lactation: Use caution

Elderly: Lower dose recommended initially

Hepatic impairment: Use caution

Renal impairment: No dose adjustment necessary

Important notes:

- At higher doses, it can cause some dopamine-reuptake inhibition
- Desirable choice for patients with cardiac problems

Serotonin Norepinephrine Reuptake Inhibitors (SNRIs)[19,23,28,39,44,45,46,59]

Class Profile

Overview: SNRIs are a class of antidepressant drugs that are mainly used in the treatment of MDD and various anxiety disorders. Some of the commonly used SNRIs are desvenlafaxine, duloxetine, levomilnacipran, milnacipran, and venlafaxine.[45]

MOA: SNRIs block serotonin and norepinephrine reuptake, thereby increasing serotonergic and noradrenergic neurotransmission and prompting a rapid downregulation of β-adrenergic receptors.

Warnings:

- **Black box warning:** All antidepressants carry a black box warning for increased risk of suicidal thinking and behavior in children, adolescents, and young adults
- May result in clinical worsening and increased risk of suicide
- Can lower seizure threshold, trigger angle-closure glaucoma, and interfere with cognitive/motor performance
- Risk of abnormal bleeding, hyponatremia (due to SIADH), and serotonin syndrome

- Can activate mania/hypomania; screen for bipolar disorder
- Can cause urinary hesitation/retention and elevate BP

Drug interactions:
- Risk of serotonin syndrome when combined with SSRIs, SNRIs, TCAs, MAOIs, or other serotonergic agents, such as buspirone, triptans, fentanyl, lithium, tryptophan, St. John's wort, linezolid, or IV methylene blue; do not use for at least 2 weeks after stopping MAOIs
- Can cause an increase in bleeding when combined with medications such as NSAIDs, aspirin, warfarin, or other drugs that may alter hemostasis
- Use caution when combined with alcohol or other CNS acting drugs

Class side effects: Anorexia, anxiety, constipation, dizziness, dry mouth, fatigue, headache, insomnia, nausea, palpitations, sexual dysfunction, somnolence, sweating, vision problems.

Contraindications: Patients with uncontrolled angle-closure glaucoma, hypersensitivity, or taking MAOIs, IV methylene blue, or linezolid.

Overdose: Less safe than SSRIs.

Discontinuation syndrome: Abrupt cessation can lead to discontinuation syndrome. Venlafaxine, desvenlafaxine, and milnacipran may especially increase the risk of discontinuation symptoms when stopped suddenly due to relatively short half-life and low protein binding.

Important notes[45]:
- Monitor BP, particularly in the first two months of treatment at higher doses of SNRIs

Individual Drug Profiles
Desvenlafaxine[4,8,12,13,19,29,43,44,45,47,52,53,56,61]

Brand name: Pristiq, Khedezla

FDA approved for: MDD

Other potential uses (off-label): Fibromyalgia, hot flashes, migraines, panic disorder

Medication forms: *ER tab* (50, 100 mg)

Dosage:
- MDD: 50 mg/day initially, can be increased based on tolerance/response to max 100 mg/day

MOA: Similar to *SNRI Class Profile* and venlafaxine; is a more potent norepinephrine-reuptake inhibitor than venlafaxine but less potent than duloxetine

Pharmacokinetics: t_{max}=7.5 hrs, $t_{1/2}$=10–11 hrs

Warnings:
- Similar to *SNRI Class Profile*

- **Black box warning:** Increased risk of suicidal thinking and behavior in children, adolescents, and young adults; not approved for use in pediatric patients
- May cause interstitial lung disease and eosinophilic pneumonia

Drug Interactions: Similar to *SNRI Class Profile*

Common side effects: Anxiety, constipation, dizziness, dry mouth, fatigue, headache, increased sweating, insomnia, nausea, sexual dysfunction, vision problems

Contraindications: Similar to *SNRI Class Profile*

Recommended lab tests: None

Overdose: GI problems, cardiac toxicity, serotonin syndrome

Tapering/withdrawal: Gradual tapering required; take on alternate days for 2 weeks

Special populations:

Pregnancy: Risk Category C

Lactation: Use caution

Elderly: Lower dose recommended due to risk of hypotension

Hepatic impairment: 50 mg/day recommended

Renal impairment: No dose adjustment necessary in mild to moderate, 50 mg/day recommended in severe

Important notes:

- Is an active metabolite of venlafaxine
- Onset of action for vasomotor symptoms is much faster than for depression
- For withdrawal and smooth tapering, cross-tapering with a long-acting SSRI can be useful

Duloxetine[4,8,11,12,13,19,29,43,44,45,47,52,53,56]

Brand name: Cymbalta

FDA approved for: MDD, GAD, chronic musculoskeletal pain, diabetic peripheral neuropathic pain, fibromyalgia

Other potential uses (off-label): Migraines, stress incontinence

Medication forms: *DR cap* (20, 30, 60 mg)

Dosage:

- MDD: 60 mg qd or 30 mg bid initially, can be increased based on tolerance/response to max 120 mg/day
- GAD: 60 mg qd initially, can be increased based on tolerance/response to max 120 mg/day
- Fibromyalgia/chronic musculoskeletal pain: 30–60 mg/day

MOA: Similar to *SNRI Class Profile;* most noradrenergic of available SNRIs

Pharmacokinetics: t_{max}=6–10 hrs, $t_{1/2}$=8–17 hrs (average 12 hrs)

Warnings:
- Similar to *SNRI Class Profile*
- **Black box warning:** Increased risk of suicidal thinking and behavior in children, adolescents, and young adults; not approved for use in pediatric patients
- May cause hepatotoxicity, orthostatic hypotension, syncope, and severe skin reactions
- Use caution in conditions which reduce gastric emptying
- Can increase fasting blood glucose in diabetic peripheral neuropathic pain patients

Drug interactions:
- Similar to *SNRI Class Profile*
- Avoid concomitant use with thioridazine or with other CYP1A2 inhibitors (e.g., fluvoxamine and quinolone-based antibiotics)
- Potent inhibitors of CYP2D6 can increase drug concentrations
- Can increase concentrations of drugs metabolized by CYP2D6 (e.g., TCAs); use caution when combined

Common side effects: Constipation, decreased appetite, diarrhea, dizziness, dry mouth, fatigue, headache, insomnia, nausea, somnolence

Contraindications:
- Similar to *SNRI Class Profile*
- Do not prescribe in patients with liver disease due to increased serum transaminases

Recommended lab tests: None

Overdose: GI problems, cardiac toxicity, serotonin syndrome

Tapering/withdrawal: Slow tapering recommended (50% reduction per week)

Special populations:
Pregnancy: Risk Category C
Lactation: Use caution
Elderly: Lower dose recommended
Hepatic impairment: Contraindicated
Renal impairment: No dose adjustment necessary in mild to moderate, avoid in severe

Important notes:
- Due to risk of hepatotoxicity, avoid in patients with history of chronic alcohol use or liver disease

Levomilnacipran[4,8,12,13,15,19,29,43,44,45,47,52,53,56]
Brand name: Fetzima
FDA approved for: MDD
Other potential uses (off-label): Anxiety disorders, fibromyalgia
Medication forms: *ER cap* (20, 40, 80, 120 mg)
Dosage:
- MDD: 20 mg/day initially, can be increased based on tolerance/response to max 120 mg/day

MOA: Similar to *SNRI Class Profile*
Pharmacokinetics: t_{max}=6–8 hrs, $t_{1/2}$=12 hrs
Warnings:

- Similar to *SNRI Class Profile*
- **Black box warning:** Increased risk of suicidal thinking and behavior in children, adolescents, and young adults; not approved for use in pediatric patients
- Use caution in patients with history of cardiovascular disease or tachyarrhythmia

Drug Interactions:

- Similar to *SNRI Class Profile*
- Lower dose recommended when used with CYP3A4 inhibitors (e.g., ketoconazole, clarithromycin, ritonavir)

Common side effects: Constipation, erectile dysfunction, increased sweating, nausea, palpitations, tachycardia, vomiting
Contraindications: Similar to *SNRI Class Profile*
Recommended lab tests: LFTs
Overdose: Data limited
Tapering/withdrawals: Slow tapering recommended
Special populations:
Pregnancy: Risk Category C
Lactation: Avoid
Elderly: Lower dose recommended
Hepatic impairment: No dose adjustment necessary
Renal impairment: 80 mg qd recommended in mild to moderate, 40 mg qd recommended in severe
Important notes:

- Capsules should be swallowed whole
- May be a more potent norepinephrine inhibitor than serotonin inhibitor

Milnacipran[4,8,12,13,17,19,29,43,44,45,47,52,53,56]
Brand name: Savella
FDA approved for: Fibromyalgia
Other potential uses (off-label): MDD, migraines
Medication forms: *Cap* (25, 50 mg); *tab* (12.5, 25, 50, 100 mg)
Dosage:

- Fibromyalgia: 100 mg bid
- MDD (adults): 25–50 mg bid

MOA: Similar to *SNRI Class Profile*; also causes dopamine reuptake
Pharmacokinetics: t_{max}=2–4 hrs, $t_{1/2}$=6–8 hrs
Warnings:

- Similar to *SNRI Class Profile*

- **Black box warning:** Increased risk of suicidal thinking and behavior in children, adolescents, and young adults; not approved for use in pediatric patients
- May cause tachycardia and hepatotoxicity

Drug interactions: Similar to *SNRI Class Profile*

Common side effects: Constipation, dizziness, dry mouth, headache, hot flashes, increased sweating, insomnia, nausea, palpitations

Contraindications: Similar to *SNRI Class Profile*

Recommended lab tests: LFTs

Overdose: Seizures, serotonin syndrome; OD rare

Tapering/withdrawal: Slow tapering recommended (25% per week)

Special populations:

Pregnancy: Risk Category C

Lactation: Avoid

Elderly: Lower dose recommended (15–25 mg bid)

Hepatic impairment: No dose adjustment necessary in mild to moderate, use caution in severe and lower dose if LFTs are elevated 5x normal

Renal impairment: No dose adjustment necessary in mild to moderate, lower dose recommended in severe

Important notes:

- Monitor LFTs and avoid prescribing in patients with history of chronic alcohol use or liver disease

Venlafaxine[4,8,12,13,19,29,30,43,44,45,47,52,53,56,60]

Brand name: Effexor, Effexor XR

FDA approved for: MDD, GAD, social anxiety disorder, panic disorder

Other potential uses (off-label): ADHD, fibromyalgia, hot flashes, migraines, OCD, PMDD, PTSD

Medication forms: *Tab* (25, 37.5, 50, 75, 100 mg); *XR tab* (37.5, 75, 150, 225 mg); *XR cap* (37.5, 75, 150 mg)

Dosage:

- Depression:
  - *IR:* 75 mg initially, can be increased based on tolerance/response to max 375 mg/day
  - *XR:* 37.5 mg initially, can be increased based on tolerance/response to max 225 mg/day
- GAD: 37.5 mg (*XR*) initially, can be increased based on tolerance/response to max 225 mg/day
- Social Anxiety: 75 mg qd (*XR*)

- Panic Disorder: 37.5 mg qd (*XR*) initially, can be increased based on tolerance/response to max 225 mg/day

MOA: Similar to *SNRI Class Profile;* also inhibits dopamine reuptake

Pharmacokinetics: t_{max}=1–2 hrs, $t_{1/2}$=5 hrs

Warnings:

- Similar to *SNRI Class Profile*
- **Black box warning**: Increased risk of suicidal thinking and behavior in children, adolescents, and young adults; not approved for use in pediatric patients
- May cause interstitial lung disease and eosinophilic pneumonia

Drug interactions:

- Similar to *SNRI Class Profile*
- Use caution with cimetidine in elderly, hepatic dysfunction, or pre-existing HTN
- Use caution with diuretics and metoprolol
- Decreases plasma levels of indinavir and imipramine
- Increases haloperidol, risperidone, and desipramine plasma levels
- Use caution with potent CYP3A4 and CYP2D6 inhibitors

Common side effects: Anorexia, anxiety, asthenia, constipation, decreased libido, dizziness, dry mouth, ejaculation disorder, fatigue, headache, insomnia, nausea, nervousness

Contraindications: Similar to *SNRI Class Profile*

Recommended lab tests: BP

Overdose: GI problems, cardiac toxicity, serotonin syndrome

Tapering/withdrawal: Very slow taper recommended (20–25% reduction per week); can be cross-tapered with longer acting agent like fluoxetine

Special populations:

Pregnancy: Risk Category C

Lactation: Use caution

Elderly: Reduce dose by 50% initially

Hepatic impairment: Reduce dose by 50% in mild to moderate, use caution in severe

Renal impairment: Reduce dose by 25% in mild to moderate, reduce dose by 50% in severe

Important notes:

- Advise patients against sudden discontinuation because of severe withdrawal symptoms
- Favorable choice for severe treatment-resistant depression when combined with other antidepressants like mirtazapine[19]
- May cause false positive on instant urine tests for PCP

Serotonin Antagonist and Reuptake Inhibitors (SARIs)[19,23,28,39,44,45,46,59]

Class Profile

Overview: Drugs of this class include nefazodone, trazodone, and to some extent vilazodone. The side-effect profile and potential toxicity of SARIs differ considerably from those of other antidepressants. These drugs should not be taken alongside MAOIs, TCAs, or SSRIs.

MOA: Inhibits the neuronal reuptake of serotonin and norepinephrine and antagonizes $5\text{-HT}_{2A/2C}$ receptors.

Warnings:

- **Black box warning:** All antidepressants carry a black box warning for increased risk of suicidal thinking and behavior in children, adolescents, and young adults; not approved for use in pediatric patients
- May result in clinical worsening and increased risk of suicide
- Can lower seizure threshold, trigger angle-closure glaucoma, and interfere with cognitive/motor performance
- Risk of abnormal bleeding, hyponatremia (due to SIADH), and serotonin syndrome
- Can activate mania/hypomania; screen for bipolar disorder

Drug interactions:

- Risk of serotonin syndrome when combined with SSRIs, SNRIs, TCAs, MAOIs, or other serotonergic agents, such as buspirone, triptans, fentanyl, lithium, tryptophan, St. John's wort, linezolid, or IV methylene blue; do not use for at least 2 weeks after stopping MAOIs
- Can cause increased bleeding when combined with medications such as NSAIDs, aspirin, warfarin, or other drugs that alter hemostasis
- Can moderately increase digoxin levels
- Use caution when combined with alcohol or other CNS acting drugs

Class side effects: Blurred vision, constipation, dizziness, dry mouth, headache, nausea, somnolence, vomiting.

Contraindications: Patients with hypersensitivity or taking MAOIs, IV methylene blue, or linezolid.

Discontinuation syndrome: Abrupt cessation can lead to discontinuation syndrome.

Individual Drug Profiles

Nefazodone[4,8,12,13,19,29,40,43,44,45,47,52,53,56]

Brand name: Serzone

FDA approved for: Depression

Other potential uses (off-label): Akathisia, panic disorder, social anxiety disorder

Medication forms: *Tab* (50, 100, 150, 200, 250 mg)

Dosage:
- Depression: 100 mg bid initially, can be increased based on tolerance/response to max 600 mg

MOA: Similar to *SARI Class Profile*

Pharmacokinetics: t_{max}=1 hr, $t_{1/2}$=2–4 hrs

Warnings:
- Similar to *SARI Class Profile*
- **Black box warning:**
  - Increased risk of suicidal thinking and behavior in children, adolescents, and young adults; not approved for use in pediatric patients
  - May cause life-threatening hepatic failure leading to transplant and/or death
- May cause orthostatic hypotension and priapism

Drug interactions:
- Similar to *SARI Class Profile*
- Increases concentration of buspirone, cyclosporine, tacrolimus, triazolam, alprazolam, terfenadine, astemizole, cisapride, and pimozole
- Combination with anti-arrhythmics, pimozide, or ziprasidone may enhance cardiotoxicity
- Caution should be used administered in combination with simvastatin, atorvastatin, or lovastatin, as there have been cases of rhabdomyolysis
- Use caution with highly protein bound drugs, as displacement could increase levels of either drug

Common side effects: Abnormal/blurred vision, confusion, constipation, dizziness, dry mouth, headache, nausea, somnolence

Contraindications:
- Similar to *SARI Class Profile*
- History of liver injury with nefazodone

Recommended lab tests: LFTs

Overdose: CNS depression, nausea/vomiting, seizures; OD rare

Tapering/withdrawal: Slow taper recommended but discontinuation syndrome uncommon

Special populations:

Pregnancy: Risk Category C

Lactation: Avoid

Elderly: Lower doses recommended

Hepatic impairment: Avoid in patients with active liver disease

Renal impairment: No dose adjustment necessary

Important notes[45]:

- In May 2004, Serzone was withdrawn from manufacturing and marketing in the US, although generic products remain available[45]
- No effects on sexual functioning, unlike other antidepressants
- Stop drug if transaminase levels increase >3x, due to risk of life-threatening hepatic failure
- Useful as adjunctive agent in treating negative symptoms of schizophrenia

Trazodone[4,6,8,12,13,19,29,43,44,45,47,52,53,56]

Brand name: Desyrel, Desyrel Dividose, Oleptro

FDA approved for: MDD

Other potential uses (off-label): Alcoholism, insomnia, panic disorder

Medication forms: *Tab* (50, 100, 150, 300 mg); *ER tab* (150, 300 mg)

Dosage:
- MDD:
  - *IR*: 150 mg/day initially divided bid or tid, can be increased based on tolerance/response to max 400 mg/day
  - *ER (Oleptro)*: 150 mg hs initially, can be increased based on tolerance/response to max 375 mg/day

MOA: Similar to *SARI Class Profile*

Pharmacokinetics: t_{max}=1–2 hrs, $t_{1/2}$=7–10 hrs

Warnings:
- Similar to *SARI Class Profile*
- **Black box warning:** Increased risk of suicidal thinking and behavior in children, adolescents, and young adults; not approved for use in pediatric patients
- Avoid during initial recovery phase of MI and discontinue before elective surgery
- Risk of neuroleptic malignant syndrome-like reactions
- May cause QT prolongation, orthostatic hypotension, priapism

Drug interactions:
- Similar to *SARI Class Profile*
- Use lower dose with potent CYP3A4 inhibitors (e.g., ritonavir, ketoconazole, indinavir, itraconazole, nefazodone)
- Concurrent use with CYP3A4 inducers (e.g., carbamazepine) may require higher dose of trazodone
- Can potentiate the effects of phenytoin by increasing serum levels
- Can enhance the effects of alcohol, barbiturates, and other CNS depressants

Common side effects: Blurred vision, constipation, dizziness, drowsiness, dry mouth, fatigue, headache, sedation, vomiting

Contraindications: Similar to *SARI Class Profile*

Recommended lab tests: None

Overdose: Drowsiness, ataxia, nausea/vomiting, tinnitus, lethargy, seizures, coma, bradycardia, hypotension, and priapism can develop; OD rare

Tapering/withdrawal: Slow tapering recommended

Special populations:

Pregnancy: Risk Category C

Lactation: Use caution (<100 mg/day recommended)

Elderly: Lower dose recommended

Hepatic impairment: Use caution

Renal impairment: No dose adjustment necessary

Important notes[45]:

- Inform patients about the symptoms and risk of priapism
- Commonly used sedating antidepressant for insomnia
- May augment response in SSRIs and treat SSRI- or MAOI-induced insomnia

Vilazodone[4,8,12,13,18,19,29,43,44,45,47,52,53,56]

Brand name: Viibryd

FDA approved for: MDD

Other potential uses (off-label): Social anxiety disorder

Medication forms: *Tab* (10, 20, 40 mg)

Dosage:

- MDD: 10 mg/day initially, can be increased based on tolerance/response to max 40 mg/day

MOA: Selective serotonin reuptake inhibitor and partial agonist of $5HT_{1A}$ receptors

Pharmacokinetics: t_{max}=4–5 hrs, $t_{1/2}$=25 hrs

Warnings:

- Similar to *SARI Class Profile*
- **Black box warning:** Increased risk of suicidal thinking and behavior in children, adolescents, and young adults; not approved for use in pediatric patients

Drug interactions:

- Similar to *SARI Class Profile*
- Interacts more severely with any drugs that can potentiate serotonin syndrome
- In concomitant use with CYP3A4 inhibitors, reduce dose to 20 mg
- In concomitant use with CYP3A4 inducers, increase dose 2x to max 80 mg

Common side effects: Diarrhea, dizziness, dry mouth, headache, insomnia, nausea, vomiting

Contraindications: Similar to *SARI Class Profile*

Recommended lab tests: None

Overdose: Seizures, serotonin syndrome; OD rare

Tapering/withdrawal: Slow tapering recommended (over a week or longer)

Special populations:

Pregnancy: Risk Category C
Lactation: Avoid
Elderly: No dose adjustment necessary
Hepatic impairment: No dose adjustment necessary in mild to moderate, reduce dose in severe
Renal impairment: No dose adjustment necessary
Important notes:
- Reportedly causes less sexual dysfunction and weight gain than other antidepressants
- Should always be taken with food

Other Medications
Agomelatine[29,47,52,53,56]
Brand name: Valdoxan, Melitor, Thymanax
FDA approved for: None (approved for MDD in Europe)
Other potential uses (off-label): GAD, insomnia, MDD
Medication forms: *Tab* (25 mg)
Dosage:
- MDD: 25 mg/day hs initially, can be increased based on tolerance/response to max 50 mg/day

MOA: Agonist at MT_1 and MT_2 receptors, antagonizes $5\text{-}HT_{2C}$ receptors
Pharmacokinetics: t_{max}=0.5–4 hrs, $t_{1/2}$=1–2 hrs
Warnings:
- Contraindicated for use in patients with galactose intolerance, lactase enzyme deficiency, or glucose-galactose malabsorption

Drug interactions:
- Risk of serotonin syndrome when combined with SSRIs, SNRIs, TCAs, MAOIs, or other serotonergic agents
- Plasma concentration increased with potent CYP1A2 inhibitors (e.g., fluvoxamine, ciprofloxacin)

Common side effects: Abdominal pain, anxiety, back pain, constipation, diarrhea, dizziness, headache, increased sweating, nausea, sleepiness, somnolence, vomiting
Contraindications:
- Severe renal and hepatic impairment
- Patients taking CYP1A2 inhibitors (e.g., fluvoxamine, ciprofloxacin) and/or MAOIs

Recommended lab tests: LFTs
Overdose: Somnolence, abdominal pain; OD rare
Tapering/withdrawal: Tapering generally not required

Special populations:
Pregnancy: No data in humans
Lactation: Avoid
Elderly: Not recommended for ages 74+
Hepatic impairment: Contraindicated in severe
Renal impairment: Use caution in mild to moderate, contraindicated in severe
Important notes:
- Instruct patient to report any symptoms of liver injury immediately
- Should be taken at night time due to sedative effects

Bupropion[4,8,12,13,19,21,29,43,44,45,47,52,53,56]
Brand name: Aplenzin, Buproban, Budeprion SR & XL, Forfivo XL, Wellbutrin, Wellbutrin XL, Wellbutrin SR, Zyban
FDA approved for: MDD, smoking cessation, seasonal affective disorder
Other potential uses (off-label): ADHD, bipolar depression, sexual side effects of psychotropic medications, weight loss
Medication forms: *Tab* (75, 100 mg); *SR tab* (100, 150, 200 mg); *ER tab* (150, 174, 300, 348, 450, 522 mg)
Dosage:
- MDD:
  - *IR:* 100 mg bid initially, can be increased based on tolerance/response to max 450 mg/day
  - *SR:* 150 mg/day initially, can be increased based on tolerance/response to max 400 mg/day
  - *ER:* 150 mg/day initially, can be increased based on tolerance/response to max 450 mg/day
  - *Aplenzin (bupropion hydrobromide):* 174–348 mg/day initially, can be increased based on tolerance/response to max 522 mg/day
  - *Forfivo XL:* 450 mg/day
- Seasonal Affective Disorder:
  - *Wellbutrin XL* (September–November): 150 mg/day initially, can be increased based on tolerance/response to max 300 mg/day
  - *Aplenzin:* 174 mg/day initially, can be increased based on tolerance/response to max 348 mg/day
- Smoking Cessation (*Zyban*): 150 qd for 3 days, then increase to 150 mg bid for 2–3 months

MOA: Weakly inhibits the neuronal reuptake of dopamine and norepinephrine but does not inhibit monoamine oxidase or the reuptake of serotonin
Pharmacokinetics: t_{max}=2–5 hrs, $t_{1/2}$=14–21 hrs

Warnings:
- **Black box warning:**
  - Increased risk of suicidal thinking and behavior in children, adolescents, and young adults; not approved for use in pediatric patients
  - Serious neuropsychiatric events observed in patients using bupropion for smoking cessation
- May result in clinical worsening and increased risk of suicide
- Can lower seizure threshold, cause hypertension, trigger angle-closure glaucoma, and activate mania/hypomania

Drug interactions:
- Increased risk of hypertensive crisis with MAOIs
- Can lower seizure threshold with anti-psychotics, TCAs, theophylline, opioids, or cocaine
- Increased dose may be needed if used concomitantly with CYP2B6 inducers; decreased dose recommended if used with CYP2B6 inhibitors
- Can increase concentrations of drugs metabolized by CYP2D6
- Increased CNS toxicity in combination with dopaminergic drugs
- Can create false-positive urine test results for amphetamines

Common side effects: Agitation, anxiety, constipation, dizziness, dry mouth, increased sweating, headache, insomnia, nausea, tachycardia, vomiting, weight loss

Contraindications:
- Hypersensitivity, CNS tumor, recent head injury, history of seizure
- Do not use in patients with anorexia or bulimia, or withdrawing from alcohol or benzodiazepines, because of increased seizure risk
- Do not use concomitantly with MAOIs, linezolid, or IV methylene blue

Recommended lab tests: None

Overdose: Tremor, paresthesias, slurred speech, lethargy, confusion, hallucinations, seizure; OD rare

Tapering/withdrawal: Slow tapering recommended

Special populations:
Pregnancy: Risk Category C
Lactation: Use caution (reported case of seizure in 6-month-old baby)
Elderly: Lower dose recommended
Hepatic impairment: Reduce dose by 50%
Renal impairment: No dose adjustment necessary

Important notes:
- Risk of seizure seems dose dependent
- First medicine approved for seasonal affective disorder
- May be effective for SSRI-induced sexual side effects

- May increase cognition, energy, and memory
- Zyban is a good choice for patients who have not set a quit date for smoking

Mirtazapine[4,8,12,13,19,29,37,43,44,45,47,52,53,56]
Brand name: Remeron, Remeron SolTab
FDA approved for: MDD
Other potential uses (off-label): Anxiety disorder, insomnia, loss of appetite, SSRI-induced sexual side effects
Medication forms: *Tab* (7.5, 15, 30, 45 mg); *ODT* (15, 30, 45 mg)
Dosage:
- MDD: 15 mg qhs initially, can be increased based on tolerance/response to max 45 mg qhs

MOA: Blocks presynaptic α_2 receptors, enhancing both noradrenaline and serotonin release; also blocks H_1 receptors for strong sedative action
Pharmacokinetics: t_{max}=1.5–2 hrs, $t_{1/2}$=26–37 hrs
Warnings:
- **Black box warning:** Increased risk of suicidal thinking and behavior in children, adolescents, and young adults; not approved for use in pediatric patients
- May result in clinical worsening and increased risk of suicide
- Can lower seizure threshold, trigger angle-closure glaucoma, and interfere with cognitive/motor performance
- Risk of discontinuation symptoms, akathisia, hyponatremia (due to SIADH), serotonin syndrome, somnolence, dizziness, increased appetite, and weight gain
- Can activate mania/hypomania; screen for bipolar disorder
- May cause agranulocytosis; monitor regularly for signs of infection (e.g., sore throat)
- May increase cholesterol/triglycerides and transaminase levels

Drug interactions:
- Risk of serotonin syndrome when combined with SSRIs, SNRIs, TCAs, MAOIs, or other serotonergic agents
- Concomitant use with alcohol, other CNS depressants, or diazepam can further impair motor and cognitive functions
- Hepatic enzyme inducers (e.g., carbamazepine, phenytoin, rifampicin) increase clearance and may require a dosage increase of mirtazapine if used concomitantly
- Concomitant use with cimetidine can increase levels over 50%; reduction of mirtazapine dosage is recommended

- Use caution when using with potent CYP3A4 inhibitors, HIV protease inhibitors, azole antifungals, erythromycin, nefazodone, or warfarin

Common side effects: Asthenia, constipation, dizziness, dry mouth, increased appetite, somnolence, weight gain

Contraindications: Patients with hypersensitivity or taking MAOIs, linezolid, or IV methylene blue

Recommended lab tests: Lipid profile, weight

Overdose: Drowsiness, disorientation, tremor, headache, nausea/vomiting, ataxia, and rhabdomyolysis; fairly safe in OD with no reported fatalities

Tapering/withdrawal: Tapering recommended

Special populations:

Pregnancy: Risk Category C

Lactation: Use caution

Elderly: Lower dose recommended

Hepatic impairment: Use caution

Renal impairment: Lower dose recommended

Important notes:

- Possibly useful in depressed patients with coexisting anxiety disorder
- Lower risk of drug interactions; good choice for medically ill patients
- Lower sexual dysfunction than other antidepressant agents
- Lower doses are more sedating than higher doses

Reboxetine[29,47,52,53,56]

Brand name: Edronax, Prolift

FDA approved for: None

Other potential uses (off-label): MDD, drug-induced weight gain, eating disorder

Medication forms: *Tab* (2, 4 mg)

Dosage: 4 mg bid

MOA: Selective norepinephrine reuptake inhibitor and α_2-adrenergic receptor antagonist

Pharmacokinetics: t_{max}=1.5–2 hrs, $t_{1/2}$=12–14 hrs

Warnings:

- Use caution in patients with urinary retention, prostatic hypertrophy, glaucoma, cardiac problems, hypertension, or seizure disorder

Drug interactions:

- Risk of serotonin syndrome when combined with SSRIs, SNRIs, TCAs, MAOIs, or other serotonergic agents
- Increases concentration of thioridazine and pimozide; can cause cardiac arrhythmias

- Increases levels of alprazolam, buspirone, triazolam, simvastatin, atorvastatin, lovastatin, TCAs, and some beta blockers

Common side effects: Constipation, diaphoresis, dizziness, dry mouth, headache, increased sweating, insomnia, nausea, sedation, urinary retention

Contraindications: Hypersensitivity

Recommended lab tests: None

Overdose: Hypertensive crisis, confusion, seizures

Tapering/withdrawal: Tapering recommended

Special populations:

Pregnancy: Data not available

Lactation: Avoid

Elderly: Lower dose recommended

Hepatic/Renal impairment: Lower dose recommended

Important notes:

- May be effective for patients with cognitive problems

Vortioxetine[4,8,12,13,19,29,43,44,45,47,48,52,53,56]

Brand name: Brintellix

FDA approved for: MDD

Other potential uses (off-label): Anxiety disorders

Medication forms: *Tab* (5, 10, 15, 20 mg)

Dosage:

- MDD: 10 mg/day initially, can be increased based on tolerance/response to max 20 mg/day

MOA: Inhibits the reuptake of serotonin; antagonizes 5-HT_3, 5-HT_{1D}, and 5-HT_7 receptors; agonizes 5-HT_{1A} receptors; and is a 5-HT_{1B} receptor partial agonist

Pharmacokinetics: t_{max}=7–11 hrs, $t_{1/2}$=66 hrs

Warnings:

- **Black box warning**: Increased risk of suicidal thinking and behavior in children, adolescents, and young adults; not approved for use in pediatric patients
- May result in clinical worsening and increased risk of suicide
- May lower seizure threshold and trigger angle-closure glaucoma
- Risk of abnormal bleeding, hyponatremia (due to SIADH), and serotonin syndrome
- May activate mania/hypomania; screen for bipolar disorder
- May cause various types of HSRs

Drug interactions:

- Risk of serotonin syndrome when combined with SSRIs, SNRIs, TCAs, MAOIs, or other serotonergic agents

- Reduce dosage by half when used with strong inhibitors of CYP2D6 (e.g., bupropion, fluoxetine, paroxetine, quinidine)

Common side effects: Constipation, diarrhea, dizziness, dry mouth, flatulence, nausea, puritus, sexual dysfunction, vomiting

Contraindications: Patients with hypersensitivity or taking MAOIs, linezolid, or IV methylene blue

Recommended lab tests: Monitor for weight and BMI changes

Overdose: Abdominal pain, diarrhea, serotonin syndrome

Tapering/withdrawal: Slow taper recommended

Special populations:

Pregnancy: Risk Category C

Lactation: Avoid

Elderly: No dose adjustment necessary

Hepatic impairment: No dose adjustment necessary in mild to moderate, avoid in severe

Renal impairment: No dose adjustment necessary

Important notes:

- Monitor patients for symptoms of bleeding
- Being investigated as a treatment for GAD

Monoamine Oxidase Inhibitors (MAOIs)[19,23,28,39,44,46,56,59]

Class Profile

Overview: MAOIs are used for atypical depression and are also useful for Parkinson's disease and several other disorders. However, MAOIs have serious side effects, especially hypertensive crisis. Because of potentially lethal dietary and drug interactions, they are reserved as the last line of treatment for depression. The MAOIs commonly in use include:

- Nonselective MAO-A/MAO-B inhibitors
  - Hydrazines (e.g., isocarboxazid, phenelzine)
  - Non-hydrazines (tranylcypromine)
- Selective MAO-A inhibitors (moclobemide)
- Selective MAO-B inhibitors (selegiline)

MOA: Enhance norepinephrine, serotonin, and dopamine by irreversibly blocking monoamine oxidase from breaking down these neurotransmitters.

Warnings:

- **Black box warning:** All antidepressants carry a black box warning for increased risk of suicidal thinking and behavior in children, adolescents, and young adults; not approved for use in pediatric patients
- May cause severe hypertensive crisis (possibly fatal)
- Requires a low-tyramine diet due to risk of hypertensive crisis with improper diet restriction; avoid intake of tyramine-rich foods, including aged cheeses, cured meats, sauerkraut, liver, yeast extract, pods of broad beans, yogurt,

marmite, vegemite, aged fish, beer, wine, and large amounts of chocolate or caffeine[45]

- Interaction with alcohol is harmful and strictly prohibited
- Discontinue 10 days prior to elective surgery
- Use caution in patients with DM due to risk of hypoglycemia
- May result in clinical worsening and increased suicide risk
- Can activate mania/hypomania; screen for bipolar disorder

Drug interactions:

- Risk of serotonin syndrome when combined with SSRIs, SNRIs, TCAs, MAOIs, or other serotonergic agents, such as buspirone, triptans, fentanyl, lithium, tryptophan, St. John's wort, linezolid, or IV methylene blue; wait at least 2 weeks before beginning another serotonergic agent or MAOI
- Hypertensive crisis may result from use with sympathomimetic drugs such as amphetamines, methylphenidate, cocaine, dopamine, epinephrine, norepinephrine, methyldopa, levodopa, L-tryptophan, and phenylalanine, or from combining with other MAOIs
- Seizures, delirium, coma, or death may result when combined with meperidine or dextromethorphan
- Avoid cold/cough medicines, sinus medications, asthma inhalants, and weight-reducing OTC drugs
- Wait 5 weeks after discontinuing fluoxetine before starting MAOI therapy

Class side effects: Blurred vision, dizziness, dry mouth, headache, orthostatic hypotension, rash, sexual dysfunction, weight gain.

Contraindications: Patients with hypersensitivity, severe liver/kidney impairment, severe or frequent headaches, cardiovascular/cerebrovascular diseases, uncontrolled hypertension, thyroid disorders, or pheochromocytoma.

Recommended lab tests: BP, LFTs, RFTs.

Overdose: Hypertension, diaphoresis, delirium, seizures, multi-organ failure; OD can be fatal.

Tapering/withdrawal: Tapering not necessary.

Special populations:

Pregnancy: Risk Category C

Lactation: Avoid

Elderly: Lower dose recommended

Hepatic impairment: Avoid

Renal impairment: No dose adjustment necessary in mild to moderate, avoid in severe

Important notes:

- Wait 2 weeks before starting another antidepressant or other MAOIs
- Due to severe dietary restrictions, MAOIs are rarely used these days
- Blood pressure should be monitored closely during treatment

Individual Drug Profiles
Isocarboxazid[4,8,12,13,19,29,43,44,45,47,52,53]

Brand name: Marplan

FDA approved for: Depression

Other potential uses (off-label): Anxiety, bulimia, obesity, panic disorder

Medication forms: *Tab* (10 mg)

Dosage:
- Depression: 10 mg bid initially, can be increased based on tolerance/response to max 60 mg/day divided (use caution with dosages ⊠40 mg/day)

MOA: Non-selectively inhibits MAO in the brain, heart, and liver; mechanism in depression is unknown but may be due to increased levels of biogenic amines in the brain

Pharmacokinetics: t_{max}=5–10 days, $t_{1/2}$=1–3 hrs

Warnings:
- Similar to *MAOI Class Profile*
- **Black box warning:** Increased risk of suicidal thinking and behavior in children, adolescents, and young adults; not approved for use in pediatric patients
- Can exacerbate anxiety and agitation; use caution in hyperactive, agitated, or schizophrenic patients

Common side effects: Agitation, anxiety, constipation, dizziness, dry mouth, drowsiness, headache, insomnia, nausea, orthostatic hypotension, sexual dysfunction, tremor

Important notes:
- May have some use in the treatment of bulimia

Moclobemide[29,47,52,53]

Brand name: Aurorix, Clobemix, Manerix

FDA approved for: None

Other potential uses (off-label): Depression, bulimia, PTSD

Medication forms: *Tab* (150, 300 mg)

Dosage:
- Depression: 300 mg/day initially, can be increased based on tolerance/response to max 600 mg/day

MOA: Reversibly blocks MAO-A from breaking down

Pharmacokinetics: t_{max}=1.2 hrs, $t_{1/2}$=2 hrs

Common side effects: Blurred vision, dizziness, dry mouth, headache, hypotension, sexual dysfunction, weight gain

Important notes:
- No significant rise in BP when combined with tyramine-containing foods

Phenelzine[4,8,12,13,19,29,38,43,44,45,47,52,53]

Brand name: Nardil

FDA approved for: Depression (atypical, non-endogenous, or neurotic)

Other potential uses (off-label): Agoraphobia, bulimia, migraines, selective mutism

Medication forms: *Tab* (15 mg)

Dosage:

- Depression: 15 mg tid initially, can be increased based on tolerance/response to max 90 mg/day divided

MOA: Non-selective inhibition of MOA, other pharmacologic actions, or both may result in clinical effect

Pharmacokinetics: t_{max}=43 min, $t_{1/2}$=11–13 hrs

Warnings:

- Similar to *MAOI Class Profile*
- **Black box warning:** Increased risk of suicidal thinking and behavior in children, adolescents, and young adults; not approved for use in pediatric patients

Common side effects: Blurred vision, constipation, dizziness, dry mouth, fatigue, headache, myoclonus, sexual dysfunction, weight gain

Important notes:

- "Newcastle cocktail," previously used for treatment-refractory depression, used a combination of clomipramine or phenelzine, lithium, and tryptophan[45]

Tranylcypromine[4,8,9,12,13,19,29,43,44,45,47,52,53]

Brand name: Parnate

FDA approved for: MDD without melancholia

Other potential uses (off-label): Anxiety, panic disorder

Medication forms: *Tab* (10 mg)

Dosage:

- MDD: 30 mg divided tid initially, can be increased based on tolerance/response to max 60 mg/day

MOA: Non-selective inhibition of MAO increases serotonin levels in the brain

Pharmacokinetics: t_{max}=0.67–3.5 hrs, $t_{1/2}$=1.5–3.5 hrs

Warnings:

- Similar to *MAOI Class Profile*
- **Black box warning:** Increased risk of suicidal thinking and behavior in children, adolescents, and young adults; not approved for use in pediatric patients
- Possibility of dependence, even if used within therapeutic range

Common side effects: Blurred vision, drowsiness, dry mouth, headache, insomnia, sexual dysfunction

Selegiline[4,8,12,13,19,29,33,43,44,45,47,52,53]

Brand name: Emsam, Zelapar, Eldepryl

FDA approved for: MDD (transdermal), Parkinsonism (oral, as adjunctive)

Other potential uses (off-label): ADHD, dementia, Parkinson's disease

Medication forms: *Transdermal patch* (20mg/20cm^2[6mg/24 hrs], 30mg/30cm^2 [9mg/24 hrs], 40mg/40cm^2 [12 mg/24 hrs]); *tab* (1.25, 5 mg); *cap* (1.25, 5 mg)

Dosage:

- MDD: One 6 mg/24 hr patch qd initially, can be increased based on tolerance/ response to max 12 mg/24hr qd

MOA: Irreversible MOAI, inhibiting both MOA-A and MAO-B at antidepressant doses

Pharmacokinetics: t_{max}=40–90 min, $t_{1/2}$=18–25 hrs (transdermal)

Warnings:

- Similar to *MAOI Class Profile*
- **Black box warning:** Increased risk of suicidal thinking and behavior in children, adolescents, and young adults; not approved for use in pediatric patients
- Monitor patients for melanoma

Common side effects: Application-site reactions (transdermal), dizziness, dry mouth, nausea, rash

Important notes:

- Has neuroprotective effects and is reported to increase longevity in rodents and dogs
- Reduced risk of hypertensive crisis at low oral doses compared to other MAOIs
- No requirement on dietary restrictions at lower doses

Tricyclic Antidepressants (TCAs)[19,23,28,39,44,46,59]

Class Profile

Overview: TCAs are a group of medications used primarily in the treatment of depression. In the past few years, TCAs have been replaced in clinical use by newer antidepressants with more favorable side-effect profiles. The following TCAs are the most commonly used: amitriptyline, amoxapine, clomipramine, desipramine, doxepin, imipramine, mianserin, maprotiline, nortriptyline, protriptyline, and trimipramine.

Warnings:

- **Black box warning:** All antidepressants carry a black box warning for increased risk of suicidal thinking and behavior in children, adolescents, and young adults; not approved for use in pediatric patients

- May result in clinical worsening and increased suicide risk
- Use caution with history of seizure, urinary retention, angle-closure glaucoma or increased IOP, thyroid disorders, cardiovascular disorder, and suicidal tendency
- Discontinue before elective surgery
- Can alter blood glucose levels, exacerbate psychosis or schizophrenia, and lower seizure threshold
- Can activate mania/hypomania; screen for bipolar disorder
- Abrupt cessation may cause anticholinergic side effects and withdrawal symptoms

Drug interactions:

- Risk of serotonin syndrome when combined with SSRIs, SNRIs, TCAs, MAOIs, or other serotonergic agents, such as buspirone, triptans, fentanyl, lithium, tryptophan, St. John's wort, linezolid, or IV methylene blue; do not use for at least two weeks after stopping MAOIs
- Use with anticholinergic agents increases anticholinergic effects (e.g., paralytic ileus, tachycardia)
- Reduces antihypertensive effects of guanethidine
- Antipsychotics exacerbate the sedative, anticholinergic, epileptogenic, and pyretic effects of TCAs and increase risk of NMS
- Can cause delirium when combined with disulfiram
- Increases effects of alcohol, barbiturates, and other CNS depressants
- Use caution with anticoagulants; can increase warfarin levels
- Can cause arrhythmias, hypertension, and tachycardia when combined with sympathomimetics
- Allow five weeks after discontinuing fluoxetine before starting TCA therapy
- Levels raised by concurrent use with CYP2D6 inhibitors; use caution when combined

Class side effects: Blurred vision, constipation, dizziness, drowsiness, dry mouth, headache, insomnia, nausea, orthostatic hypotension, taste problems, tingling, tremor, urinary retention, weight gain.

Contraindications: Hypersensitivity, history of arrhythmias, heart disease, mania, severe liver disease, children <7 yrs, MAOIs taken within prior 14 days.

Recommended lab tests: EKG, LFTs.

Overdose: Coma, seizures, dysrhythmias, respiratory failure, hypotension, and death; OD common.

Tapering/withdrawal: Slow taper recommended.

Individual Drug Profiles

Amitriptyline[1,4,8,12,13,19,29,43,44,45,47,52,53,56]

Brand name: Elavil, Amitid

FDA approved for: Depression in adults and adolescents (ages 12–17 yrs)

Other potential uses (off-label): ADHD, bulimia, chronic pain, dysthymia, fibromyalgia, IBS, migraines, PTSD

Medication forms: *Tab* (10, 25, 50, 75, 100, 150 mg); *IM injection* (10mg/ml sol)

Dosage:

- Depression: 25–50 mg qhs initially, can be increased based on tolerance/response to max 300 mg/day
- Dysthymia: 150–300 mg/day
- PTSD: 150–300 mg/day

MOA: Promotes neuronal activity by blocking the membrane pump mechanism which is responsible for the absorption of serotonin and norepinephrine in serotonergic and adrenergic neurons; also has sedative properties

Pharmacokinetics: t_{max}=4 hrs, $t_{1/2}$=15 hrs

Warnings:

- Similar to *TCA Class Profile*
- **Black box warning:** Increased risk of suicidal thinking and behavior in children, adolescents, and young adults; not approved for use in pediatric patients
- May cause serious side effects: MI, prolonged QT interval, sudden cardiac death, bone marrow depression, coma, agranulocytosis, hepatotoxicity, NMS, stroke, paralytic ileus, hyperpyrexia, testicular swelling, gynecomastia, alopecia, edema, arrhythmia

Drug Interactions:

- Similar to *TCA Class Profile*
- Cimetidine can increase plasma levels

Common side effects: Dizziness, drowsiness, dry mouth, hallucinations, increased appetite, tachycardia, tingling, urinary retention, weight gain

Contraindications:

- Similar to *TCA Class Profile*
- Concomitant use with cisapride

Special populations:

Pregnancy: Risk Category C

Lactation: Use caution

Elderly: Lower dose recommended (10 mg tid)

Hepatic impairment: Use caution

Renal impairment: Lower dose recommended

Important notes:

- Used for migraines and chronic pain by primary care physicians and neurologists

Amoxapine[2,4,8,12,13,19,29,43,44,45,47,52,53,56]

Brand name: Asendin

FDA approved for: Depressive disorder with neurotic symptoms, psychotic depression, depression with anxiety and agitation

Other potential uses (off-label): Schizophrenia

Medication forms: *Tab* (25, 50, 100, 150 mg); *cap* (25, 50, 100 mg)

Dosage:

- Depression: 50 mg bid–tid initially, can be increased based on tolerance/response to max 400 mg/day

MOA: Reduces norepinephrine and serotonin reuptake and antagonizes dopamine receptors

Pharmacokinetics: t_{max}=90 min, $t_{1/2}$=8 hrs

Warnings:

- Similar to *TCA Class Profile*
- **Black box warning:** Increased risk of suicidal thinking and behavior in children, adolescents, and young adults; not approved for use in pediatric patients
- Discontinue if NMS, rash, or drug fever develops
- Can cause tardive dyskinesia (TD) and sedation/drowsiness

Drug Interactions: Similar to *TCA Class Profile*

Common side effects: Ataxia, blurred vision, constipation, dizziness, drowsiness, dry mouth, increased appetite, nausea, prolactinemia, sweating

Contraindications: Similar to *TCA Class Profile*

Special populations:

Pregnancy: Risk Category C

Lactation: Avoid

Elderly: Lower dose recommended (10 mg tid)

Hepatic impairment: Use caution

Renal impairment: Lower doses recommended

Important notes:

- Good choice for depression with severe anxiety or agitation

Clomipramine[4,8,12,13,19,26,29,43,44,45,47,52,53,56]

Brand name: Anafranil

FDA approved for: OCD in adults and children/adolescents (ages 10–17 yrs)

Other potential uses (off-label): Depression, chronic pain, panic disorder

Medication forms: *Cap* (25, 50, 75 mg)

Dosage:

- OCD: 25 mg/day initially, can be increased based on tolerance/response to max 250 mg/day

MOA: Increases serotonin and norepinephrine in the synaptic cleft

Pharmacokinetics: t_{max}=4–6 hrs, $t_{1/2}$=32 hrs

Warnings:
- Similar to *TCA Class Profile*
- **Black box warning**: Increased risk of suicidal thinking and behavior in children, adolescents, and young adults; not approved for use in pediatric patients except for patients with OCD
- Can cause elevation of liver enzymes, weight gain, and sexual dysfunction

Drug Interactions:
- Similar to *TCA Class Profile*
- Increased levels with haloperidol, methylphenidate, and highly protein bound drugs

Common side effects: Constipation, dizziness, drowsiness, dry mouth, headache, indigestion, increased appetite, nausea, sweating, weight gain

Contraindications:
- Similar to *TCA Class Profile*
- Patients receiving ECT

Special populations:

Pregnancy: Risk Category C

Lactation: Avoid

Elderly: Lower dose recommended

Hepatic impairment: Use caution

Renal impairment: Lower dose recommended

Desipramine[3,4,8,12,13,19,29,43,44,45,47,52,53,56]

Brand name: Norpramin

FDA approved for: Depression

Other potential uses (off-label): ADHD, bulimia, cocaine abuse, fibromyalgia, IBS, panic disorder

Medication forms: *Tab* (10, 25, 50, 75, 100, 150 mg)

Dosage:
- Depression: 100–200 mg/day, max 300 mg/day

MOA: Inhibits reuptake of norepinephrine and serotonin

Pharmacokinetics: $t_{1/2}$=17 hrs

Warnings:
- Similar to *TCA Class Profile*
- **Black box warning:** Increased risk of suicidal thinking and behavior in children, adolescents, and young adults; not approved for use in pediatric patients

- May cause serious agranulocytosis, decreased neutrophil count, leucopenia, and SIADH

Drug Interactions: Similar to *TCA Class Profile*

Common side effects: Dizziness, drowsiness, dry mouth, insomnia, tachycardia, tingling, weight gain

Contraindications:

- Similar to *TCA Class Profile*
- Patients receiving ECT

Therapeutic levels: 100–300 ng/mL

Special populations:

Pregnancy: Risk Category C

Lactation: Use caution

Elderly: Lower dose recommended (max 150 mg/day)

Hepatic impairment: Use caution

Renal impairment: Lower dose recommended

Important notes:

- Reportedly associated with increased risk of breast cancer in women

Doxepin [4,8,12,13,19,29,31,43,44,45,47,52,53,56]

Brand name: Silenor, Sinequan

FDA approved for: Depression, anxiety, insomnia, depression and anxiety associated with alcoholism

Other potential uses (off-label): Chronic pain, urticaria

Medication forms: *Tab* (3, 6 mg); *cap* (10, 25, 50, 75, 100, 150 mg); *oral conc* (10 mg/ml)

Dosage:

- Depression/anxiety: 25 mg bid initially, can be increased based on tolerance/response to max 300 mg/day
- Insomnia: 10-15 mg qhs (Silenor: 3–6 mg qhs)

MOA: Blocks H_1 and H_2 receptors; prevents norepinephrine deactivation

Pharmacokinetics: t_{max}=3.5 hrs, $t_{1/2}$=15.3 hrs

Warnings:

- Similar to *TCA Class Profile*
- **Black box warning**: Increased risk of suicidal thinking and behavior in children, adolescents, and young adults; not approved for use in pediatric patients
- Can cause drowsiness, TD, and EPS

Drug interactions:

- Similar to *TCA Class Profile*
- Use with cimetidine can increase plasma levels
- Avoid use with tolazamide

Common side effects: Dizziness, drowsiness, dry mouth, hypotension, taste problems

Contraindications:

- Similar to *TCA Class Profile*
- Patients with glaucoma and urinary retention

Special populations:

Pregnancy: Risk Category C

Lactation: Avoid

Elderly: Lower dose recommended (15–200 mg)

Hepatic impairment: Lower dose recommended

Renal impairment: Lower dose recommended

Important notes:

- Very sedating antidepressant; may help patients resistant to other hypnotics
- Not recommended in cardiac disease due to cardiotoxic properties

Imipramine[4,8,12,13,19,25,29,43,44,45,47,52,53,56]

Brand name: Tofranil, Tofranil-PM

FDA approved for: Depression in adults and adolescents (ages 12–17 yrs), enuresis (bedwetting) for ages ≥6 yrs

Other potential uses (off-label): ADHD, anxiety, bulimia, chronic pain, migraines

Medication forms: *Tab* (10, 25, 50 mg); *cap* (75, 100, 125, 150 mg)

Dosage:

- Depression: 75 mg/day initially, can be increased based on tolerance/response to max 300 mg/day
- Enuresis: 25 mg qhs (≥ 6 yrs) initially, can be increased based on tolerance/response to max 75 mg/day

MOA: Similar to *TCA Class Profile*

Pharmacokinetics: t_{max}=1–2 hrs, $t_{1/2}$=6–18 hrs

Warnings:

- Similar to *TCA Class Profile*
- **Black box warning:** Increased risk of suicidal thinking and behavior in children, adolescents, and young adults; not approved for use in pediatric patients
- May cause serious side effects: agranulocytosis, decreased neutrophil count, EPS, leukopenia, photosensitization, thrombocytopenia, and SIADH

Drug Interactions:

- Similar to *TCA Class Profile*
- Increased levels with methylphenidate
- Decreased levels with enzyme inducers (e.g., barbiturates, phenytoin)

Common side effects: Dry mouth, insomnia, orthostatic hypotension, tachycardia

Contraindications:
- Similar to *TCA Class Profile*
- Patients receiving ECT

Special populations:
Pregnancy: No information available; consider risks/benefits
Lactation: Safe/preferred among TCAs
Elderly: Lower dose recommended (initiate at 30–40 mg, max 100 mg)
Hepatic impairment: Lower dose recommended
Renal impairment: Lower dose recommended

Important notes:
- Some efficacy in bedwetting in children
- Avoid in patients with cardiac problems

Maprotiline[4,8,12,13,19,29,32,43,44,45,47,52,53]
Brand name: Ludiomil
FDA approved for: Depression
Other potential uses (off-label): Anxiety, enuresis, tension headaches
Medication forms: *Coated tab* (20, 50, 75 mg)
Dosage:
- Depression: 75–150 mg/day initially, can be increased based on tolerance/response to max 225 mg/day

MOA: Selectively inhibits norepinephrine reuptake into the presynaptic neuron but does not affect reuptake of serotonin
Pharmacokinetics: t_{max}=12 hrs, $t_{1/2}$=51 hrs
Warnings:
- Similar to *TCA Class Profile*
- **Black box warning:** Increased risk of suicidal thinking and behavior in children, adolescents, and young adults; not approved for use in pediatric patients
- Use caution in patients with BPH

Drug interactions:
- Similar to *TCA Class Profile*
- Can cause prolonged QTc syndrome with concomitant use of cisapride or pimozide
- Can enhance cardiotoxicity when used with thyroid medication

Common side effects: Allergic reaction, anxiety, blurred vision, constipation, dizziness, drowsiness, dry mouth, headache, hives, insomnia, nausea, nervousness, tremor, weakness
Important notes:
- Only TCA with pregnancy risk Category B

Mianserin[29,47,52,53,56]
Brand name: None—not available in US
FDA approved for: None
Other potential uses (off-label): Depression, chronic pain, EPS
Medication forms: *Tab* (10, 30, 60 mg)
Dosage:
• Depression: 30–60 mg/day
MOA: Inhibits α_2 and H_1 receptors but has minimal effect on serotonin and no effect on norepinephrine reuptake
Pharmacokinetics: t_{max}=2–3 hrs, $t_{1/2}$=biphasic half life

Nortriptyline[29,47,52,53,56]
Brand name: Pamelor, Aventyl
FDA approved for: MDD
Other potential uses (off-label): ADHD, chronic pain, enuresis, fibromyalgia, migraines, smoking cessation
Medication forms: *Cap* (10, 25, 50, 75 mg); *oral sol* (10 mg/5 ml)
Dosage:
• MDD: 25 mg tid initially, can be increased based on tolerance/response to max 150 mg/day
MOA: Inhibits the reuptake of norepinephrine
Pharmacokinetics: t_{max}=1 hr, $t_{1/2}$=15–39 hrs
Warnings:
• Similar to *TCA Class Profile*
• **Black box warning:** Increased risk of suicidal thinking and behavior in children, adolescents, and young adults; not approved for use in pediatric patients
• May cause serious side effects: agranulocytosis, arrhythmia, eosinophilia, leukopenia, MI, stroke, SIADH
Drug interactions:
• Similar to *TCA Class Profile*
• Can cause hypoglycemia with chlorpropamide and stimulating effects with reserpine
• Increased risk of arrhythmia when used with thyroid agent
• Plasma levels increased when used with cimetidine
Common side effects: Arrhythmia, dizziness, drowsiness, dry mouth, insomnia, orthostatic hypotension, tingling, tachycardia, weight gain

Protriptyline[29,47,52,53,56]
Brand name: Vivactil
FDA approved for: Depression
Other potential uses (off-label): Bulimia, chronic pain
Medication forms: *Tab* (5, 10 mg)
Dosage:
- Depression: 15–60 mg/day

MOA: Inhibits the reuptake of norepinephrine
Pharmacokinetics: t_{max}=4–12 hrs, $t_{1/2}$=54–198 hrs
Warnings:
- Similar to *TCA Class Profile*
- **Black box warning:** Increased risk of suicidal thinking and behavior in children, adolescents, and young adults; not approved for use in pediatric patients

Drug interactions: Similar to *TCA Class Profile*
Contraindications: Similar to *TCA Class Profile*
Common side effects: Dizziness, drowsiness, dry mouth, fatigue, headache, lack of coordination, nausea, nightmares, restlessness, stomach pain, tinnitus, unpleasant taste, vomiting

Trimipramine[29,47,52,53,56]
Brand name: Surmontil
FDA approved for: Depression
Other potential uses (off-label): Bulimia, chronic pain, insomnia
Medication forms: *Cap* (25, 50, 100 mg)
Dosage:
- Depression: 50–150 mg/day

MOA: Has an unknown MOA; does not act primarily by central nervous system stimulation
Pharmacokinetics: t_{max}=12 hrs, $t_{1/2}$=23 hrs
Warnings:
- Similar to *TCA Class Profile*
- **Black box warning:** Increased risk of suicidal thinking and behavior in children, adolescents, and young adults; not approved for use in pediatric patients
- May cause serious arrhythmia, blood dyscrasias, confusion, and incoordination
- May impair ability to operate machinery

Drug interactions:
- Similar to *TCA Class Profile*

Common side effects: Blurred vision, changes in appetite/weight, constipation, difficulty urinating, dizziness, drowsiness, dry mouth, headache, increased appetite, weakness

References:

1. Accord Healthcare, Inc. 2014. "AMITRIPTYLINE HYDROCHLORIDE- amitriptyline hydrochloride tablet, film coated." US National Library of Medicine: DailyMed. Accessed January 6, 2015. http://dailymed.nlm.nih.gov/dailymed/drugInfo.cfm?setid=1 e6d2c80-fbc8-444e-bdd3-6a91fe1b95bd.

2. Actavis Pharma, Inc. 2014. "AMOXAPINE- amoxapine tablet." US National Library of Medicine: DailyMed. October 18, 2014. http://dailymed.nlm.nih.gov/dailymed/drugInfo. cfm?setid=a16297df-3158-48db-85e5-5cd506885556.

3. Actavis Pharma, Inc. 2014. "DESIPRAMINE HYDROCHLORIDE- desipramine hydrochloride tablet, film coated." US National Library of Medicine: DailyMed. Accessed January 6, 2015. http://dailymed.nlm.nih.gov/dailymed/drugInfo.cfm?setid=ba02a95d-d82e-4a13-90b4-a219abc0249a.

4. Albers, Lawrence J., Rhoda K. Hahn, and Christopher Reist. 2010. *Handbook of Psychiatric Drugs*. 2011 ed. 8–38. Current Clinical Strategies Publishing.

5. American Psychiatric Association (APA). 2013. *Diagnostic and Statistical Manual of Mental Disorders*. 5th ed. (DSM-5®). Washington, DC: American Psychiatric Publishing.

6. Angelini Pharma, Inc. 2014. "OLEPTRO - trazodone hydrochloride tablet, extended release." US National Library of Medicine: DailyMed. Accessed October 24, 2014. http://dailymed.nlm.nih.gov/ dailymed/drugInfo.cfm?setid=88c45123-f475-4dd0-bbac-c261868924ef.

7. Apotex Corp. 2014. "PAXIL- paroxetine hydrochloride hemihydrate tablet, film coated." US National Library of Medicine: DailyMed. Accessed October 23, 2014. http://dailymed.nlm.nih.gov/ dailymed/drugInfo.cfm?setid=584ace29-6e40-432f-950f-ab7e98653d32.

8. Center Watch. 2015. "FDA Approved Drugs by Therapeutic Area." Accessed February 3, 2015. http://www.centerwatch.com/drug-information/fda-approved-drugs/therapeutic-area/17/ psychiatry-psychology.

9. Covis Pharmaceuticals, Inc. 2013. "PARNATE- tranylcypromine sulfate tablet, film coated." US National Library of Medicine: DailyMed. Accessed October 19, 2014. http://dailymed.nlm.nih.gov/ dailymed/drugInfo.cfm?setid=2e7350bd-ab32-4619-a3f9-12fdf56fc5e2.

10. Dista Products. 2014. "PROZAC- fluoxetine hydrochloride capsule." US National Library of Medicine: DailyMed. Accessed January 5, 2015. http://dailymed.nlm.nih.gov/dailymed/drugInfo. cfm?setid=c88f33ed-6dfb-4c5e-bc01-d8e36dd97299.

11. Eli Lilly & Co. 2014. "CYMBALTA- duloxetine hydrochloride capsule, delayed release." US National Library of Medicine: DailyMed. Accessed January 5, 2015. http://dailymed.nlm.nih.gov/ dailymed/drugInfo.cfm?setid=2f7d4d67-10c1-4bf4-a7f2-c185fbad64ba.

12. Elsevier Gold Standard, Inc. 2015. "Clinical Pharmacology." Accessed March 12, 2015. https:// www.clinicalpharmacology.com.

13. Epocrates. 2015. Accessed March 25, 2015. https://online.epocrates.com.

14. Forest Laboratories, Inc. 2014. "CELEXA- citalopram hydrobromide tablet, film coated." US National Library of Medicine: DailyMed. Accessed October 23, 2014. http://dailymed.nlm.nih.gov/dailymed/drugInfo.cfm?setid=4259d9b1-de34-43a4-85a8-41dd214e9177.

15. Forest Laboratories, Inc. 2014. "FETZIMA- levomilnacipran hydrochloride capsule, extended release." US National Library of Medicine: DailyMed. Accessed October 24, 2015. http://dailymed.nlm.nih.gov/dailymed/drugInfo.cfm?setid=f371258d-91b3-4b6a-ac99-434a1964c3af.

16. Forest Laboratories, Inc. 2014. "LEXAPRO- escitalopram oxalate tablet, film coated." US National Library of Medicine: DailyMed. Accessed January 5, 2015. http://dailymed.nlm.nih.gov/dailymed/drugInfo.cfm?setid=13bb8267-1cab-43e5-acae-55a4d957630a.

17. Forest Laboratories, Inc. 2014. "SAVELLA- milnacipran hydrochloride tablet, film coated." US National Library of Medicine: DailyMed. Accessed January 5, 2015. http://dailymed.nlm.nih.gov/dailymed/drugInfo.cfm?setid=16a4a314-f97e-4e91-95e9-576a3773d284.

18. Forest Laboratories, Inc. 2014. "VIIBRYD- vilazodone hydrochloride tablet." US National Library of Medicine: DailyMed. Accessed October 24, 2014. http://dailymed.nlm.nih.gov/dailymed/drugInfo.cfm?setid=4c55ccfb-c4cf-11df-851a-0800200c9a66.

19. Gabbard, Glen O., ed. 2007. *Gabbard's Treatments of Psychiatric Disorders.* 4th ed. 5–28, 381–466. Washington, DC: American Psychiatric Publishing.

20. Genpharm, Inc. 2007. "FLUVOXAMINE MALEATE- fluvoxamine maleate tablet, coated." US National Library of Medicine: DailyMed. Accessed October 23, 2014. http://dailymed.nlm.nih.gov/dailymed/drugInfo.cfm?setid=9c16f853-1a0b-4ce3-8e17-e2bf666c4292.

21. GlaxoSmithKline, LLC. 2014. "WELLBUTRIN- bupropion hydrochloride tablet, film coated." US National Library of Medicine: DailyMed. Accessed January 6, 2015. http://dailymed.nlm.nih.gov/dailymed/drugInfo.cfm?setid=60525754-0d2b-4ba4-918a-1c9d3eff89b2.

22. Greenberg, P.E., A.A. Fournier, T. Sisitsky, C.T. Pike, and R.C. Kessler. 2015. "The economic burden of adults with major depressive disorder in the United States (2005 and 2010)." *J Clin Psychiatry* 76(2):155–162. doi: 10.4088/JCP.14m09298.

23. Hales, Robert. E., S. Yudofsky, and L. Roberts, eds. 2014. *The American Psychiatric Publishing Textbook of Psychiatry.* 6th ed. 353–390. Washington, DC: American Psychiatric Publishing.

24. Hasler, Gregor. 2010. "Pathophysiology of Depression: Do We Have Any Solid Evidence." *World Psychiatry* 9(3):155–161.

25. Lupin Pharmaceuticals, Inc. 2014. "IMIPRAMINE HYDROCHLORIDE- imipramine hydrochloride tablet, film coated." US National Library of Medicine: DailyMed. Accessed January 6, 2015. http://dailymed.nlm.nih.gov/dailymed/drugInfo.cfm?setid=55311747-710c-43c4-821d-76323ff2520e.

26. Mallinckrodt, Inc. 2014. "ANAFRANIL- clomipramine hydrochloride capsule." US National Library of Medicine: DailyMed. Accessed October 21, 2014. http://dailymed.nlm.nih.gov/dailymed/drugInfo.cfm?setid=4074b555-7635-41a9-809d-fae3b3610059.

27. Mallinckrodt, Inc. 2014. "TOFRANIL- imipramine hydrochloride tablet, sugar coated." US National Library of Medicine: DailyMed. Accessed October 21, 2014. http://dailymed.nlm.nih.gov/dailymed/drugInfo.cfm?setid=1827a5aa-733a-49d9-89d9-48ea0367b230.

28. Medscape. 2015. "Psychiatry and Mental Health." Accessed March 12, 2015. http://www.medscape.com/psychiatry.

29. Medscape: Drugs & Diseases. 2015. "Psychiatrics." Accessed February 3, 2015. http://reference.medscape.com/drugs/psychiatrics.

30. Medscape: Drugs & Diseases. 2015. "Venlafaxine (Rx): Effexor, Effexor XR." Accessed January 13, 2015. http://reference.medscape.com/drug/effexor-venlafaxine-342963.

31. Mylan Institutional, Inc. 2014. "DOXEPIN HYDROCHLORIDE- doxepin hydrochloride capsule." US National Library of Medicine: DailyMed. October 21, 2014. http://dailymed.nlm.nih.gov/dailymed/drugInfo.cfm?setid=137a953b-3c48-405f-86a6-ff778cb7f5f2.

32. Mylan Pharmaceuticals, Inc. 2014. "MAPROTILINE HYDROCHLORIDE- maprotiline hydrochloride tablet, film coated." US National Library of Medicine: DailyMed. Accessed October 23, 2014. http://dailymed.nlm.nih.gov/dailymed/drugInfo.cfm?setid=c3ca69e6-1ea0-4c2c-abcb-7264b2e79a87.

33. Mylan Specialty. 2012. "ELDEPRYL- selegiline hydrochloride capsule." US National Library of Medicine: DailyMed. Accessed October 15, 2014. http://dailymed.nlm.nih.gov/dailymed/drugInfo.cfm?setid=106429ad-859a-4b29-babf-42cb85f7236e.

34. National Alliance on Mental Illness (NAMI). 2006. "Many Americans Know Little about Mental Illnesses, Most Agree Knowing Warnings Signs Would Help, New Survey Shows." Accessed March 10, 2015. http://www2.nami.org/Content/NavigationMenu/Top_Story/Public_Still_Lacks_Mental_Health_Knowledge.htm.

35. National Institute of Mental Health (NIMH). 2015a. "Antidepressant Medications for Children and Adolescents: Information for Parents and Caregivers." Accessed March 25, 2015. http://www.nimh.nih.gov/health/topics/child-and-adolescent-mental-health/antidepressant-medications-for-children-and-adolescents-information-for-parents-and-caregivers.shtml.

36. National Institute of Mental Health (NIMH). 2015b. "What is Depression?" Accessed April 21, 2015. http://www.nimh.nih.gov/health/topics/depression/index.shtml.

37. Organon USA, Inc. 2014. "REMERON- mirtazapine tablet, film coated." US National Library of Medicine: DailyMed. Accessed October 16, 2014. http://dailymed.nlm.nih.gov/dailymed/drugInfo.cfm?setid=010f9162-9f7f-4b6d-a6e4-4f832f26f38e.

38. Parke-Davis Division of Pfizer, Inc. 2014. "NARDIL- phenelzine sulfate tablet, film coated." US National Library of Medicine: DailyMed. Accessed October 24, 2014. http://dailymed.nlm.nih.gov/dailymed/drugInfo.cfm?setid=513a41d0-37d4-4355-8a6d-a2c643bce6fa.

39. Preston, John D., and James Johnson. 2011. *Clinical Psychopharmacology Made Ridiculously Simple.* 7th ed. 2–19. Miami: MedMaster Inc.

40. Ranbaxy Pharmaceuticals, Inc. 2009. "NEFAZODONE HYDROCHLORIDE- nefazodone hydrochloride tablet." US National Library of Medicine: DailyMed. Accessed October 24, 2014. http://dailymed.nlm.nih.gov/dailymed/drugInfo.cfm?setid=b1d149db-ad43-4f3f-aef1-fb0395ba4191.

41. Roerig. 2014. "ZOLOFT- sertraline hydrochloride tablet, film coated." US National Library of Medicine: DailyMed. Accessed October 23, 2014. http://dailymed.nlm.nih.gov/dailymed/drugInfo. cfm?setid=fe9e8b7d-61ea-409d-84aa-3ebd79a046b5.

42. Roxane Laboratories, Inc. 2014. "PROTRIPTYLINE HYDROCHLORIDE- protriptyline hydrochloride tablet." US National Library of Medicine: DailyMed. Accessed October 21, 2014. http:// dailymed.nlm.nih.gov/dailymed/drugInfo.cfm?setid=700abc58-9362-4ef5-9d7a-dd3c4d364d0a.

43. RxList. 2015. "Drugs A-Z List." Accessed March 25, 2015. http://www.rxlist.com/drugs/alpha_a. htm.

44. Schatzberg, A.F., and Charles B. Nemeroff, eds. 2009. *The American Psychiatric Publishing Textbook of Psychopharmacology*. 4th ed. 261–530. Washington, DC: American Psychiatric Publishing.

45. Schatzberg, A.F., Jonathan O. Cole, and Charles DeBattista. 2010. *Manual of Clinical Psychopharmacology*. 7th ed. 37–145. Washington, DC: American Psychiatric Publishing.

46. Stahl, S.M. 2008. *Essential Psychopharmacology: Neuroscientific Basis and Practical Applications*. 3rd ed. 284–369. New York: Cambridge Press.

47. Stahl, S.M. 2011. *Essential Psychopharmacology: the Prescriber's Guide*. 4th ed. 5–8, 21–27, 29–34, 71–76, 103–108, 109–115, 145–151, 153–158, 171–176, 177–183, 185–190, 191–196, 213–218, 235–240, 343–348, 373–376, 381–386, 387–391, 393–397, 413–417, 419–425, 451–457, 469–474, 491–496, 513–517, 533–540, 547–553, 597–601, 603–607, 619–624, 635–640, 641–645. Cambridge: Cambridge University Press.

48. Takeda Pharmaceuticals America, Inc. 2014. "BRINTELLIX- vortioxetine hydrobromide tablet, film coated." US National Library of Medicine: DailyMed. Accessed October 16, 2014. http://dailymed.nlm.nih.gov/dailymed/drugInfo.cfm?setid=4b0700c9-b417-4c3a-b36f-de461e125bd3.

49. Taro Pharmaceuticals U.S.A., Inc. 2014. "NORTRIPTYLINE HYDROCHLORIDE- nortriptyline hydrochloride capsule." US National Library of Medicine: DailyMed. Accessed October 21, 2014. http://dailymed.nlm.nih.gov/dailymed/drugInfo.cfm?setid=aee2c1a1-d848-4c3b-8c6d-8a4f6ce94c28.

50. Teva Women's Health, Inc. 2014. "SURMONTIL- trimipramine maleate capsule." US National Library of Medicine: DailyMed. Accessed October 21, 2014. http://dailymed.nlm.nih.gov/dailymed/drugInfo.cfm?setid=0177d783-773c-41bf-9db9-eb7e5c64474a.

51. Teva Women's Health, Inc. 2014. "VIVACTIL- protriptyline hydrochloride tablet, film coated." US National Library of Medicine: DailyMed. Accessed October 21, 2014. http://www.dailymed.nlm. nih.gov/dailymed/archives/fdaDrugInfo.cfm?archiveid=142322.

52. Truven Health Analytics. 2015. *Micromedex 2.0*. Accessed March 20, 2015. http://www.micromedexsolutions.com/home/dispatch.

53. UpToDate. 2015. Accessed March 12, 2015. http://www.uptodate.com/home.

54. US Food and Drug Administration (FDA). 2007. *FDA Proposes New Warnings About Suicidal Thinking, Behavior in Young Adults Who Take Antidepressant Medications*. Last accessed March 25, 2015. http://www.fda.gov/NewsEvents/Newsroom/PressAnnouncements/2007/ucm108905.htm.

55. US Food and Drug Administration (FDA). 2009. "Labeling Change Request Letter for Antidepressant Medications." Center for Drug Evaluation and Research. Accessed March 24, 2015. http://www.fda.gov/Drugs/DrugSafety/InformationbyDrugClass/ucm096352.htm.

56. US National Library of Medicine. 2015. "Drugs and Lactation Database (LactMed)." Accessed February 3, 2015. http://toxnet.nlm.nih.gov/newtoxnet/lactmed.htm.

57. US National Library of Medicine. 2015. "Toxicology Data Network." Accessed March 17, 2015. http://toxnet.nlm.nih.gov.

58. Warner, C. H., W. Bobo, C. Warner, S. Reid, and J. Rachal. 2006. "Antidepressant discontinuation syndrome." *Am Fam Physician* 74(3):449–456.

59. Wegmann, J. 2008. *Psychopharmacology: Straight Talk on Mental Health Medications.* 29–60. Eau Claire: Pesi, LLC.

60. Wyeth Pharmaceuticals, Inc. 2014. "EFFEXOR XR- venlafaxine hydrochloride capsule, extended release." US National Library of Medicine: DailyMed. Accessed January 5, 2015. http://dailymed.nlm.nih.gov/dailymed/drugInfo.cfm?setid=53c3e7ac-1852-4d70-d2b6-4fca819acf26.

61. Wyeth Pharmaceuticals, Inc. 2014. "PRISTIQ EXTENDED-RELEASE- desvenlafaxine succinate tablet, extended release. US National Library of Medicine: DailyMed. Accessed October 24, 2014. http://dailymed.nlm.nih.gov/dailymed/drugInfo.cfm?setid=0f43610c-f290-46ea-d186-4f998ed99fce.

Chapter 5
Bipolar Disorder And Mood Stabilizers

Bipolar disorder, also known as manic-depressive illness, is a common, recurrent, and often severe psychiatric illness that is genetically inherited.[11,22] This disorder is characterized by periods of severe depression with alternating periods of elevated or irritable mood (manic episodes).[12] Bipolar disorder affects approximately 5.7 million people in the US (2.6% of the US population); globally, it is the sixth leading cause of disability.[31] It is equally prevalent in males and females, but rapid-cycling bipolar disorder is four times more prevalent in females.[16] Approximately 25–50% of bipolar patients attempt suicide, and 11% of those attempts result in completed suicides.[13,16]

The etiology of bipolar disorder is complex and multifactorial and involves genetic, neurophysiological, biochemical, psychodynamic, and environmental factors.[16] This disorder is the most heritable of all psychiatric disorders. First-degree relatives of bipolar type 1 (BP-1) patients are seven times more likely to develop the disorder.[16] The offspring of a bipolar parent has a 50% chance of developing the same disorder, and identical twins demonstrate a 33–90% concordance rate for BP-1.[12,16]

The goals for managing this disorder include the rapid, full remission of acute episodes, prevention of new episodes, and optimization of daily functioning.[22] Psychopharmacology complemented by other supporting modalities such as psychotherapy and psychosocial interventions is the mainstay form of treatment.[3,22] Additionally, lifestyle management is critical for patient stability.[20]

DSM-5 Types[3,4]
Bipolar disorder can be categorized into mild, moderate, and severe, and includes:
- Bipolar I Disorder
    - Episodes
        - Current or most recent episode manic
        - Current or most recent episode hypomanic
        - Current or most recent episode depressed
        - Current or most recent episode unspecified
    - Specifiers
        - With anxious distress
        - With mixed features
        - With rapid cycling
        - With melancholic features
        - With atypical features

- With mood-congruent psychotic features
- With mood-incongruent psychotic features
- With catatonia
- With per partum onset
- With seasonal pattern
- Bipolar II Disorder
  - Current or most recent episode hypomanic
  - Current or most recent episode depressed
- Cyclothymic Disorder with anxious distress
- Substance/Medication-Induced Bipolar and Related Disorder
- Bipolar and Related Disorder Due to Another Medical Condition
- Other Specified Bipolar and Related Disorder
- Unspecified Bipolar and Related Disorder

Mood Stabilizers

As a group, mood-stabilizing medications are used in the treatment of bipolar disorder[3]; 13 of these medications are currently approved by the FDA.[6,23] For treating acute bipolar depression, however, only three medications are FDA approved: quetiapine, olanzapine plus fluoxetine, and lurasidone.[9]

Mood stabilizers are grouped into two main classes: anticonvulsants and second-generation antipsychotics. Lithium and chlorpromazine (Thorazine) also carry bipolar-related indications.[22]

Lithium
Lithium[2,5,6,7,8,9,12,17, 21,22,23,25,26,27,28,29]
Brand name: Eskalith, Eskalith CR, Lithobid
FDA approved for: Acute treatment of manic episodes, maintenance therapy for bipolar depression
Other potential uses (off-label): Agitation, MDD, migraine, neutropenia, treatment-resistant depression, SIADH, suicidal prevention
Medication forms: *Tab* (300); *ER tab* (300, 450 mg); *cap* (150, 300, 600 mg); *liq* (8mEq/5ml)
Dosage:
- Acute mania:
  - *IR:* 900–2400 mg/day divided tid-qid
  - *ER:* 900–1800 mg/day divided bid
  - *Liq:* 10 mL tid **or** 5 mL tid–qid
- Maintenance:
  - *IR:* 900–1200 mg/day divided tid-qid
  - *ER:* 900–1200 mg/day divided bid

MOA: Exact mechanism unknown; changes sodium transport across cell membranes, influences reuptake of serotonin and/or norepinephrine, and balances excitatory and inhibitory neurotransmitters

Pharmacokinetics: t_{max}=0.5–2 hrs, $t_{1/2}$=18–30 hrs, renal excretion 89–98%

Warnings:

- **Black box warning:** Toxicity is closely related to serum lithium levels and can occur at doses close to therapeutic levels; facilities for prompt and accurate serum lithium determinations should be available before initiating therapy
- Chronic therapy is associated with diminution of renal-concentrating ability, glomerular and interstitial fibrosis, and nephron atrophy
- May cause encephalopathic syndrome in combination with a neuroleptic
- May impair physical/mental abilities
- Use caution in patients with thyroid disorders or significant cardiovascular impairment

Drug interactions:

- Interacts with various medications; use utmost care when prescribing
- Can enhance adverse/toxic effects of other serotonin modulators; use caution with SSRIs and other serotonergic agents
- Can prolong the effects of neuromuscular blocking agents
- Can decrease the effects of amphetamines
- Bupropion may increase seizure risk in combination
- Iodide salts increase hypothyroidism with concurrent use
- Increased risk of neurotoxicity with calcium channel blockers, diuretics, metronidazole
- Increased plasma levels with indomethacin, piroxicam, other NSAIDs, COX-2 inhibitors, ACE inhibitors, and angiotensin II receptor antagonists
- Decreased levels with theophylline, acetazolamide, urea, xanthine agents, and alkalinizing agents
- Use with carbamazepine can increase risk of neurotoxic side effects
- Lithium plasma levels can increase or decrease when used with fluoxetine

Common side effects: Affects most body systems—anorexia, ataxia, cogwheel rigidity, coma, confusion, diabetes insipidus, diarrhea, dizziness, drowsiness, folliculitis, hair loss, hallucination, lethargy, muscle weakness, nausea, polyuria, polydipsia, psoriasis, seizure, sick sinus node syndrome, slowed intellectual functioning, tremor, vomiting

Contraindications: Severe renal impairment or cardiovascular disorder, Addison's disease, diarrhea, pregnancy, sick sinus syndrome, sodium depletion, hypersensitivity

Recommended lab tests: CBC, CMP, serum electrolytes, serum lithium concentrations

Therapeutic levels: 0.8 to 1.4 mEq/L (0.4–0.8 mEq/L for augmentation/maintenance)

Overdose: Dizziness, nausea, stomach pain, vomiting, muscular weakness, ataxia, agitation, confusion, hand tremors, seizures, slurred speech, nystagmus, tinnitus, blurred vision, kidney failure, hyperthermia, seizure, coma, rigidity, myoclonus, serotonin syndrome

Tapering/withdrawal: Tapering recommended over a period of 3 months
Special populations:
Pregnancy: Risk Category D
Lactation: Contraindicated
Elderly: Lower dose recommended (150–300 mg/day)
Hepatic impairment: No dose adjustment necessary
Renal impairment: Lower dose recommended in mild to moderate, avoid in severe
Important notes[22,23]:

- "Miracle" medication with various uses including manic depression, unipolar depression, SIADH, neutropenia, thyrotoxic crisis, migraine and cluster headaches
- Has a very narrow therapeutic index; levels should be monitored regularly
- Due to delay in onset of action, therapy with antipsychotic for acute mania may be necessary
- One of only two medications that decrease suicidal ideations/attempts
- Adjunctive agent to augment antidepressants for treatment-resistant unipolar depression
- Encourage patients to drink plenty of fluids to avoid dehydration while taking lithium

Anticonvulsants

Anticonvulsants are a group of drugs originally used in the treatment of seizures. They are also utilized increasingly as mood stabilizers in treating bipolar disorder.[23] The drugs included in this class with indications in the treatment of bipolar disorder are[22,23]:

- Carbamazepine
- Gabapentin
- Oxcarbazepine

- Lamotrigine
- Topiramate
- Valproate

Carbamazepine[2,6,7,8,9,12,17,21,22,23,25,26,27,28,29,30]
Brand name: Tegretol, Tegretol XR, Carbatrol, Equetro, Epitol
FDA approved for: Acute manic or mixed episodes associated with bipolar 1 disorder (Equetro), partial seizures, generalized tonic-clonic seizures, mixed seizures, trigeminal neuralgia
Other potential uses (off-label): Bipolar maintenance, aggressive outbursts, alcohol or benzodiazepine withdrawal, impulsivity, RLS, PTSD
Medication forms: *IR tab* (200 mg); *SR tab* (100, 200, 400 mg); *ER tab* (100, 200, 400 mg); *chew tab* (100 mg); *cap* (100, 200, 300 mg); *ER cap* (100, 200, 300 mg); *liq* (100 mg/5 mL [450 ml bottle]); *suspension* (100mg/5ml)
Dosage:

- Bipolar mania *(Equetro):* 200 mg bid, can be increased based on tolerance/response to max 1600 mg/day (maintain serum level of 4–12 g/ml)

MOA: Stabilizes voltage-gated sodium channels, reduces cell excitability, potentiates GABA receptors, may act on temporal lobe and limbic system

Pharmacokinetics: t_{max}=4–5 hrs, $t_{1/2}$=25–65 hrs initially and then 12–17 hrs

Warnings:

- **Black box warning:**
  - Serious and sometimes fatal dermatologic reactions (including SJS/TEN) have been reported, especially in patients with the inherited allelic variant HLA-B*1502 found almost exclusively in patients of Asian descent; screen genetically at-risk patients prior to treatment, and do not start in patients who test positive for this allele
  - Aplastic anemia and agranulocytosis have been reported; obtain pretreatment hematological testing and periodically monitor CBC
- May increase the risk of suicidal ideation or behavior
- Consider drug discontinuation if significant bone marrow depression develops or if serious dermatologic reactions occur
- May cause drug reaction with eosinophilia and systemic symptoms (DRESS)
- Do not discontinue abruptly due to increased risk of seizure
- May cause hyponatremia, hepatic porphyria, increased IOP, and cognitive or motor impairment

Drug interactions:

- CYP3A4 inhibitors (e.g., fluoxetine, nefazodone) or epoxide hydrolase inhibitors increase serum levels
- CYP3A4 inducers lower serum levels
- Enhances metabolism of many drugs: clozapine, haloperidol, benzodiazepines, OCPs, methadone, valproate, clomipramine, warfarin, nefazodone, and other CYP1A2 or CYP3A4 substrates
- Use with diuretics may cause hyponatremia
- Concomitant use with lithium can increase the risk of neurotoxic side effects
- Can potentiate sedative effects of other CNS depressants (e.g., alcohol, barbiturates)
- Avoid use with other medications that can cause bone marrow suppression
- Discontinue MAOIs for at least 2 weeks before starting carbamazepine

Common side effects: Asthenia, ataxia, blurred vision, constipation, dizziness, drowsiness, nausea, pruritus, rash, somnolence, vomiting

Contraindications:

- Bone marrow suppression, lactation, pregnancy
- Hypersensitivity to drug or to TCAs
- Concomitant use with nefazodone or MOAIs

Recommended lab tests: CBC, LFTs, serum carbamazepine concentrations, serum cholesterol profile, urinalysis

Overdose: CNS/respiratory depression, coma, seizures, rhabdomyolysis and renal failure, oliguria, cardiac conduction abnormalities, hypotension; OD potentially fatal

Tapering/withdrawal: Gradual tapering recommended (25% reduction per week for 1 month)

Special populations:

Pregnancy: Risk Category D due to neural tube defects

Lactation: Contraindicated

Elderly: No dose adjustment necessary

Hepatic impairment: Use caution in mild to moderate, avoid in severe

Renal impairment: No dose adjustment necessary

Important notes:

- More effective in rapid-cycling and mixed episodes; third-line agent after lithium and valproate for bipolar
- Warn patients about signs of bone marrow suppression requiring prompt medical attention
- May be helpful in combination with another mood stabilizer or atypical antipsychotic
- Recommended to monitor blood levels at least weekly for first 8 weeks of treatment

Gabapentin[2,6,7,8,9,12,17,19,21,22,23,25,26,27,28,29]

Brand name: Gralise, Neurontin

FDA approved for: Partial seizures, post-herpetic neuralgia

Other potential uses (off-label): Bipolar disorder, alcohol withdrawal, ALS, chronic pain, hot flashes, insomnia, migraines, orthostatic tremor, social anxiety disorder, spasticity

Medication forms: *Tab* (400, 600, 800 mg); *cap* (100, 300, 400 mg); *oral sol* (250mg/5ml)

Dosage:

- Bipolar disorder: 900–2700 mg/day divided tid, higher doses can be given near bedtime

MOA: Modulates release of excitatory neurotransmitters; does not bind to $GABA_A$ or $GABA_B$ receptor

Pharmacokinetics: t_{max}=8 hrs, $t_{1/2}$=6 hrs

Warnings:

- Can cause rhabdomyolysis; regular monitoring of blood CPK level is recommended
- May increase the risk of suicidal ideation or behavior
- May cause drug reaction with eosinophilia and systemic symptoms (DRESS)
- Can cause somnolence, sedation, impaired driving, and dizziness

Drug interactions:
- Combination of propranolol and gabapentin may induce dystonia
- Antacids can decrease levels
- Can potentiate sedative effects of other CNS depressants (e.g., alcohol, barbiturates)

Common side effects: Abnormal thinking, asthenia, ataxia, blurred vision, constipation, diarrhea, dizziness, drowsiness, fatigue, fever, headache, infection, malaise, somnolence, tremor, weight gain

Contraindications: Hypersensitivity

Recommended lab tests: None

Overdose: Sedation, ataxia, movement disorders, nystagmus, slurred speech, profound CNS depression; no reported fatalities

Tapering/withdrawal: Gradual taper recommended

Special populations:

Pregnancy: Risk Category C

Lactation: Use caution and monitor for side effects

Elderly: Lower dose recommended

Hepatic impairment: No dose adjustment necessary

Renal impairment: 200–300 mg/day recommended in mild to moderate, 100–150 mg/day recommended in severe

Important notes:
- More useful in treatment of anxiety disorders and pain than in mood disorders[25]
- Possibly helpful for fibromyalgia and chronic neuropathic pain syndromes
- Promising agent for addiction, anxiety, pain, and insomnia

Lamotrigine[2,6,7,8,9,10,12,17,21,22,23,25,26,27,28,29]

Brand name: Lamictal, Lamictal ODT, Lamictal XR

FDA approved for: Maintenance of bipolar I disorder, partial seizures, generalized seizures of Lennox-Gastaut syndrome, primary generalized tonic-clonic seizures

Other potential uses (off-label): Bipolar disorder, migraines, obesity, treatment-resistant depression

Medication forms: *Tab* (25, 100, 150, 200 mg); *chew tab* (2, 5, 25 mg); *ODT* (25, 50, 100, 200 mg); *ER tab* (25, 50, 100, 200, 250, 300 mg)

Dosage:
- Bipolar Disorder:
  - 25 mg/day initially for first week, can be increased by 25–50 mg every two weeks to max 200 mg/day
  - *With valproic acid:* 25 mg/day initially for 2 weeks, can be increased by 25 mg for two weeks and then increased by 50 mg for one week to max 100 mg/day

MOA: Effects sodium channels that modulate release of glutamate, decreasing levels of glutamate and aspartate; also has weak inhibitory effect on $5\text{-}HT_3$ receptors and blocks uptake of dopamine

Pharmacokinetics: t_{max}=1.4–4.8 hrs, $t_{1/2}$=25 hrs

Warnings:

- **Black box warning:** Can cause serious hypersensitivity reactions (including SJS/TEN); medication should be immediately discontinued with appearance of any rash
- May increase risk of suicidal ideation or behavior
- May cause drug reaction with eosinophilia and systemic symptoms (DRESS)
- Use in early pregnancy is associated with cleft palate and lip in neonates
- Use caution in patients with hepatic or renal function impairment
- May cause blood dyscrasias (e.g., neutropenia, thrombocytopenia, pancytopenia)
- Risk of aseptic meningitis; monitor for signs of meningitis

Drug interactions:

- Phenobarbital, carbamazepine, phenytoin, and OCP lower serum concentration
- Valproate doubles lamotrigine levels; lamotrigine decreases valproate levels slightly
- Decreased levels with protease inhibitors lopinavir/ritonavir and atazanavir/lopinavir

Common side effects: Abdominal pain, accidental injury, agitation, amnesia, ataxia, blurred vision, confusion, depression, diarrhea, diplopia, dizziness, emotional lability, fatigue, fever, headache, infection, insomnia, irritability, nausea, pharyngitis, rash, rhinitis, somnolence, tremor, vomiting, weight gain

Contraindications: Hypersensitivity

Overdose: Delirium, periorbital edema, generalized erythema, hepatitis, renal failure

Tapering/withdrawal: Gradual taper recommended over 2 weeks

Special populations:

Pregnancy: Risk Category C

Lactation: Can be used if not using other psychotropics; use caution and monitor closely

Elderly: Lower dose recommended

Hepatic impairment: No dose adjustment necessary in mild to moderate, reduce dose 25–50% in severe

Renal impairment: Lower dose recommended

Important notes:

- Has more favorable side-effect profile than other anticonvulsants
- Must be titrated very slowly to decrease risk of associated rash and SJS
- Restart the initial dosage titration if missed for >5 half lives
- Not indicated for treatment of acute mania or MDD
- Inform patient about the possibility of rash before starting treatment[25]

- Educate patients about avoiding new foods, deodorants, detergents, cosmetics, and fabric softeners for first 3 months of treatment[25]

Oxcarbazepine[2,6,7,8,9,12,17,18,21,22,23,25,26,27,28,29]

Brand name: Trileptal, Oxtellar XR

FDA approved for: Monotherapy or adjunctive therapy in the treatment of partial seizures

Other potential uses (off-label): Bipolar disorder, chronic pain, migraines,

Medication forms: *Tab* (150, 300, 600 mg), *XR tab* (150, 300, 600 mg), *oral suspension* (300mg/5mL [60mg/mL])

Dosage:
- Bipolar disorder: 300 mg bid initially, can be increased based on tolerance/response to max 2400 mg/day (target dose 1200 mg/day)

MOA: Active metabolite 10-Monohydroxy metabolite (MHD) blocks voltage-gated sodium channels of hyper-excited neurons

Pharmacokinetics: t_{max}=4.5 hrs, $t_{1/2}$=2–11 hrs

Warnings:
- May cause anaphylactic reactions, angioedema, and serious dermatological reactions (including SJS/TEN); avoid in patients with HSR to carbamazepine
- May cause drug reaction with eosinophilia and systemic symptoms (DRESS)
- May increase risk of suicidal ideation or behavior
- May cause cognitive/neuropsychiatric/hematological adverse events or hyponatremia
- Avoid in seizure control during pregnancy

Drug interactions:
- Increases phenytoin levels
- Decreased plasma levels with carbamazepine and phenobarbital
- Decreases effectiveness of OCP

Common side effects: Abdominal pain, abnormal gait, abnormal vision, ataxia, diplopia, dizziness, dyspepsia, fatigue, headache, indigestion, nausea, nystagmus, somnolence, tremor, vomiting

Contraindications: Hypersensitivity

Recommended lab tests: Serum sodium, CBC, LFTs

Overdose: Vomiting, somnolence; relatively safe in OD

Tapering/withdrawal: Gradual taper recommended

Special populations:

Pregnancy: Risk Category C

Lactation: Use caution and monitor

Elderly: Lower dose preferred

Hepatic impairment: No dose adjustment necessary in mild to moderate, avoid in severe

Renal impairment: Lower dose recommended in mild to moderate, reduce dose 50% in severe and avoid XR

Important notes:
- Is similar to carbamazepine but with fewer drug interactions and less frequent monitoring required
- In 2010, the US Department of Justice charged Novartis with illegally marketing Trileptal as psychiatric or pain-management drug[32]

Topiramate[2,6,7,8,9,12,14,17,21,22,23,25,26,27,28,29]

Brand name: Qudexy XR, Topamax, Topamax Sprinkle, Topiragen, Trokendi XR

FDA approved for: Partial-seizures, tonic–clonic seizures, migraine prophylaxis

Other potential uses (off-label): Bipolar disorder, alcoholism, eating disorder, obesity, psychotropic drug-induced weight gain, tremor

Medication forms: *Tab* (25, 50, 100, 200 mg); *cap sprinkle* (15, 25 mg); *ER cap* (25, 50, 100, 200 mg)

Dosage:
- Bipolar disorder: 50–300 mg/day
- Weight loss: 50–100 mg qhs
- Migraine headache (Topamax): 50–200 mg

MOA: Blocks sodium channels, inhibits release of glutamate and carbonic anhydrase, augments activity of GABA

Pharmacokinetics: t_{max}=1.5–4 hrs, $t_{1/2}$=21 hrs

Warnings:
- ER form contraindicated within 6 hours of ETOH use and in patients with metabolic acidosis taking metformin
- Risk of fetal toxicity, including increased risk of craniofacial defects
- May increase the risk of suicidal ideation or behavior
- Increased kidney-stone risk with failure to maintain adequate fluid intake
- May cause life-threatening hyperchloremic metabolic acidosis
- May increase IOP and visual-field defects; use caution in patients with history of angle-closure glaucoma
- Can cause oligohidrosis and hyperthermia, paresthesia, cognitive/neuropsychiatric impairment, and hyperammonemia/encephalopathy (with or without use with valproic acid)

Drug interactions:
- Increased clearance and decreased levels with CYP450 inducers (e.g., phenytoin, carbamazepine)
- Concurrent use with citalopram can increase risk of QTc prolongation
- May potentiate the sedative effects of alcohol or other CNS depressants
- Use with valproic acid increases risk of encephalopathy

- Avoid with other carbonic anhydrase inhibitors as it can cause metabolic acidosis
- Avoid with anticholinergics due to risk of heart disorders (CHF)
- Decreases contraceptive efficacy when combined with OCP
- Concurrent use with metformin may cause metabolic acidosis
- Monitor lithium levels when combined

Common side effects: Ataxia, confusion, dizziness, fatigue, fever, hypoesthesia, kidney stones, memory difficulty, nervousness, painful periods, paresthesia, psychomotor retardation, somnolence, speech disorder, taste perversion, weight loss

Contraindications: Hypersensitivity, alcohol use

Recommended lab tests: Serum bicarbonate, serum creatinine/BUN, serum electrolytes

Overdose: Severe metabolic acidosis and coma reported; OD rare

Tapering/withdrawal: Gradual tapering recommended

Special populations:

Pregnancy: Risk Category D

Lactation: Use caution and monitor

Elderly: Lower dose may be indicated depending on creatinine clearance

Hepatic impairment: No dose adjustment necessary in mild to moderate, lower dose in severe

Renal impairment: Lower dose recommended (50–100 mg/day max)

Important notes[23]:

- Uniquely associated with weight loss in some patients
- Patients should be advised to drink plenty of water to prevent kidney-stone formation
- Warn patients about potential confusion and cognitive side effects

Valproate[1,2,6,7,8,9,12,17,21,22,23,25,26,27,28,29]

(valproic acid, valproate sodium, divalproex sodium)

Brand name: Depakene, Depacon, Depakote, Depakote ER, Depakote Sprinkles, Stavzor

FDA approved for: Acute mania and mixed bipolar episodes, complex partial seizures, migraine prophylaxis

Other potential uses (off-label): Bipolar prophylaxis, agitation, BPD, dementia, impulsivity, PTSD, substance abuse

Medication forms: *SR tab* (250, 500 mg); *enteric-coated tab* (125, 250, 500 mg); *cap* (250 mg); *DR cap* (125, 250, 500 mg); *liq* (250 mg/5 mL [480 ml bottle]); *injection* (100 mg/ml [5 ml vial])

Dosage:

- Bipolar mania: 15mg/kg/day initially, can be increased based on tolerance/response to max 60 mg/kg/day (average dose 1000–1500 mg/day)

MOA: Increases GABA levels in the brain and enhances/mimics GABA action at post-synaptic receptors

Pharmacokinetics: t_{max}=4–17 hrs, $t_{1/2}$=8–10 hrs

Therapeutic levels: 50–125 mcg/ml

Warnings:

- **Black Box Warnings:**
  - May cause serious or fatal hepatotoxicity, usually during first six months of treatment
  - Increased risk of acute liver failure and resultant deaths in patients with hereditary neurometabolic syndromes caused by mitochondrial DNA polymerase gamma (POLG) gene mutations
  - May cause major congenital malformations including neural tube defects
  - Cases of life-threatening pancreatitis reported
- Risk of bleeding and thrombocytopenia with continuous use; monitor platelet count and coagulation tests before initiating therapy and during follow-up
- Do not discontinue abruptly due to increased risk of seizure
- May cause drug reaction with eosinophilia and systemic symptoms (DRESS)
- May increase risk of suicidal ideation or behavior
- Risk of hyperammonemia, hyperammonemic encephalopathy, and hypothermia with topiramate

Drug interactions:

- Aspirin, cimetidine, ibuprofen, SSRIs, erythromycin, and felbamate inhibit drug metabolism and increase serum levels
- Serum concentration lowered with phenytoin, phenobarbital, carbamazepine, rifampin, primidone, ritonavir, and carbapenem antibiotics
- Can decrease serum concentration of olanzapine
- Decreases metabolism of AZT, diazepam, amitriptyline, nortriptyline, carbamazepine, ethosuximide, primidone, lamotrigine, phenobarbital, phenytoin, tolbutamide, zidovudine, lorazepam and increases their serum levels
- Can displace warfarin from protein binding; monitor INR and PT
- Risk of CNS depression when used with alcohol or other CNS depressants

Common side effects: Abdominal pain, alopecia, amblyopia, anorexia, asthenia, ataxia, blurred vision, bronchitis, constipation, decreased blood platelet count, depression, diarrhea, diplopia, dizziness, fever, flu syndrome, fluid retention, headache, hemorrhage, increased appetite, insomnia, involuntary eye movement, nausea, nervousness, rash, somnolence, throat irritation, tinnitus, tremor, vomiting, weight gain

Contraindications: Hepatic dysfunction, mitochondrial disorders, urea cycle disorders, pregnancy, hypersensitivity

Recommended lab tests: LFTs, CBC, blood levels

Overdose: CNS depression, coma, miotic pupils, tachycardia, hypotension, QTc prolongation, and respiratory depression

Tapering/withdrawal: Slow tapering recommended

Special populations:

Pregnancy: Risk Category D due to neural tube defects

Lactation: Secreted in breast milk in low quantities; use caution due to hepatotoxicity

Elderly: Lower dose recommended (range 250–750 mg)

Hepatic impairment: Avoid

Renal impairment: No dose adjustment necessary

Important notes[23]:

- Inform patient about early symptoms of liver disease[23]
- When switching from enteric-coated tab to ER, increase dose by 8–20%
- Should not be prescribed to women of child-bearing age because of risk of PCOS
- If prescribed, monitor female patients for symptoms of PCOS: weight gain, hirsutism, menstrual irregularities, and acne
- Do not use to prevent migraine headaches in pregnant women[23]

Atypical Antipsychotics (Second Generation)

Atypical or second generation antipsychotics (SGAs) are frequently prescribed for mood stabilization in patients with acute manic symptoms and are also used for bipolar depression.[15,22] They can be taken alone or in combination with other mood stabilizers.[15,22]

Currently, SGAs are considered the drug of choice for bipolar disorders, as they have a rapid onset of action, few side effects, and are effective for treating bipolar depression and the agitation and impulsivity that frequently characterize the presentation of bipolar disorder.[15,25]

These medications include:

- Aripiprazole
- Asenapine
- Lurasidone
- Olanzapine
- Quetiapine
- Risperidone
- Ziprasidone

For full details, please refer to *Chapter 8: Psychotic Disorders and Antipsychotics.* The dosages that are usually prescribed for mood stabilization are provided below.[9]

Aripiprazole[7,17,25]

Bipolar-related indications: Acute treatment and maintenance of mania or mixed episodes of bipolar I disorder (as monotherapy or as adjunct to lithium/valproate), acute treatment of agitation associated with bipolar I disorder (IM)

Dosage:

- Bipolar I disorder:

- *Adjunctive to lithium/valproate:* 10–15 mg po qd initially, can be increased based on tolerance/response to max 30 mg/day (target 15 mg qd)
- *Monotherapy, manic or mixed episodes:* 15 mg po qd initially, can be increased based on tolerance/response to max 30 mg/day
- Bipolar disorder agitation:
  - 9.75 mg IM initially (range 5.25–15 mg), second dose may be required, max 30 mg/day
  - For ongoing therapy, replace injection with oral aripiprazole 10–30 mg/day as soon as possible

Asenapine[7,17,25]
Bipolar-related indications: Acute mania or mixed episodes associated with bipolar I disorder (as monotherapy or in combination with lithium/valproate)
Dosage:
- Bipolar disorder (manic or mixed):
  - *Monotherapy:* 5 mg bid initially, can be increased based on tolerance/response to max 10 mg bid
  - *Combination therapy (with lithium/valproate):* 5 mg bid initially, can be increased based on tolerance/response to max 10 mg bid

Lurasidone[7,17,25]
Bipolar-related indications: Depressive episodes associated with bipolar I disorder
Dosage:
- Bipolar depression: 20 mg/day initially with food, can be increased based on tolerance/response to max 120 mg/day

Olanzapine[7,17,25]
Bipolar-related indications: Acute treatment and maintenance of mania or mixed episodes of bipolar I disorder (as monotherapy or as adjunct to lithium/valproate) acute agitation associated with bipolar I mania (IM), bipolar depression (in combination with fluoxetine), treatment-resistant depression (in combination with fluoxetine)
Dosage:
- Bipolar mania:
  - *Monotherapy:* 10–15 mg/day po initially, can be increased based on tolerance/response to max 20 mg/day
  - *Adjunct to lithium/valproate:* 10 mg/day po initially, can be increased based on tolerance/response to max 20 mg/day
- Bipolar-related agitation: 10 mg IM (short-acting), consider 5–7.5 mg for geriatric, max 30 mg/day

- Treatment-resistant depression, depression associated with bipolar I disorder (*see package insert for Symbax when used in combination with fluoxetine*): 25 mg fluoxetine/6 mg olanzapine po each evening, can be increased based on tolerance/response to max 75 mg/18 mg per day

Quetiapine[7,17,25]

Bipolar-related indications: Acute mania or mixed episodes associated with bipolar I disorder (as monotherapy or in combination with lithium/valproate), maintenance of bipolar I disorder (adjunctive to lithium/valproate), bipolar depression

Dosage:
- Bipolar I disorder, mania (as monotherapy or as adjunct to lithium/ valproate):
  - *IR:* 50 mg bid initially, can be increased based on tolerance/response to max 800 mg/day (usual range 400–800 mg/day)
  - *XR:* 300 mg qd initially, can be increased based on tolerance/response to max 800 mg/day
- Bipolar I maintenance (IR or ER): 400–800 mg/day, max 800 mg/day
- Bipolar I disorder, depressive episodes associated with bipolar I or II disorder
  - *IR:* 50 mg qd hs initially, can be increased based on tolerance/response to max 300 mg/day
  - *XR:* 50 mg qd hs initially, can be increased based on tolerance/ response to max 300 mg/day

Risperidone[7,17,25]

Bipolar-related indications: Acute mania or mixed episodes of bipolar I disorder (as monotherapy or as adjunct to lithium/valproate), bipolar I disorder maintenance (IM, in monotherapy or as adjunct to lithium/valproate)

Dosage:
- Bipolar I mania: 2–3 mg po qd initially, range 1–6 mg daily
- Bipolar I maintenance: 25 mg IM in deltoid/gluteal muscle every 2 weeks initially, max 50 mg every 2 weeks

Ziprasidone[7,17,25]

Bipolar-related indications: Acute mania or mixed episodes of bipolar I disorder, maintenance in bipolar I disorder (as adjunct to lithium/valproate)

Dosage:
- Bipolar I disorder: 40 mg po bid initially, can be increased based on tolerance/ response to max 120–160 mg/day

Other Medications

Chlorpromazine[7,17,25]

(Refer to *Chapter 8: Psychotic Disorders and Antipsychotics* for further details)

Bipolar-related indications: Manic episodes in bipolar disorder

Dosage:

- Bipolar disorder, manic episode, outpatient:
  - *Oral:* 10 mg tid–qid or 25 mg bid–tid
  - *IM:* 25 mg, can repeat in 1 hr if needed
- Bipolar disorder, manic episode, inpatient:
  - *Oral:* 25–50 mg tid
  - *IM:* 25 mg, can repeat with additional 25–50 mg in 1 hr if needed

References:

1. AbbVie, Inc. 2014. "DEPAKOTE- divalproex sodium tablet, delayed release." US National Library of Medicine: DailyMed. Accessed January 7, 2015. http://dailymed.nlm.nih.gov/dailymed/drugInfo. cfm?setid=08a65cf4-7749-4ceb-6895-8f4805e2b01f.

2. Albers, Lawrence J., Rhoda K. Hahn, and Christopher Reist. 2010. *Handbook of Psychiatric Drugs.* 2011 ed. 75–78. Current Clinical Strategies Publishing.

3. American Psychiatric Association (APA). 2002. "Practice guideline for the treatment of patients with bipolar disorder (revision)." *Am J Psychiatry* 159(4 suppl):1–50. Accessed April 29, 2013.

4. American Psychiatric Association (APA). 2013. *Diagnostic and Statistical Manual of Mental Disorders.* 5th ed. (DSM-5®). Washington, DC: American Psychiatric Publishing.

5. ANI Pharmaceuticals, Inc. 2005. "LITHOBID- lithium carbonate tablet, film coated, extended release." US National Library of Medicine: DailyMed. Accessed October 29, 2014. http://dailymed. nlm.nih.gov/dailymed/drugInfo.cfm?setid=f7f5b69a-c2a1-4586-a189-1475d41387c0.

6. Center Watch. 2015. "FDA Approved Drugs by Therapeutic Area." Accessed February 3, 2015. https://www.centerwatch.com/drug-information/fda-approved-drugs/therapeutic-area/17/ psychiatry-psychology.

7. Elsevier Gold Standard, Inc. 2015. "Clinical Pharmacology." Accessed March 12, 2015. https:// www.clinicalpharmacology.com.

8. Epocrates. 2015. Accessed March 25, 2015. https://online.epocrates.com.

9. Gabbard, Glen O., ed. 2007. *Gabbard's Treatments of Psychiatric Disorders.* 4th ed. 5–28, 381–466. Washington, DC: American Psychiatric Publishing.

10. GlaxoSmithKline, LLC. 2015. "LAMICTAL- lamotrigine tablet." US National Library of Medicine: DailyMed. Accessed January 18, 2015. http://dailymed.nlm.nih.gov/dailymed/drugInfo. cfm?setid=d7e3572d-56fe-4727-2bb4-013ccca22678.

11. Goodwin, F.K., and K.R. Jamison. 2007. "Treatment: Medical Treatment of Hypomania Mania." In *Manic-Depressive Illness: Bipolar Disorders and Recurrent Depression*, 699–746. Oxford University Press, USA.

12. Hales, Robert. E., S. Yudofsky, and L. Roberts, eds. 2014. *The American Psychiatric Publishing Textbook of Psychiatry*. 6th ed. 311–352. Washington, DC: American Psychiatric Publishing.

13. Jamison, K. R. 2000. "Suicide and bipolar disorder." *J Clin Psychiatry* 61(Suppl 9):47–51.

14. Janssen Pharmaceuticals, Inc. 2014. "TOPAMAX- topiramate tablet, coated." US National Library of Medicine: DailyMed. Accessed January 8, 2015. http://dailymed.nlm.nih.gov/dailymed/drugInfo.cfm?setid=21628112-0c47-11df-95b3-498d55d89593.

15. Ketter, T.A. 2009. "Mood Stabilizers and Antipsychotics." In *Handbook of Diagnosis and Treatment of Bipolar Disorders*, 499–660. Washington, DC: American Psychiatric Publishing.

16. Medscape. 2015. "Bipolar Affective Disorder." Accessed March 12, 2015. http://emedicine.medscape.com/article/286342-overview#aw2aab6b2b3.

17. Medscape: Drugs & Diseases. 2015. "Psychiatrics." Accessed February 3, 2015. http://reference.medscape.com/drugs/psychiatrics.

18. Novartis Pharmaceuticals Co. 2014. "TRILEPTAL- oxcarbazepine tablet, film coated; TRILEPTAL- oxcarbazepine suspension." US National Library of Medicine: DailyMed. Accessed April 8, 2015. http://dailymed.nlm.nih.gov/dailymed/drugInfo.cfm?setid=4c5c86c8-ab7f-4fcf-bc1b-5a0b1fd0691b.

19. Parke-Davis Division of Pfizer, Inc. 2014. "NEURONTIN- gabapentin tablet, film coated." US National Library of Medicine: DailyMed. Accessed November 4, 2014. http://dailymed.nlm.nih.gov/dailymed/drugInfo.cfm?setid=ee9ad9ed-6d9f-4ee1-9d7f-cfad438df388.

20. Preston, John D., and James Johnson. 2011. *Clinical Psychopharmacology Made Ridiculously Simple*. 7th ed. 20–28. Miami: MedMaster Inc.

21. RxList. 2015. "Drugs A-Z List." Accessed March 25, 2015. http://www.rxlist.com/drugs/alpha_a.htm.

22. Schatzberg, A.F., and C.B. Nemeroff, eds. 2009. *The American Psychiatric Publishing Textbook of Psychopharmacology*. 4th ed. 695–808. Washington, DC: American Psychiatric Publishing.

23. Schatzberg, A.F., Jonathan O. Cole, and Charles DeBattista. 2010. *Manual of Clinical Psychopharmacology*. 7th ed. 17–19, 281–357. Washington, DC: American Psychiatric Publishing.

24. Stahl, S.M. 2008. *Essential Psychopharmacology: Neuroscientific Basis and Practical Applications*. 3rd ed. 370–387. New York: Cambridge Press.

25. Stahl, S.M. 2011. *Essential Psychopharmacology: the Prescriber's Guide*. 4th ed. 85–90, 487–490, 579–583, 591–595, 625–630. Cambridge: Cambridge University Press.

26. Truven Health Analytics. 2015. *Micromedex 2.0*. Accessed March 20, 2015. http://www.micromedexsolutions.com/home/dispatch.

27. UpToDate. 2015. Accessed March 12, 2015. http://www.uptodate.com/home.

28. US National Library of Medicine. 2015. "Drugs and Lactation Database (LactMed)." Accessed February 3, 2015. http://toxnet.nlm.nih.gov/newtoxnet/lactmed.htm.

29. US National Library of Medicine. 2015. "Toxicology Data Network." Accessed March 17, 2015. http://toxnet.nlm.nih.gov.

30. Validus Pharmaceuticals, LLC. 2013. "EQUETRO- carbamazepine capsule, extended release." US National Library of Medicine: DailyMed. Accessed October 29, 2014. http://dailymed.nlm.nih.gov/dailymed/drugInfo.cfm?setid=be478f3c-40f6-47cc-8ab9-f420a9372b1c.

31. Wegmann, J. 2008. *Psychopharmacology: Straight Talk on Mental Health Medications.* 61–82. Eau Claire: Pesi, LLC.

32. Wilson D. 2010. "Novartis pays $422.5 million in settlement." *New York Times.*   http://prescriptions.blogs.nytimes.com/2010/09/30/novartis-pays-422-5-million-in-settlement/?_r=0.

Chapter 6
Anxiety Disorders And Anxiolytics

Anxiety can be a normal reaction to stress, but when it disrupts daily functioning, it becomes a disorder. Anxiety disorders are some of the most prevalent and crippling mental health problems.[12] Despite the widespread occurrence, anxiety disorders often goes unrecognized and may therefore remain undertreated for years.[46]

According to the Epidemiological Catchment Area (ECA) in conjunction with other studies, the estimated lifetime prevalence rates for anxiety disorders are as follows[46]:

- Panic disorder (2.3–2.7%)
- GAD (4.1–6.6%)
- OCD (2.3–2.6)
- PTSD (1–9.3%)
- Social phobia (2.6–13.3%)

More females experience anxiety disorders than males, as indicated by the female to male ratio of 3:2.[46] Panic disorder has a bimodal age of onset, first in ages 15–24 and second in ages 45–54.[9] The onset of social phobia usually occurs before 20 years of age.

Anxiety disorders have multifactorial etiologies, as both genetic factors and psychosocial stressors are implicated in the development of these conditions.[25] Symptoms include constant worrying, palpitations, difficulty breathing, restlessness, fatigue, difficulty concentrating, hypervigilance, irritability, muscle tension, and trembling, among others. Risk factors include genetics, substance abuse, stressful lifestyles, and personality disorders.[46] Diagnosis is mainly clinical. Lab tests such as thyroid profiles, ECG, and urine toxicology may be necessary to exclude medical illness or substance abuse. Management includes both psychotherapy and pharmacotherapy.[46] Psychotherapy includes cognitive behavior therapy (CBT) and exposure therapy.[14] Various relaxation techniques, such as yoga and meditation, may also help to manage anxiety disorders. Clinicians should educate patients about the pathophysiology and prognosis of the disease and provide them with relevant self-help materials.[21]

Anxiolytics

Antidepressants and benzodiazepines are the two major classes of drugs used to treat anxiety disorders. Other drugs used to treat anxiety include buspirone, hydroxyzine (antihistamine), prazosin (alpha-blocker), propranolol (beta-blocker), and many other medications.[45] The APA recommends the use of SSRIs and SNRIs over benzodiazepines in the treatment of anxiety and panic disorders.[6]

Benzodiazepines
Class Profile[12,14,21,30,37,38,45,46]
Overview: Benzodiazepines (benzos) have been used widely for anxiety and various other psychiatric and medical disorders. These drugs inhibit neuronal activity in the

amygdala and the cerebral cortex, alleviating anxiety and reducing seizures.[4] Benzos with clear utility in anxiety include the following drugs[39]:

- Alprazolam
- Chlordiazepoxide
- Clonazepam
- Clorazepate
- Diazepam
- Lorazepam
- Oxazepam

Rapid onset: alprazolam, clorazepate, diazepam

Intermediate onset: chlordiazepoxide, lorazepam

Slow onset: clonazepam, oxazepam

MOA: Binds to benzodiazepine receptors at $GABA_A$, which is a major inhibitory neurotransmitter, resulting in relaxation through decreased excitability of neurons.

Warnings:

- May cause dependence, tolerance, and withdrawal symptoms with long-term use, even at therapeutic doses; gradual tapering is required due to risk of severe withdrawal symptoms, including seizure
- May cause CNS depression, impaired motor/cognitive performance, and memory loss
- Use with caution in patients with compromised pulmonary function, psychotic disorder, history of alcohol/substance abuse
- Use with caution in patients with MDD or history of suicide ideations/attempts
- Can precipitate mania/hypomania and cause paradoxical reactions (aggression, hyperactivity)
- May increase seizure severity and/or frequency
- Use with alcohol can be deadly because they are cross-tolerant

Drug interactions:

- Increased CNS depression when taken with TCAs, MAOIs, anticonvulsants, antihistamines, alcohol, narcotics, phenothiazines, phenylbutazones, methadone, barbiturates, opioid pain killers, buprenorphine, or other CNS depressants
- Use with CYP3A inhibitors increase levels, while inducers decrease levels
- Can cause seizures if used with flumazenil

Class side effects: Apnea, ataxia, confusion, depression, dizziness, drowsiness, dry mouth, fatigue, hangover, headache, memory impairment, muscle weakness, nausea, nervousness, psychomotor retardation, respiratory depression, slurred speech, somnolence.

Contraindications: Angle-closure glaucoma, sleep apnea, myasthenia gravis, hypersensitivity, acute alcohol intoxication, concomitant sodium oxybate use.

Recommended lab tests: CBC, LFTs.

Overdose: Usually safe when used alone but can be fatal when combined with opiates or other CNS depressants. Symptoms of overdose include sedation, drowsiness, ataxia, slurred speech, and hypotonia.

Tapering/withdrawal: Tapering necessary to reduce chances of withdrawal symptoms.

Individual Drug Profiles

Alprazolam[1,7,10,11,12,14,20,29,34,36,37,39,40,41,42,43]

Brand name: Niravam, Xanax, Xanax XR, Alprazolam Intensol

FDA approved for: GAD, panic disorder

Other potential uses (off-label): Agitation, depression, insomnia

Medication forms: *Tab* (0.25, 0.5, 1, 2 mg); *ODT* (0.25, 0.5, 1, 2 mg); *ER tab* (0.5, 1, 2, 3 mg); *oral sol* (1 mg/ml)

Dosage:
- GAD: 0.25–0.5 mg tid–qid initially, can be increased based on tolerance/response to max 4 mg/day
- Panic Disorder:
  - *IR:* 0.5 mg tid, may require up to 10 mg/day divided tid (average 5–6 mg/day)
  - *ER:* 0.5–1 mg/day, average 3–6 mg/day
- Anxiety associated with depression: 1–4 mg/day divided tid

MOA: Similar to *Benzo Class Profile*; also likely alters noradrenergic systems by causing downregulation of postsynaptic β-adrenergic receptors

Pharmacokinetics: t_{max}=1–2 hrs, $t_{1/2}$=12–15 hrs, works within 20 minutes

Warnings:
- Similar to *Benzo Class Profile*
- High abuse potential, especially in substance-abuse populations
- May cause interdose anxiety and has weak uricosuric effect

Drug interactions:
- Similar to *Benzo Class Profile*
- Increases plasma levels of imipramine, desipramine, and digoxin
- Use caution with sertraline, paroxetine, diltiazem, isoniazid, macrolides, cyclosporine, amiodarone, nicardipine, nifedipine, and grapefruit juice
- Use caution with CYP3A inhibitors, including nefazodone, fluvoxamine, cimetidine, HIV protease inhibitors, fluoxetine, propoxyphene, and OCP, as they can increase levels
- Carbamazepine (CYP3A inducer) decreases levels

Common side effects: Cognitive disorder, confusion, constipation, decreased or increased libido, depression, drowsiness, dry mouth, dysarthria, fatigue, headache, increased appetite, irritability, light-headedness, memory impairment, rash, weight gain

Contraindications:
- Similar to *Benzo Class Profile*
- Concomitant use with ketoconazole or itraconazole (potent CYP3A inhibitors)

Recommended lab tests: Similar to *Benzo Class Profile*

Overdose: CNS depression, AV block, and coma

Tapering/withdrawal: Slowly taper by 10% every month (taper higher doses by 50% initially, then by 10% every month); withdrawal occurs within first 1–6 days

Special populations:

Pregnancy: Risk Category D

Lactation: Avoid

Elderly: Lower initial dose recommended

Hepatic impairment: No dose adjustment necessary in mild to moderate, use caution in severe

Renal impairment: 0.25–0.5 mg tid

Important Notes:
- One of the few benzos to exhibit antidepressant properties
- Popular benzo among primary care physicians for panic episodes and anxiety disorders

Chlordiazepoxide[1,7,10,11,12,14,20,22,34,36,37,39,40,41,42,43]

Brand name: Librium, Librax

FDA approved for: Anxiety disorder, alcohol withdrawal, pre-operative apprehension

Other potential uses (off-label): Insomnia, opioid withdrawal

Medication forms: *Cap* (5, 10, 25 mg)

Dosage:
- Anxiety: 5-10 mg tid–qid in mild to moderate, 20–25 mg tid–qid in severe

MOA: Similar to *Benzo Class Profile*

Pharmacokinetics: t_{max}=1–2 hrs, $t_{1/2}$=24–48 hrs

Warnings:
- Similar to *Benzo Class Profile*
- Can lead to acute HSR
- May cause anterograde amnesia
- Can lead to ataxia and over-sedation, although rare

Drug interactions: Similar to *Benzo Class Profile*

Common side effects: Ataxia, dizziness, drowsiness, muscle weakness

Contraindications: Similar to *Benzo Class Profile*

Recommended lab tests: Similar to *Benzo Class Profile*

Overdose:
- Similar to *Benzo Class Profile*

- Respiratory depression/arrest with large overdoses, fatalities reported

Tapering/withdrawal: Slow taper recommended

Special populations:

Pregnancy: Risk Category D

Lactation: Avoid

Elderly: Lower dose by 50%

Hepatic Impairment: 5 mg qid

Renal Impairment: Lower dose by 50%

Clonazepam[1,7,10,11,12,13,14,20,34,36,37,39,40,41,42,43]

Brand name: Klonopin

FDA approved for: Panic disorder, seizure disorder

Other potential uses (off-label): Alcohol withdrawal, bipolar disorder, essential tremor, insomnia, RLS, sleepwalking

Medication forms: *Tab* (0.125, 0.25, 0.5, 1, 2 mg); *wafer* (0.125, 0.25, 0.5, 1, 2 mg)

Dosage:

- Panic disorder: 0.25 mg bid initially, can be increased based on tolerance/response to 4 mg/day max

MOA: Similar to Benzo Class Profile

Pharmacokinetics: t_{max}=1–4 hrs, $t_{1/2}$=30–40 hrs

Warnings:

- Similar to *Benzo Class Profile*
- Can cause hypersalivation

Drug interactions:

- Similar to *Benzo Class Profile*
- Use with valproate may cause seizure

Common side effects: Ataxia, depression, dizziness, fatigue, sinusitis, somnolence

Contraindications:

- Similar to *Benzo Class Profile*
- Severe liver disease

Recommended lab tests: Similar to *Benzo Class Profile*

Overdose: Similar to *Benzo Class Profile*

Tapering/withdrawal: Slow taper recommended

Special populations:

Pregnancy: Risk Category D

Lactation: Use caution

Elderly: Lower dose recommended

Hepatic impairment: Use caution in mild to moderate, avoid in severe

Renal impairment: Use caution

Important notes:

- Has anxiolytic, hypnotic, sedative, muscle-relaxant, anticonvulsant, and amnestic properties
- Tolerance to sedation develops faster than antianxiety effect
- Easy to taper; may be used to cross-taper other short-acting benzos

Clorazepate[1,7,10,11,12,14,19,20,23,34,36,37,39,40,41,42,43]

Brand name: Tranxene, Tranxene T-Tab, Gen-Xene

FDA approved for: Anxiety disorder, adjuvant therapy in management of partial seizure, symptomatic relief of acute alcohol withdrawal

Other potential uses (off-label): Agitation, insomnia

Medication forms: *Tab* (3.75, 7.5, 11.25, 15, 22.5 mg)

Dosage:

- Anxiety: 15–30 mg/day in divided doses (range 15–60 mg/day)
- Acute alcohol withdrawal:
  - *Day 1:* 30 mg once initially, max 90 mg in divided doses
  - *Day 2:* 45–90 mg in divided doses
  - *Day 3:* 22.5–45 mg in divided doses
  - *Day 4:* 15–30 mg in divided doses
  - *Day 5 and onward:* 7.5–15 mg in divided doses, discontinue when stable

MOA: Similar to *Benzo Class Profile*

Pharmacokinetics: t_{max}=1–4 hrs, $t_{1/2}$= approx 40–50 hrs

Warnings:

- Similar to *Benzo Class Profile*
- Do not use in depressive neuroses or in psychotic reactions

Drug interactions: Similar to *Benzo Class Profile*

Common side effects: Confusion, dizziness, drowsiness, fatigue, headache, nervousness, slurred speech

Contraindications: Similar to *Benzo Class Profile*

Overdose: CNS depression, hypotension, coma; OD can be fatal

Tapering/withdrawal: Slow taper recommended

Special populations:

Pregnancy: Risk Category D

Lactation: Avoid

Elderly: Lower dose recommended (7.5–15 mg initially)

Hepatic impairment: Specific guidelines not available; use caution

Renal impairment: Specific guidelines not available; use caution

Diazepam[1,7,10,11,12,14,20,33,34,36,37,39,40,41,42,43]

Brand name: Diastat, Diastat AcuDial, Valium

FDA approved for: Anxiety disorder, short-term relief of symptoms of anxiety, acute alcohol withdrawal, skeletal muscle spasm, convulsive disorder (adjunctive)

Other potential uses (off-label): Agitation, benzodiazepine withdrawal, insomnia

Medication forms: *Tab* (2, 5, 10 mg); *oral sol* (5mg/5ml, 5mg/ml); *injectable* (5mg/ml), *rectal gel* (2.5, 10, 20 mg)

Dosage:
- Anxiety: 2–10 mg po bid–tid **or** 2–10 mg IV/IM bid–tid, max 30 mg/8 hours
- Alcohol withdrawal:
    - 10 mg po q3–4hr during first 24 hr, reduce to 5 mg po tid–qid prn
      or
    - 10 mg IV/IM, may give additional doses as needed

MOA: Similar to Benzo Class Profile

Pharmacokinetics: t_{max}=1.5 hrs, $t_{1/2}$=20–50 hrs

Warnings:
- Similar to *Benzo Class Profile*
- Decreased WBC count and neutropenia reported; monitor WBC count with differential regularly

Drug interactions:
- Similar to *Benzo Class Profile*
- Increased and prolonged sedation with CYP3A inhibitors cimetidine, ketoconazole, fluvoxamine, fluoxetine, and omeprazole

Common side effects: Ataxia, dizziness, drowsiness, fatigue, muscle weakness, slurred speech

Contraindications:
- Similar to *Benzo Class Profile*
- Patients under 6 months of age
- Severe hepatic insufficiency

Overdose: Respiratory depression, coma; OD can be fatal

Tapering/Withdrawal: Slow taper recommended

Special populations:

Pregnancy: Risk Category D

Lactation: Avoid

Elderly: 2–2.5 mg po qd–bid

Hepatic impairment: Use caution and decrease usual dose by 50%

Renal impairment: No dose adjustment necessary

Important notes:
- Only benzo available in oral, liquid, injectable, and rectal formulations

Lorazepam[1,6,7,10,11,12,14,20,34,36,37,39,40,41,42,43]

Brand name: Ativan, Lorazepam Intensol

FDA approved for: Anxiety disorder, short-term relief of symptoms of anxiety, anxiety associated with depressive symptoms, insomnia

Other potential uses (off-label): Agitation, alcohol withdrawal, catatonia, muscle spasms, myoclonus, RLS

Medication form: *Tab* (0.5, 1, 2 mg); *oral conc* (2 mg/ml); *injectable* (2 mg/ml)

Dosage:
- Anxiety disorders: 2–3 mg po bid–tid prn initially, can be increased based on tolerance/response to max 10 mg/day, maintenance 2–6 mg/day po divided bid–tid
- Insomnia: 2–4 mg po qhs

MOA: Similar to *Benzo Class Profile*

Pharmacokinetics: t_{max}=3 hrs, $t_{1/2}$=12–14 hrs, metabolized primarily by liver

Warnings: Similar to *Benzo Class Profile*

Drug interactions:
- Similar to *Benzo Class Profile*
- Valproate and probenecid reduce drug clearance and raise levels
- Can cause sedation, hallucinations, and irrational behavior with scopolamine
- Can cause sedation, excessive salivation, hypotension, ataxia, delirium, and respiratory arrest with clonazepam
- Level reduced with theophylline, aminophylline, or OCP

Common side effects: Dizziness, drowsiness, headache, respiratory depression, sedation, weakness

Contraindications:
- Similar to *Benzo Class Profile*
- Intra-arterial route of administration

Overdose: Respiratory depression, hypotension, hypothermia, coma, rhabdomyolysis; OD rare

Tapering/withdrawal: Slow taper recommended

Special populations:

Pregnancy: Risk Category D

Lactation: Safe/preferred option

Elderly: 1–2 mg po divided

Hepatic impairment: No dose adjustment necessary in mild to moderate, lower dose recommended in severe

Renal impairment: No dose adjustment necessary in mild to moderate, avoid in severe

Important notes:
- Used for a variety of medical and psychiatric conditions

Oxazepam[1,7,10,11,12,14,20,34,35,36,37,39,40,41,42,43]

Brand name: Serax

FDA approved for: Anxiety disorder, short-term relief of symptoms of anxiety, anxiety associated with depression, alcohol withdrawal; tension, agitation, and irritability in older patients

Other potential uses (off-label): Insomnia

Medication forms: *Cap* (10, 15, 30 mg)

Dosage:

- Anxiety:
  - *Mild/moderate:* 10–15 mg tid–qid
  - *Severe anxiety, agitation, or anxiety associated with depression:* 15–30 mg tid–qid prn
- Alcohol withdrawal: 15–30 mg tid–qid prn

MOA: Similar to *Benzo Class Profile*

Pharmacokinetics: t_{max}=3 hrs, $t_{1/2}$=8.2 hrs

Warnings:

- Similar to *Benzo Class Profile*
- May cause hypotension

Drug interactions: Similar to *Benzo Class Profile*

Common side effects: Confusion, dizziness, drowsiness, muscle weakness, paradoxical reactions, psychomotor retardation

Contraindications:

- Similar to *Benzo Class Profile*
- Psychosis

Overdose: Similar to *Benzo Class Profile*

Tapering/withdrawal: Slow taper recommended

Special populations:

Pregnancy: Risk Category D

Lactation: Safe/preferred option

Elderly: 10 mg tid

Hepatic impairment: No dose adjustment necessary

Renal impairment: No dose adjustment necessary

Important notes:

- Used extensively since 1960s; more moderate effects than other benzos
- Preferred in liver disease, along with lorazepam and temazepam

Non-Benzodiazepine Medications

Buspirone[1,7,10,11,12,14,20,34,36,37,39,40,41,42,43,44]

Brand name: Buspar

FDA approved for: GAD, management of anxiety disorders

Other potential uses (off-label): Autism, bruxism, depression (augmentation of other treatments), smoking cessation

Medication forms: *Tab* (5, 7.5, 10, 15, 30 mg); *cap* (5, 7.5, 10, 15 mg)

Dosage:
- Anxiety disorders: 10–15 mg/day divided, can be increased based on tolerance/response to max 60 mg/day
- Smoking cessation: 30–60 mg/day for 9–13 weeks beginning 2–3 weeks before quit date

MOA: Agonist at $5\text{-}HT_{1A}$ and D_2 receptors; no effect on GABA

Pharmacokinetics: t_{max}=40–90 min, $t_{1/2}$=2–3 hrs

Warnings:
- May interfere with cognitive/motor performance
- When switching from a sedative/hypnotic, taper gradually before starting buspirone due to potential of withdrawal reaction

Drug interactions:
- Can elevate BP when used with MAOIs; avoid with MAOIs or up to 2 weeks after stopping MAOIs
- Avoid with furazolidone, procarbazine, or alcohol; use caution with other CNS-active drugs
- LFT results may show increased levels when combined with trazodone
- CYP3A4 inducers (e.g., rifampin) decrease plasma levels; CYP3A4 inhibitors increase plasma levels (e.g., diltiazem, verapamil, erythromycin, grapefruit juice, itraconazole, nefazodone)
- Increases levels of haloperidol

Common side effects: Dizziness, drowsiness, excitement, headache, nausea, nervousness

Contraindications: Hypersensitivity

Recommended lab tests: None

Overdose: No fatalities reported

Tapering/withdrawal: Not required

Special populations:

Pregnancy: Risk Category B

Lactation: Avoid

Elderly: No dose adjustment necessary

Hepatic impairment: Lower dose recommended in mild to moderate, avoid in severe

Renal impairment: No dose adjustment necessary in mild to moderate, avoid in severe

Important notes:
- No documented dependence, tolerance, or withdrawal issues
- Can be used as augmentation strategy with SSRIs for depression and anxiety
- Does not alter alertness, attention, memory, and reaction time
- Takes 2–6 weeks to show effect in patients with GAD

Hydroxyzine[1,7,10,11,12,14,20,28,34,36,37,39,40,41,42,43]

Brand name: Atarax, Vistaril

FDA approved for: Anxiety, pruritus, premedication sedation, nausea/vomiting

Other potential uses (off-label): GAD, agitation, alcohol/opioid withdrawal, insomnia

Medication forms: *Tab* (10, 25, 50 mg); *cap* (25, 50, 100 mg); *syrup/oral suspension* (25 mg/5 ml); *injectable sol* (25, 50 mg/ml)

Dosage:
- Anxiety:
  - 50–100 mg po tid-qid
    or
  - 50–100 mg IM tid-qid

MOA: Antagonist at H_1 receptors; has skeletal-muscle-relaxing, bronchodilating, anti-histaminic, antiemetic, and analgesic properties

Pharmacokinetics: t_{max}=2 hrs, $t_{1/2}$=20 hrs

Warnings:
- May cause excessive morning drowsiness after intake the prior evening
- Use with caution in patients requiring intact cognitive function or in patients with reduced respiratory function (e.g., asthma, COPD)

Drug interactions:
- May cause CNS depression if combined with cetirizine, sodium oxybate, iso-carboxazid, tranylcypromine, or other anxiolytics, sedatives, hypnotics or CNS depressants

Common side effects: Drowsiness, dry mouth, hallucinations, fatigue, pruritus, rash

Contraindications:
- Hypersensitivity, pregnancy
- Inter-arterial, subcutaneous, or IV administration

Recommended lab tests: None

Overdose: Hypotension, sedation; no fatalities reported

Tapering/withdrawal: Tapering generally not required

Special populations:

Pregnancy: Risk Category C (not assigned by FDA), contraindicated

Lactation: Avoid

Elderly: Initiate dose at lowest recommended

Hepatic impairment: No dose adjustment necessary in mild to moderate, use caution in severe

Renal impairment: No dose adjustment necessary in mild to moderate, reduce dose by 50% in severe

Important notes:
- May be used for agitation and anxiety in children

Antidepressants

SSRIs

(Refer to *Chapter 4: Depressive Disorders and Antidepressants* for further details)

SSRIs are the treatment of choice for the long-term management of anxiety disorders. However, they may require 4–6 weeks to relieve the symptoms of anxiety.[12,36,46] SSRIs are helpful for treating GAD, panic disorder, OCD, social phobia, PTSD, separation anxiety disorder, selective mutism, and anxiety associated with eating disorders.[5,30]

Escitalopram[10,20,39]

Anxiety-related indications: GAD in adults

Dosage:
- GAD: 10 mg qd initial/max

Important notes:
- Maintain at lowest effective dose and assess periodically

Fluoxetine[10,20,39]

Anxiety-related indications: OCD in adults and children/adolescents (ages 7–17 yrs), panic disorder

Dosage:
- OCD:
  - Prozac: 20–60 mg/day
  - Prozac Weekly: 90 mg/week
- Panic disorder: 10 mg/day initially, can be increased based on tolerance/response to max 20 mg/day

Important notes:
- Not as well tolerated as other SSRIs for panic disorder or other anxiety disorders

Fluvoxamine[10,20,39]

Anxiety-related indications: OCD in adults and children/adolescents (ages 8–17 yrs), social anxiety disorder

Dosage:
- OCD: 50 mg qhs (**or** 100 mg/day *ER cap*) initially, can be increased based on tolerance/response to max 300 mg/day
- Social anxiety disorder: 100 mg *ER cap* qhs, can be increased based on tolerance/response to max 300 mg/day

Paroxetine[10,20,39]
Anxiety-related indications: OCD, panic disorder, social anxiety disorder, GAD, PTSD
Dosage:
- OCD: 20 mg/day initially, can be increased based on tolerance/response to max 60 mg/day
- Panic disorder:
  - *IR:* 10 mg/day initially, can be increased based on tolerance/response to max 60 mg/day
    or
  - *Paxil CR:* 12.5 mg/day initially, can be increased based on tolerance/response to max 75 mg/day
- Social anxiety disorder:
  - *IR:* 20 mg/day
    or
  - *Paxil CR:* 12.5 mg/day initially, can be increased based on tolerance/response to max 37.5 mg/day
- GAD: 20 mg/day initially, can be increased based on tolerance/response to max 50 mg/day
- PTSD: 20 mg/day initially, can be increased based on tolerance/response to max 50 mg/day

Important notes:
- Adjust to maintain lowest effective dosage

Sertraline[10,20,39]
Anxiety-related indications: OCD in adults and children/adolescents (ages 6–17 yrs), panic disorder, PTSD, social anxiety disorder
Dosage:
- OCD: 50 mg qam initially, can be increased based on tolerance/response to max 200–300 mg/day
- Panic disorder/PTSD/social anxiety disorder: 25 mg qam initially, can be increased based on tolerance/response to max 200 mg/day

SNRIs
(Refer to *Chapter 4: Depressive Disorders and Antidepressants* for further details)

Duloxetine[10,23,39]
Anxiety-related indications: GAD
Dosage:
- GAD: 60 mg qd initially, can be increased based on tolerance/response to max 120 mg/day

Venlafaxine[10,20,39]
Anxiety-related indications: GAD, social anxiety disorder, panic disorder
Dosage:
- GAD: 37.5 mg qd (*XR*) initially, can be increased based on tolerance/response to max 225 mg/day
- Social Anxiety: 75 mg qd (*XR*)
- Panic Disorder: 37.5 mg qd (*XR*) initially, can be increased based on tolerance/response to max 225 mg/day

TCAs
(Refer to *Chapter 4: Depressive Disorders and Antidepressants* for further details)
Limit the use of TCAs to cases where SSRIs and SNRIs are ineffective.[5]

Clomipramine[10,20,39]
Anxiety-related indications: OCD in adults and children/adolescents (ages 10–17 yrs)
Dosage:
- OCD: 25 mg/day initially, can be increased based on tolerance/response to max 250 mg/day

Doxepin[10,20,39]
Anxiety-related indications: Anxiety
Dosage:
- Anxiety: 25 mg bid initially, can be increased based on tolerance/response to max 300 mg/day

Alpha-Blockers

Alpha-blockers act as antagonists of central α-adrenergic receptors. They are also used to treat anxiety disorders such as GAD, panic disorder, and PTSD. The alpha-blockers used for the treatment of anxiety are prazosin and clonidine hydrocloride.[32]

Clonidine hydrochloride[10,20,39]
(Refer to *Chapter 7: ADHD and Its Treatment* for further details)

Other potential uses (off-label): Anxiety, insomnia, severe agitation
Dosage:
- *IR tab:* 0.05–0.1 mg hs initially, can be increased based on tolerance/response to max 0.6 mg divided
- *Transdermal:* same dose as oral

Prazosin[1,7,10,11,12,14,20,27,32,34,36,37,39,40,41,42,43]
Brand name: Minipress
FDA approved for: Hypertension
Other potential uses (off-label): PTSD, nightmares
Medication forms: *Cap* (1, 2, 5 mg)
Dosage:
- PTSD-related nightmares and sleep disruption: 1 mg qhs initially, maintenance 2–15 mg qhs

MOA: Causes vasodilation, decreasing total peripheral resistance and diastolic BP
Pharmacokinetics: t_{max}=0.5–3 hrs, $t_{1/2}$=2–3 hrs
Warnings:
- May cause syncope after first dose
- Can increase symptoms of narcolepsy
- May cause marked urinary retention in elderly patients
- May cause Intraoperative Floppy Iris Syndrome (IFIS) and priapism

Drug interactions:
- Avoid use with nintedanib due to fatal side effects
- Can cause marked vasodilation and low BP with vasodilators (e.g., nitrates, sildenafil)

Common side effects: Blurred vision, constipation, diarrhea, dizziness, drowsiness, fatigue, first dose effect, fluid retention, headache, nasal congestion, nausea, palpitations, weakness

Contraindications: Hypersensitivity, concomitant use with amifampridine, elderly patients with orthostatic hypotension
Recommended lab tests: BP
Overdose: Hypotension, torsades de pointes, agitation, seizures, priapism; OD rare
Tapering/withdrawal: Slow taper recommended
Special populations:
Pregnancy: Risk Category C
Lactation: Use caution
Elderly: No dose adjustment necessary
Hepatic impairment: Lower dose recommended

Renal impairment: No dose adjustment necessary
Important Notes:
- Used for treating symptoms of PTSD

Beta-Blockers

Beta-blockers interfere with the receptor binding of epinephrine, weakening the effects of stress hormones.[45] Beta-blockers effectively treat anxiety disorders by significantly reducing the physiological symptoms of the fight-or-flight response.[15] The beta-blocker used to treat anxiety is propranolol.[15]

Propranolol[1,7,10,11,12,14,16,20,34,36,37,39,40,41,42,43]

Brand name: Hemangeol, Inderal, Inderal LA, InnoPran XL

FDA approved for: Various cardiac conditions, tremor, migraine prophylaxis, hypertension

Other potential uses (off-label): Performance anxiety, agitation, akathisia, alcohol withdrawal, tremor, hyperthyroidism

Medication forms: *Tab* (10, 20, 40, 60, 80 mg); *ER cap* (60, 80, 120, 160 mg); *oral sol* (20, 40mg/5 ml); *injectable sol* (1mg/ml)

Dosage:
- Performance anxiety: 10–40 mg prn
- Essential tremor: 40 mg po bid initially, 120–320 mg/day po divided bid–tid for maintenance
- Antipsychotic-induced akathisia: 10–30 mg tid

MOA: Helps to control physical symptoms of anxiety by blocking β-adrenergic receptors

Pharmacokinetics: t_{max}=1.5–2 hrs (IR)/12–15 hrs (ER), $t_{1/2}$=3–6 hrs (IR)/8–20 hrs (ER)

Warnings:
- May cause HSR including severe skin reactions (including SJS/TEN)
- Discontinue use before major surgery
- May exacerbate angina pectoris and symptoms of hyperthyroidism upon abrupt withdrawal
- Use with extreme caution in patients with pheochromocytoma, cardiac failure, Wolf-Parkinson-White syndrome, or bronchospastic lung disease
- May cause misregulation of glucose metabolism and can mask signs of hypoglycemia

Drug interactions:
- Use caution with drugs that affect CYP2D6, 1A2, or 2C19 pathways
- Avoid use with nintedanib due to fatal side effects
- Use caution with ACE inhibitors, alpha-blockers, reserpine, NSAIDs, MAOIs, TCAs, anesthetics, neuroleptics, warfarin, thyroxine, or other antiarrhythmics

Common side effects: Bone pain, bronchospasm, depression, fatigue, hypotension, insomnia, low energy, sleep problems

Contraindications: CHF, cardiogenic shock, sinus bradycardia, sick sinus syndrome, heart block, compromised pulmonary function, hypersensitivity

Recommended lab tests: RFTs, LFTs

Overdose: AV block, intraventricular conduction delay, CHF; OD uncommon but potentially severe

Tapering/withdrawal: Slow tapering necessary

Special populations:

Pregnancy: Risk Category C

Lactation: Safe/preferred option

Elderly: Lower doses recommended

Hepatic impairment: Lower doses recommended

Renal impairment: No dose adjustment necessary

Important notes:

- Effective in treatment of social phobias (dose 10–40 mg)
- Effective in alleviating performance anxiety

Anticonvulsants

Gabapentin[10,20,39]

(Refer to *Chapter 5: Bipolar Disorder and Mood Stabilizers* for further details)

Other potential uses (off-label): Social anxiety disorder

Dosage:

- Social anxiety disorder: 900-2700 mg/day divided tid, higher doses can be given at bedtime

Pregabalin[1,7,10,11,12,14,20,26,34,36,37,39,40,41,42,43]

Brand name: Lyrica

FDA approved for: Diabetic neuropathy, fibromyalgia, neuropathic pain, partial seizure, post-herpetic neuralgia

Other potential uses (off-label): GAD, hot flashes, insomnia, RLS

Medication forms: *Cap* (25, 50, 75, 100, 150, 200, 225, 300 mg); *oral sol* (20 mg/ml)

Dosage:

- GAD: 300–450 mg/day divided bid–tid

MOA: Strongly binds to alpha-2 subunit of voltage-gated calcium channels in CNS, is a GABA analogue, reduces the calcium-dependent release of pro-nociceptive neurotransmitters

Pharmacokinetics: t_{max} =1.5 hrs, $t_{1/2}$=5–7 hrs

Warnings:
- May cause HSR and angioedema
- May increase risk of suicidal ideation or behavior
- Use caution in patients with renal/cardiovascular disorders
- Can cause peripheral edema, weight gain, dizziness, and somnolence

Drug interactions:
- Can potentiate the sedative effects of alcohol, buprenorphine, cannabis, and other CNS depressants
- Avoid concomitant use with ACE inhibitors and statins
- Can cause peripheral edema when used with thiazolidinedione

Common side effects: Abnormal thinking, asthenia, ataxia, blurred vision, constipation, dizziness, dry mouth, edema, headache, incoordination, increased appetite, somnolence, tremor, weight gain

Contraindications: Hypersensitivity

Lab test recommended: RFTs

Tapering/withdrawal: Gradual taper recommended

Special populations:

Pregnancy: Risk Category C

Lactation: Avoid

Elderly: Lower dose preferred

Hepatic impairment: No dose adjustment necessary

Renal impairment: Lower and divided dose recommended

Important notes:
- Useful for various painful nerve conditions

Tiagabine[1,7,8,10,11,12,14,20,34,36,37,39,40,41,42,43]

Brand name: Gabitril

FDA approved for: Partial seizure

Other potential uses (off-label): Anxiety disorders

Medication forms: *Tab* (2, 4, 12, 16 mg)

Dosage:
- Chronic pain and anxiety: 2–12 mg/day

MOA: Inhibits neuronal and glial uptake of GABA

Pharmacokinetics: t_{max}=45 min, $t_{1/2}$=7–9 hours

Warnings:
- May cause HSR, angioedema, and serious rash
- May increase the risk of suicidal ideation or behavior
- Can induce seizure in non-epileptic patients or during withdrawal
- Can cause cognitive/neuropsychiatric impairment and exacerbate EEG abnormalities

Drug interactions:
- May potentiate sedative effects of alcohol, buprenorphine, cannabis, and other CNS depressants
- Level increased considerably with potent CYP3A4 inhibitors (idelalisib, ivacaftor)
- Decreases steady-state valproate concentration
- Clearance 60% greater with carbamazepine, phenytoin, and phenobarbital
- Replaces protein-bound drugs and increases their free plasma concentration

Common side effects: Asthenia, ataxia, depression, diarrhea, difficulty with attention/concentration, dizziness, ecchymosis, flu-like syndrome, nausea, nervousness, somnolence, tremors, vomiting

Contraindications: Hypersensitivity

Recommended lab tests: LFTs

Overdose: Limited data; seizures, CNS depression, agitation, hallucinations, coma

Tapering/withdrawal: Gradual tapering recommended

Special populations:

Pregnancy: Risk Category C

Lactation: Unknown risk; avoid

Elderly: Lower dose recommended

Hepatic Impairment: Lower dose recommended

Renal Impairment: No dose adjustment necessary

Important notes:
- Secondary treatment option for anxiety disorders; used to augment SSRIs, SNRIs, benzos

Antipsychotics
(Refer to *Chapter 8: Psychotic Disorders and Antipsychotics* for further details)

Olanzapine[10,20,39]
Other potential uses (off-label): OCD, PTSD
Dosage:
- OCD/PTSD: 7.5–15 mg/day

Quetiapine[10,20,39]
Other potential uses (off-label): Anxiety, OCD
Dosage:
- OCD/anxiety: 50–300 mg/day

Risperidone[10,20,39]
Other potential uses (off-label): OCD, PTSD
Dosage:
- OCD/PTSD: 1–2 mg/day

References:

1. Albers, Lawrence J., Rhoda K. Hahn, and Christopher Reist. 2010. *Handbook of Psychiatric Drugs*. 2011 ed. 60–66. Current Clinical Strategies Publishing.

2. American Psychiatric Association (APA). 2009. "Practice guideline for the treatment of patients with panic disorder." Accessed March 16, 2015. http://psychiatryonline.org/content.aspx?bookid=28&sectionid=1680635.

3. American Psychiatric Association (APA). 2013. *Diagnostic and Statistical Manual of Mental Disorders*. 5th ed. (DSM-5®). Washington, DC: American Psychiatric Publishing.

4. Ashton, Heather C. 2002. "Benzodiazepines: How They Work & How to Withdraw." Accessed February 23, 2015. http://benzo.org.uk/manual/bzcha01.htm#26.

5. Bandelow, B., L. Sher, R. Bunevicius, E. Hollander, S. Kasper, J. Zohar, and H.J. Moller. 2012. "Guidelines for the pharmacological treatment of anxiety disorders, obsessive-compulsive disorder and posttraumatic stress disorder in primary care." *Int J Psychiatry Clin Pract* 16(2):77–84. doi: 10.3109/13651501.2012.667114.

6. BTA Pharmaceuticals, Inc. 2014. "ATIVAN- lorazepam tablet." US National Library of Medicine: Daily Med. Accessed November 12, 2014. http://dailymed.nlm.nih.gov/dailymed/drugInfo.cfm?setid=07cae057-a593-4e4d-a478-2d7fc9f06857.

7. Center Watch. 2015. "FDA Approved Drugs by Therapeutic Area." Accessed February 3, 2015. http://www.centerwatch.com/drug-information/fda-approved-drugs/therapeutic-area/17/psychiatry-psychology.

8. Cephalon, Inc. 2012. "GABITRIL- tiagabine hydrochloride tablet." US National Library of Medicine: DailyMed. Accessed November 4, 2014. http://dailymed.nlm.nih.gov/dailymed/drugInfo.cfm?setid=cf97a72e-951e-a7db-a574-adac12a6b189.

9. Eaton, W.W., R.C. Kessler, H.U. Wittchen, and W.J. Magee. 1994. "Panic and panic disorder in the United States." *Am J Psychiatry* 151(3):413–420.

10. Elsevier Gold Standard, Inc. 2015. "Clinical Pharmacology." Accessed March 12, 2015. https://www.clinicalpharmacology.com.

11. Epocrates. 2015. Accessed March 25, 2015. https://online.epocrates.com.

12. Gabbard, Glen O., ed. 2007. *Gabbard's Treatments of Psychiatric Disorders*. 4th ed. 29–38, 477–580. Washington, DC: American Psychiatric Publishing.

13. Genentech, Inc. 2013. "KLONOPIN- clonazepam tablet." US National Library of Medicine: Daily Med. Accessed November 12, 2014. http://dailymed.nlm.nih.gov/dailymed/drugInfo.cfm?setid=542f22e8-dad2-47a8-93b6-30936715d73b.

14. Hales, Robert. E., S. Yudofsky, and L. Roberts, eds. 2014. *The American Psychiatric Publishing Textbook of Psychiatry*. 6th ed. 388–419. Washington, DC: American Psychiatric Publishing.

15. Hayes, P.E., and S.C. Schulz. 1987. "Beta-blockers in anxiety disorders." *J Affect Disord* 13(2):119–130.

16. Heritage Pharmaceuticals Inc. 2014. "PROPRANOLOL HYDROCHLORIDE- propranolol hydrochloride tablet." US National Library of Medicine: Daily Med. Accessed November 12, 2014. http://dailymed.nlm.nih.gov/dailymed/drugInfo.cfm?setid=976077df-038b-4b01-bc4e-751cd70d4441.

17. Hofmann, Stefan G., and Jasper A. J. Smits. 2008. "Cognitive-Behavioral Therapy for Adult Anxiety Disorders: a Meta-Analysis of Randomized Placebo-Controlled Trials." *Journal of Clinical Psychiatry* 69(4):621–632.

18. Kessler, R. C., W. Chiu, O. Demler, and E. E. Walters. 2005. "Prevalence, severity, and comorbidity of 12-month dsm-iv disorders in the national comorbidity survey replication." *Archives of General Psychiatry* 62(6):617–627. doi: 10.1001/archpsyc.62.6.617.

19. Medscape: Drugs & Diseases. 2015. "Clorazepate (Rx): Tranxene SD, Tranxene T-Tab." Accessed January 13, 2015. http://reference.medscape.com/drug/tranxene-sd-tranxene-t-tab-clorazepate-342901.

20. Medscape: Drugs & Diseases. 2015. "Psychiatrics." Accessed February 3, 2015. http://reference.medscape.com/drugs/psychiatrics.

21. Medscape. 2015. "Psychiatry and Mental Health." Accessed March 12, 2015. http://www.medscape.com/psychiatry.

22. Mylan Pharmaceuticals, Inc. 2014. "CHLORDIAZEPOXIDE HYDROCHLORIDE- chlordiazepoxide hydrochloride capsule." US National Library of Medicine: Daily Med. Accessed November 12, 2014. http://dailymed.nlm.nih.gov/dailymed/drugInfo.cfm?setid=68c7d8a7-08b3-4a1a-acbd-09bbe67b8d4a.

23. Mylan Pharmaceuticals, Inc. 2014. "CLORAZEPATE DIPOTASSIUM- clorazepate dipotassium tablet." US National Library of Medicine: Daily Med. Accessed November 12, 2014. http://dailymed.nlm.nih.gov/dailymed/drugInfo.cfm?setid=9acbb3f4-4bf6-40ae-89e3-303ec167912c.

24. National Institute of Mental Health (NIMH). 2015. "Introduction: Mental Health Medications." Accessed March 16, 2015. http://www.nimh.nih.gov/health/publications/mental-health-medications/index.shtml.

25. Nolte, Tobias, Jo Guiney, Peter Fonagy, Linda C. Mayes, and Patrick Luyten. 2011. "Interpersonal stress regulation and the development of anxiety disorders: an attachment-based developmental framework." *Frontiers in Behavioral Neuroscience* 5:55. doi: 10.3389/fnbeh.2011.00055.

26. Parke-Davis Division of Pfizer Inc. 2014. "LYRICA- pregabalin capsule." US National Library of Medicine: DailyMed. Accessed January 18, 2015. http://dailymed.nlm.nih.gov/dailymed/drugInfo.cfm?setid=60185c88-ecfd-46f9-adb9-b97c6b00a553.

27. Pfizer, Inc. 2014. "MINIPRESS- prazosin hydrochloride capsule." US National Library of Medicine: Daily Med. Accessed November 12, 2014. http://dailymed.nlm.nih.gov/dailymed/drugInfo.cfm?setid=36c4da56-502e-4da1-acf7-8e81ee453dcc.

28. Pfizer, Inc. 2014. "VISTARIL- hydroxyzine pamoate capsule." US National Library of Medicine: Daily Med. Accessed November 12, 2014. http://dailymed.nlm.nih.gov/dailymed/drugInfo.cfm?setid=c271f97f-040e-492b-9194-2c8b74675a95.

29. Pharmacia and Upjohn Company. 2014. "XANAX- alprazolam tablet." US National Library of Medicine: Daily Med. Accessed November 12, 2014. http://dailymed.nlm.nih.gov/dailymed/drugInfo.cfm?setid=388e249d-b9b6-44c3-9f8f-880eced0239f.

30. Preston, John D., and James Johnson. 2011. *Clinical Psychopharmacology Made Ridiculously Simple.* 7th ed. 29–39. Miami: MedMaster Inc.

31. Rappa, Leonard, and James Viola. 2012. Condensed Psychopharmacology 2013: A Pocket Reference for Psychiatry and Psychotropic Medications. 1-46 RXPSYCH, LLC.

32. Raskind, M.A., E.R. Peskind, D.J. Hoff, K.L. Hart, H.A. Holmes, D. Warren, J. Shofer, J. O'Connell, F. Taylor, C. Gross, K. Rohde, and M.E. McFall. 2007. "A parallel group placebo controlled study of prazosin for trauma nightmares and sleep disturbance in combat veterans with post-traumatic stress disorder." *Biol Psychiatry* 61(8):928–934. doi: 10.1016/j.biopsych.2006.06.032.

33. Roche Products, Inc. 2013. "VALIUM- diazepam tablet." US National Library of Medicine: Daily Med. Accessed November 12, 2014. http://dailymed.nlm.nih.gov/dailymed/drugInfo.cfm?setid=554baee5-b171-4452-a50a-41a0946f956c.

34. RxList. 2015. "Drugs A-Z List." Accessed March 25, 2015. http://www.rxlist.com/drugs/alpha_a.htm.

35. Sandoz, Inc. 2011. "OXAZEPAM- oxazepam capsule." US National Library of Medicine: Daily Med. Accessed November 12, 2014. http://dailymed.nlm.nih.gov/dailymed/drugInfo.cfm?setid=140d8f61-912b-449a-9c34-b52e08b3d819.

36. Schatzberg, A.F., and C.B. Nemeroff, eds. 2009. *The American Psychiatric Publishing Textbook of Psychopharmacology.* 4th ed. 965–986, 1171–1200. Washington, DC: American Psychiatric Publishing.

37. Schatzberg, A.F., Jonathan O. Cole, and Charles DeBattista. 2010. *Manual of Clinical Psychopharmacology.* 7th ed. 23–27, 375–422. Washington, DC: American Psychiatric Publishing.

38. Stahl, S.M. 2008. *Essential Psychopharmacology: Neuroscientific Basis and Practical Applications.* 3rd ed. 388–419. New York: Cambridge Press.

39. Stahl, S.M. 2011. *Essential Psychopharmacology: the Prescriber's Guide.* 4th ed. 13, 77–79, 91–95, 117–121, 129–132, 159–163, 497–500. Cambridge: Cambridge University Press.

40. Truven Health Analytics. 2015. *Micromedex 2.0.* Accessed March 20, 2015. http://www.micromedexsolutions.com/home/dispatch.

41. UpToDate. 2015. Accessed March 12, 2015. http://www.uptodate.com/home.

42. US National Library of Medicine. 2015. "Drugs and Lactation Database (LactMed)." Accessed February 3, 2015. http://toxnet.nlm.nih.gov/newtoxnet/lactmed.htm.

43. US National Library of Medicine. 2015. "Toxicology Data Network." Accessed March 17, 2015. http://toxnet.nlm.nih.gov.

44. Watson Laboratories, Inc. 2013. "BUSPIRONE HCL- buspirone hydrochloride tablet." US National Library of Medicine: Daily Med. Accessed April 8, 2015. http://dailymed.nlm.nih.gov/dailymed/drugInfo.cfm?setid=a3fe0ccd-565f-4d0a-a7ba-2fad7a819358.

45. Wegmann, J. 2008. *Psychopharmacology: Straight Talk on Mental Health Medications*. 83–108. Eau Claire: Pesi, LLC.

46. Yates, William R. 2014. "Anxiety Disorders." Accessed January 13, 2015. http://emedicine.medscape.com/article/286227-overview.

Chapter 7
ADHD And Its Treatment

Attention Deficit Hyperactivity Disorder (ADHD) is a neuro-behavioral disorder marked by inattentiveness, impulsivity, and hyperactivity.[18] This condition is a major cause of disability with a high morbidity in children and adolescents. The incidence of ADHD in children is approximately 3–7% in the US and appears much more frequently in boys (13.2%) than in girls (5.6%).[11,27,42] Girls usually display symptoms of inattentiveness whereas boys usually display symptoms of hyperactivity and impulsivity.[10]

As many as 65–75% of children with ADHD will have some residual symptoms as adults, with an estimated 15–20% of children maintaining the full diagnosis into adulthood.[34,42,53] Furthermore, adults are increasingly being diagnosed with ADD/ADHD.[8,23] According to recent research, many adults may suffer from ADHD, contradicting its stereotyping as a childhood disorder.[18,22]

Genetic, neuroanatomical, environmental, and psychosocial factors contribute to the etiology of ADHD. For example, monozygotic twin studies show a 55–90% concordance rate for this disorder.[27] Symptoms of ADHD include difficulty paying attention, lack of concentration, carelessness, hyperactivity, impulsivity, failure perform a given task, restlessness, day dreaming, excessive talking, and others. The diagnosis of ADHD is predominantly clinical—most reliably obtained by home and teacher reports. Management involves medication, psychotherapy and environmental modification like avoiding distractors.[6,13] A multidimensional approach involving healthcare providers, family, and teachers may allow an affected individual to cope with these challenges and to live a productive life.

Changes in DSM-5

The age of onset for ADHD has changed from 7 years to 12 years. Also, the definition has been updated to characterize the experience of affected adults more accurately, as previous editions of the DSM did not provide appropriate guidance for diagnosis in this population.[4,5]

The subtypes of ADHD are[4]:
- Predominantly inattentive type
- Predominantly hyperactive-impulsive type
- Combined type

Medications

Medication management is an important part of treating ADHD, along with psycho-social interventions. Stimulants have been studied extensively and used to treat ADHD for several decades. These drugs are effective for 70–80% of patients.[6] In 1995, the earliest stimulant, methylphenidate, was approved for ADHD; the latest, Quillivant XR, was approved in 2012.[18,27] In 2005, an FDA Advisory Panel suggested that a black box warning be placed on all stimulant medications entailing the increased risk of cardiovascular injuries.[49]

Amphetamine-based stimulants are approved for the treatment of ADHD in children three years and older, while methylphenidate-based stimulants are approved for children six years and older.[13]

Amphetamine-based stimulants include[18,38,53]:

- Adderall
- Adderall XR
- Dexedrine
- Dexedrine Spansule
- Dextrostat
- Vyvanse

Methylphenidate-based stimulants include[18,38,53]:

- Focalin
- Focalin XR
- Methylin
- Methylin ER
- Metadate ER
- Metadate CD
- Ritalin
- Ritalin SR
- Ritalin LA
- Concerta
- Quillivant XR
- Daytrana

CNS Stimulants (amphetamine- and methylphenidate-based)
Class Profile[18,20,25,34,38,42,43,50,51,53]

MOA: CNS stimulants (amphetamine- and methylphenidate-based) block the reuptake of norepinephrine and dopamine, increasing their concentration in the extraneuronal space.

Warnings:

- **Black box warning:** CNS stimulants (amphetamine- and methylphenidate-containing products) have a high potential for abuse and dependence; assess the risk of abuse prior to prescribing and monitor for signs of abuse and dependence while on therapy.[49] Misuse may cause sudden death or serious cardiovascular adverse events.
- May cause sudden death in pediatric patients with structural heart disease
- Can lower seizure threshold, create visual disturbances, and impair mental/physical abilities
- Can exacerbate motor/phonic tics and Tourette syndrome

- Can induce manic episodes in patients with bipolar disorder and exacerbate preexisting psychosis; emergence of new manic or psychotic symptoms is also possible
- Associated with aggressive behavior and long-term mild growth suppression in children and adolescents
- May cause a mild increase in BP and a small increase in HR
- May cause peripheral vasculopathy (e.g., Raynaud's phenomenon)
- May cause priapism (methylphenidate-based only)

Drug interactions:
- Concurrent use with other sympathomimetic agents, TCAs, or MAOIs can cause headache, arrhythmia, hypertensive crisis, and hyperpyrexia; avoid for at least 2 weeks after stopping MAOIs
- Use with beta-blockers can create excessive hypertension, reflex bradycardia, and heart block
- Reduces therapeutic effectiveness of antihypertensive medications
- Use with antacids may cause increased absorption, increasing drug effectiveness and side effects
- Decreased availability with gastric- and urinary-acidifying agents
- Chlorpromazine, haloperidol, and lithium can inhibit the stimulant effects of amphetamines
- Can intensify the effects of meperidine and norepinephrine
- Can reduce the effects of antihistamines, phenobarbital, phenytoin, veratrum alkaloids, and ethosuximide
- Methylphenidate-based stimulants:
  - Inhibit the metabolism of SSRIs, anticonvulsants, TCAs, and coumadin anticoagulants
  - Avoid use with clonidine

Class side effects: Abdominal pain, angioedema, anorexia, anxiety, decreased appetite, diarrhea, dizziness, dry mouth, dyskinesia, palpitations, fever, headache, hypertension, impotence, insomnia, irritability, loss of appetite, nausea, nervousness, tachycardia, tremors, vomiting, weight loss.

Contraindications: Hypersensitivity, extreme anxiety/agitation, structural cardiac abnormalities, atherosclerotic and arteriosclerotic vascular disease, overactive thyroid gland, bipolar disorder, hypertension, motor tics, Tourette syndrome, history of drug abuse, glaucoma, within 14 days of taking an MAOI.

Recommended lab tests: Thyroid panel, lipid panel, weight and height in children, BP (optional); assess cardiovascular status with EKG if there is historical or other evidence of a cardiac risk.

Overdose: Dilated pupils, high fever, sweating, restlessness, aggressiveness, confusion, chest pain, palpitation, vomiting, tremors, hallucination, sweating, hyperpyrexia, hypertension, arrhythmia, mydriasis, agitation, delirium, and, in severe cases, seizures, coma.

Tapering/withdrawal: No tapering required.

Special populations:

Pregnancy: Risk Category C

Lactation: Lower dose recommended

Elderly: Dose as tolerated

Hepatic impairment: Use caution

Renal Impairment: Use caution

Cardiac Impairment: Contraindicated

Important notes:

- Initiate treatment with IR, then switch to ER if tolerated and effective
- Most children require treatment well into adolescence and possibly adulthood
- May be helpful in treatment-resistant depression

Amphetamine-based Stimulants: Individual Drug Profiles

Black box warning: CNS stimulants (amphetamine- and methylphenidate-containing products) have a high potential for abuse and dependence; assess the risk of abuse prior to prescribing and monitor for signs of abuse and dependence while on therapy.[49] Misuse may cause sudden death or serious cardiovascular adverse events.

Adderall[1,7,12,16,17,18,24,36,37,38,44,45,48]

(dextroamphetamine/amphetamine)

FDA approved for: ADHD in children/adolescents (ages 3–17 yrs) and adults (ages < 65 yrs), narcolepsy

Other potential uses (off-label): Depression, weight loss, cognitive side effects of psychotropics,

Medication forms: *Tab* (2.5, 3.75, 5, 6.25, 7.5, 10, 15, 20, 30 mg)

Dosage:

- ADHD (ages >6 yrs): 5 mg/day, can be increased based on tolerance/response to max 40 mg qd or divided tid
- ADHD (ages 3–6 yrs): 2.5 mg/day, can be increased based on tolerance/response to max 40 mg/day

MOA: Similar to *Stimulant Class Profile*

Pharmacokinetics: t_{max}=3 hrs, $t_{1/2}$=10–14 hrs (adults)/11–14 hrs (adolescents)/9–11 hrs (children ages 6–12 yrs), duration of action=4–5 hrs

Warnings: Similar to *Stimulant Class Profile*

Drug interactions: Similar to *Stimulant Class Profile*

Common side effects: Angioedema, anorexia, diarrhea, dry mouth, impotence, insomnia, irritability, loss of appetite, nausea, tachycardia, weight loss, tremors, tics

Important notes:
- Lasts throughout the school day if given twice daily
- A combination of isomers D- and L-amphetamine salt in a 3:1 ratio

Adderall XR[1,12,16,17,18,24,36,37,38,39,44,45,48]
(dextroamphetamine/amphetamine extended release)
FDA approved for: Treatment of ADHD of children/adolescents (ages 6–17 yrs) and adults (ages <65 yrs)
Other potential uses (off-label): Cognitive side effects of psychotropics, depression, weight loss
Medication forms: *Cap* (5, 10, 15, 20, 25, 30 mg)
Dosage:
- ADHD (adults): 20–30 mg qam
- ADHD (children/adolescents):
  - *6–12 yrs:* 5–10 mg qam initially, can be increased based on tolerance/response to max 30 mg/day
  - *13–17 yrs:* 10 mg qam intially, can be increased based on tolerance/response to max 30 mg/day
MOA: Similar to *Stimulant Class Profile*
Pharmacokinetics: Same as Adderall, duration of action=10–12 hrs
Drug interactions: Similar to *Stimulant Class Profile*
Common side effects: Abdominal pain, agitation, angioedema, anxiety, asthenia, diarrhea, dizziness, dry mouth, fever, headache, impotence, insomnia, irritability, loss of appetite, nausea, nervousness, tachycardia, urinary tract infections, vomiting, weight loss
Important notes:
- Same specifics as Adderall; 50:50 ratio of immediate and delayed-release Adderall
- Safe and well-tolerated by both children and adults, low frequency of adverse effects
- Capsule may be broken and sprinkled over food or applesauce

Dexedrine[1,2,12,16,17,18,24,36,37,38,44,45,48]
(dextroamphetamine sulfate)
Brand names: Dexedrine, ProCentra, Zenzedi
FDA approved for: ADHD in children/adolescents (ages 3–16 yrs), narcolepsy
Other potential uses (off-label): ADHD in adults, depression, weight loss
Medication forms: *Tab* (5, 10 mg); *oral sol* (5 mg/5 ml); *ProCentra oral sol* (5 mg/5 ml); *Zenzedi tab* (2.5, 5, 7.5, 10, 15, 20, 30 mg)
Dosage:
- ADHD in children/adolescents:

- *3–5 yrs:* 2.5 mg qd initially, can be increased based on tolerance/response to max 40 mg/day
- *6–16 yrs:* 5 qd or bid initially, can be increased based on tolerance/response to max 40 mg/day
- *Maintenance:* 5–15 mg bid or 5–10 mg tid

MOA: Similar to *Stimulant Class Profile*

Pharmacokinetics: t_{max}=2–3 hrs, $t_{1/2}$=10.25 hrs, duration of action=4–6 hours

Drug interactions: Similar to *Stimulant Class Profile*

Common side effects: Angioedema, anorexia, diarrhea, dry mouth, dyskinesia, dysphoria, euphoria, hypertension, impotence, insomnia, irritability, overstimulation, palpitations, restlessness, tachycardia, tremors, urticaria, weight loss

Important notes:
- Can be used in low-weight children
- Suppresses appetite; although not approved or recommended to treat obesity
- Use cautiously in patients under 5 years of age

Dexedrine Spansule[1,3,12,16,17,18,24,36,37,38,44,45,48]

(dextroamphetamine sulfate extended release)

FDA approved for: ADHD in children/adolescents (ages 6–16 yrs), narcolepsy

Medication form: *SR bead-filled cap* (5, 10, 15 mg)

Dosage: Same as Dexedrine (for ages 6–16 yrs)

MOA: Similar to *Stimulant Class Profile*

Pharmacokinetics: t_{max}=8 hrs, $t_{1/2}$=12 hrs, duration of action=10 hours

Warnings: Similar to *Stimulant Class Profile*

Drug interactions: Similar to *Stimulant Class Profile*

Common side effects: Same as Dexedrine

Important notes:
- Helpful for children unable to swallow pills as beads can be sprinkled over soft food
- Beads should be swallowed not chewed

Dextrostat[1,2,12,16,17,18,24,36,37,38,44,45,48]

(dextroamphetamine sulfate)

FDA approved for: ADHD in children/adolescents (ages 3–16 yrs), narcolepsy

Medication forms: *Tab* (5, 10 mg)

Dosage: Same as Dexedrine

MOA: Similar to *Stimulant Class Profile*

Pharmacokinetics: t_{max}=2 hrs, $t_{1/2}$=10.25 hrs, duration of action=4 hrs

Warnings: Similar to *Stimulant Class Profile*

Drug interactions: Similar to *Stimulant Class Profile*
Common side effects: Impotence, insomnia, tachycardia, tremor
Important notes:
* A dextroisomer of amphetamine

Vyvanse[1,12,16,17,18,24,36,37,38,41,44,45,48]
(lisdexamfetamine)
FDA approved for: ADHD in children/adolescents (ages 6–17 yrs) and adults (ages < 65 yrs), binge eating disorder
Medication forms: *Cap* (10, 20, 30, 40, 50, 60, 70 mg)
Dosage:
* ADHD (ages ≥6 yrs): 20–30 mg qam initially, can be increased based on tolerance/ response to max 70 mg/day
MOA: Similar to *Stimulant Class Profile*
Pharmacokinetics: t_{max}=3.5–3.8 hrs, $t_{1/2}$= 1 hr, duration of action=10 hrs
Warnings: Similar to *Stimulant Class Profile*
Drug interactions: Similar to *Stimulant Class Profile*
Common side effects: Decreased appetite, dizziness, dry mouth, insomnia, irritability, nausea, upper abdominal pain, vomiting, weight loss
Important notes:
* Only medication approved by FDA for binge eating disorder
* In severe renal impairment, max 50 mg/day; in end-stage renal disease (ESRD), max 30 mg/day
* Therapeutically inactive product attached to lysine; activated in GI tract once lysine is cleaved
* May have relative low risk of abuse due to delayed release after IV or intranasal use

Methylphenidate-based Stimulants: Individual Drug Profiles
Black box warning: CNS stimulants (amphetamine- and methylphenidate-containing products) have a high potential for abuse and dependence; assess the risk of abuse prior to prescribing and monitor for signs of abuse and dependence while on therapy.[49]

Dexmethylphenidate
Brand name: Focalin, Focalin XR

Focalin[1,12,16,17,18,24,29,36,37,38,44,45,48]
FDA approved for: ADHD in children/adolescents (ages 6–17 yrs)
Other potential uses (off-label): ADHD in adults, depression
Medication forms: *Tab* (2.5, 5, 10 mg)

Dosage:
- ADHD (ages 6–17 yrs): 2.5 mg bid initially, can be increased based on tolerance/response to max 20 mg/day

MOA: Similar to *Stimulant Class Profile*

Pharmacokinetics: t_{max}=1.5–6.5 hrs, $t_{1/2}$= 3 hrs (adults)/2–3 hrs (children), duration of action=3–4 hrs

Warnings: Similar to *Stimulant Class Profile*

Drug interactions: Similar to *Stimulant Class Profile*

Common side effects: Abdominal pain, angina, anorexia, anxiety, arrhythmia, decreased appetite, dizziness, dry mouth, fever, headache, insomnia, nausea, palpitations, tachycardia

Important notes:
- Regular growth monitoring and psychiatric evaluation recommended

Focalin XR[1,12,16,17,18,24,30,36,37,38,44,45,48]

FDA approved for: ADHD in children/adolescents (ages 6-17 yrs) and adults

Medication forms: *Cap* (5, 10, 15, 20, 25, 30, 35, 40 mg)

Dosage:
- ADHD:
  - *Children/adolescents (ages 6–17 yrs):* 5 mg qd initially, can be increased based on tolerance/response to max 30 mg/day
  - *Adults:* 10 mg qd initially, can be increased based on tolerance/response to max 40 mg/day
  - *Switch from Focalin:* same dose
  - *Switch from methylphenidate:* half dose

MOA: Similar to *Stimulant Class Profile*

Pharmacokinetics: t_{max}=1.5–6.5 hrs, $t_{1/2}$=2–4.5 hrs, duration of action=10–12 hrs

Warnings: Similar to Stimulant Class Profile

Drug interactions: Similar to Stimulant Class Profile

Common side effects: Anxiety, decreased appetite, dizziness, dry mouth, dyspepsia, headache, pharyngeal pain, tachycardia

Important notes:
- 50:50 combination of IR and XR d-methylphenidate beads; XR beads release after 4 hours

Methylphenidate hydrochloride

Brand name: Concerta, Daytrana, Metadate CD, Metadate ER, Methylin, Methylin ER, Quillivant XR, Ritalin, Ritalin LA, Ritalin SR

Concerta[1,12,16,17,18,21,24,36,37,38,44,45,48]

FDA approved for: ADHD in children/adolescents (ages 6–17 yrs) and adults (ages < 65 yrs)

Other potential uses (off-label): Depression, fatigue in adult cancer patients, weight loss

Medication forms: *ER tab* (18, 27, 36, 54 mg)

Dosage:

- ADHD (adults): 18 or 36 mg qd initially, can be increased based on tolerance/response to max 72 mg/day
- ADHD (children/adolescents): 18 mg qd initially, can be increased based on tolerance/response to max 54 mg/day in children (ages 6–12 yrs) or 72 mg/day in adolescents (ages 13–17 yrs)

MOA: Similar to *Stimulant Class Profile*

Pharmacokinetics: t_{max}=6.8 hrs, $t_{1/2}$=3.5 hrs, duration of action=10–16 hrs

Warnings: Similar to *Stimulant Class Profile*

Drug interactions: Similar to *Stimulant Class Profile*

Common side effects: Abdominal pain, anxiety, decreased appetite, dry mouth, headache, hypertension, insomnia, irritability, nausea

Important notes:

- Risk of GI obstruction due to tablet being nondeformable; avoid use in patients with GI problems (e.g., small intestine IBD, short bowel syndrome)
- Do not open or chew tablet due to osmotic pump mechanism for extended treatment
- Causes mild appetite suppression but does not prompt sleep abnormality

Daytrana[1,12,16,17,18,24,33,36,37,38,44,45,48]

FDA approved for: ADHD in children/adolescents (ages 6–17 yrs)

Medication forms: *Transdermal patch* (10, 15, 20, 30 mg/9 hrs)

Dosage:

- ADHD (ages 6–17 yrs): Apply patch on hip 2 hours before desired onset, then remove after 9 hours; dose according to manufacturer's recommendations
  - Week 1: 10 mg/12.5 cm² patch
  - Week 2: 15 mg/18.75 cm² patch
  - Week 3: 20 mg/25 cm² patch
  - Week 4: 30 mg/37.5 cm² patch

MOA: Similar to *Stimulant Class Profile*

Pharmacokinetics: t_{max}=7.5–10 hrs, $t_{1/2}$=3–4 hrs, duration of action=9 hrs

Warnings: Similar to *Stimulant Class Profile*

Drug interactions: Similar to *Stimulant Class Profile*

Common side effects: Anxiety, decreased appetite, dizziness, insomnia (if patch worn >9 hours), mild skin reactions to patch (redness, edema), nausea, tachycardia, weight loss

Important notes:
- Transdermal formulation contains methylphenidate in multi-polymeric adhesive layer on transparent backing
- Helpful for those who cannot tolerate oral form, need a flexible schedule, or can't swallow pills
- Do not expose application site to heat
- More methylphenidate bioavailable due to bypassing first pass metabolism

Metadate CD[1,12,16,17,18,24,36,37,38,44,45,46,48]

FDA approved for: ADHD in children/adolescents (ages 6–17 yrs), narcolepsy

Other potential uses (off-label): ADHD in adults, depression

Medication forms: *Cap* (10, 20, 30, 40, 50, 60 mg)

Dosage:
- ADHD (ages 6–17 yrs): 20 mg qam before breakfast initially, can be increased based on tolerance/response to max 60 mg/day

MOA: Similar to *Stimulant Class Profile*

Pharmacokinetics: t_{max}=two distinct peaks—1.5–3 hrs (early peak)/4.5–6.6 hrs (second peak), $t_{1/2}$=2.5–6.8 hrs, duration of action=9–12 hrs

Warnings: Similar to *Stimulant Class Profile*

Drug interactions: Similar to *Stimulant Class Profile*

Common side effects: Abdominal pain, anorexia, dizziness, headache, hypertension, insomnia, nausea, nervousness, tachycardia

Important notes:
- Capsule contains 30% IR/70% DR beads
- Should not be used in patients with fructose intolerance, glucose-galactose malabsorption, or sucrase-isomaltase insufficiency
- Use with halogenated anesthetics is contraindicated

Metadate ER[1,12,16,17,18,24,36,37,38,44,45,47,48]

FDA approved for: ADHD in children/adolescents (ages 6–17 yrs), narcolepsy

Other potential uses (off-label): ADHD in adults, depression

Medication forms: *ER tab* (10, 20 mg); *cap* (10, 20 mg)

Dosage:
- ADHD (ages 6–17 yrs): 10 mg qam, can be increased to 30 mg bid (same dosing as Methylin ER)

MOA: Similar to *Stimulant Class Profile*

Pharmacokinetics: t_{max}=two distinct peaks—1.5–3 hrs (early peak)/4.5–6.6 hrs (second peak), $t_{1/2}$=2.5–6.8 hrs, duration of action=10 hrs

Warnings: Similar to *Stimulant Class Profile*

Drug interactions: Similar to *Stimulant Class Profile*

Common side effects: Abdominal pain, anorexia, dizziness, headache, hypertension, insomnia, nausea, nervousness, tachycardia

Important notes:

- Should not be used in patients with galactose intolerance, Lapp lactase deficiency, or glucose-galactose malabsorption
- Use with halogenated anesthetics is contraindicated
- Mild CNS stimulant gradually released from wax matrix
- Well-tolerated with relatively infrequent insomnia and decreased appetite

Methylin[1,12,16,17,18,19,24,36,37,38,44,45,48]

FDA approved for: ADHD in children/adolescents (ages 6–17 yrs) and adults (ages <65 yrs), narcolepsy

Medication forms: *Tab*: (5, 10, 20 mg); *chew tab* (2.5, 5, 10 mg); *oral sol* (5 mg, 10 mg/5 ml)

Dosage:

- ADHD (adults): 20–30 mg qd divided bid–tid taken 30–45 minutes before meal, can be increased based on tolerance/response to max 60 mg/day
- ADHD (ages 6–17 yrs): 2.5–5 mg bid initially, can be increased based on tolerance/response to max 60 mg/day

MOA: Similar to *Stimulant Class Profile*

Pharmacokinetics: t_{max}=1–2 hrs, $t_{1/2}$=2.7–3.5 hrs, duration of action=3–5 hrs

Warnings: Similar to *Stimulant Class Profile*

Drug interactions: Similar to *Stimulant Class Profile*

Common side effects: Anorexia, BP/HR changes, cardiac arrhythmia, dizziness, dyskinesia, headache, insomnia, nausea, nervousness

Important notes:

- Useful for patients unable to swallow tablets
- Use caution in emotionally labile patients

Methylin ER[1,12,16,17,18,19,24,36,37,38,44,45,48]

FDA approved for: ADHD in children/adolescents (ages 6-17) and adults (ages <65 yrs), narcolepsy

Medication forms: *Tab* (10, 20 mg)

Dosage:

- ADHD: 10 mg/day, can be increased based on tolerance/response to max 60 mg/day

MOA: Similar to *Stimulant Class Profile*

Pharmacokinetics: t_{max}=6.8 hrs, $t_{1/2}$=3.5 hrs, duration of action=8 hrs

Warnings: Similar to *Stimulant Class Profile*

Drug interactions: Similar to *Stimulant Class Profile*

Common side effects: Abdominal pain, anorexia, BP/HR changes, headache, insomnia, nausea

Important notes:

- May use in place of methylphenidate IR tablets

Quillivant XR [1,12,16,17,18,24,28,36,37,38,44,45,48]

FDA approved for: ADHD in children/adolescents (ages 6–17 yrs) and adults (ages <65 yrs)

Other potential uses (off-label): Depression, improving fatigue in HIV/cancer patients, narcolepsy

Medication forms: *ER oral suspension* (25 mg/5 ml [300, 600, 750, and 900 mg bottle])

Dosage:

- ADHD: 25 mg (5ml) qam initially, can be increased based on tolerance/response to max 60 mg/day (about 12 ml when reconstituted)

MOA: Similar to *Stimulant Class Profile*

Pharmacokinetics: t_{max}=4 hrs, $t_{1/2}$=5.2 hrs, duration of action=10 hrs

Warnings: Similar to *Stimulant Class Profile*

Drug interactions: Similar to *Stimulant Class Profile*

Common side effects: Abdominal pain, decreased appetite, hypertension, insomnia, nausea, vomiting

Important notes:

- Comes in powder form for reconstitution with water
- Use caution with personal/family history of cardiac problems or psychiatric disorder
- First once-daily ER liquid medication for ADHD

Ritalin[1,12,16,17,18,24,26,32,36,37,38,44,45,48]

FDA approved for: ADHD in children/adolescents (ages 6-17 yrs), narcolepsy

Other potential uses (off-label): ADHD in adults, depression, weight loss

Medication forms: *Tab* (5, 10, 20 mg)

Dosage:

- ADHD (ages 6–17 yrs): 2.5–5 mg bid initially, can be increased based on tolerance/response to max 60 mg/day

MOA: Similar to *Stimulant Class Profile*

Pharmacokinetics: t_{max}=1–2 hrs, $t_{1/2}$=2.7–3.5 hrs, duration of action=3–4 hrs

Warnings: Similar to *Stimulant Class* Profile

Drug interactions: Similar to *Stimulant Class Profile*
Common side effects: Anorexia, BP/HR changes, headache, insomnia, nausea, nervousness
Important notes:
- Short-acting, mild CNS stimulant preferred in patients with loss of appetite or insomnia
- Avoid in patients with marked symptoms of depression or fatigue
- Prolonged use can lead to tolerance and psychological dependence

Ritalin LA[1,12,16,17,18,24,31,36,37,38,44,45,48]
FDA approved for: ADHD in children/adolescents (ages 6–17 yrs), narcolepsy
Other potential uses (off-label): ADHD in adults, depression, weight loss
Medication forms: *Cap* (10, 20, 30, 40 mg)
Dosage:
- ADHD: 20 mg qam before breakfast initially, can be increased based on tolerance/response to max 60 mg/day
MOA: Similar to *Stimulant Class Profile*
Pharmacokinetics: t_{max}=two distinct peaks—1.5–3 hrs (early peak)/4.5–6.6 hrs (second peak), $t_{1/2}$=2.5–6.8 hrs, duration of action=8–12 hrs
Warnings: Similar to *Stimulant Class Profile*
Drug interactions: Similar to *Stimulant Class Profile*
Common side effects: Abdominal pain, bruxism, depression, dry mouth, headache, insomnia, loss of appetite, nausea, nervousness, tachycardia
Important notes:
- 50:50 (IR:ER beads) capsule mimics bid dose of Ritalin
- Beads may be sprinkled over soft food

Ritalin SR[1,12,16,17,18,24,26,32,36,37,38,44,45,48]
FDA approved for: None (discontinued in US)
Medication forms: *Tab* (20 mg)
Dosage: Same as Ritalin
Pharmacokinetics: t_{max}=4.7 hrs, $t_{1/2}$=3–4 hrs, duration of action=4–8 hrs
Common side effects: Abdominal pain, depression, headache, insomnia, loss of appetite, nausea, nervousness, tachycardia

Nonstimulants
At least 30% of patients cannot tolerate or respond poorly to stimulants but respond to non-stimulant medications.[1] Compared to stimulants, these drugs have a longer duration of action, do not prompt rebound or insomnia, involve a minimal risk of abuse or dependence, and may alleviate comorbid symptoms like tics.[18] Despite their

delayed onset of action (3–4 weeks), non-stimulants possess several advantages, such as[18]:

- Once-daily dosing
- No need for triplicate prescription
- Minimal addiction potential

- Effects typically last 24 hours
- Can treat comorbid depression

Notable nonstimulants include:

- Atomoxetine
- Clonidine hydrochloride/Kapvay
- Guanfacine/Intuniv
- Bupropion

- Desipramine
- Imipramine
- Nortryptyline

Notable Nonstimulants

Atomoxetine[1,12,15,16,17,18,24,36,37,38,44,45,48,50]

Brand name: Strattera

FDA approved for: Maintenance for ADHD in children and adults

Other potential uses (off-label): Binge eating, cocaine dependence, MDD with psychotic features, schizophrenia, Tourette syndrome

Medication forms: *Cap* (10, 18, 25, 40, 60, 80, 100 mg)

Dosage:

- ADHD in adults (weight >70 kg): 40 mg qd initially, can be increased based on tolerance/response to max 100 mg/day divided
- ADHD in children:
  - *Weight ≤70 kg*: 0.5 mg/kg/day initially, can be increased based on tolerance/response to max 1.4 mg/kg/day qd or bid
  - *Weight >70 kg:* 40 mg qd initially, can be increased based on tolerance/response to max 100 mg qd or bid

MOA: Inhibits noradrenergic monoamine reuptake

Pharmacokinetics: t_{max}=1–2 hrs, $t_{1/2}$=5.2 hrs

Warnings:

- **Black box warning:** Increased risk of suicidal thinking and behavior in children and adolescents
- Can cause liver damage and serious cardiovascular events; avoid in children or adolescents with serious structural cardiac abnormalities
- Can cause hypertension and tachycardia, which may result in orthostasis or syncope
- May cause emergence/worsening of aggressive behavior, psychotic or manic symptoms
- May lead to priapism, urinary hesitation/retention, and HSR
- May suppress growth

Drug Interactions:
- Reduce dose or avoid concomitant use with inhibitors of CYP3A4 (e.g., azole antifungals)
- Can increase levels of alprazolam, buspirone, and triazolam via CYP3A4 inhibition
- Plasma levels can increase with CYP2D6 inhibitors
- Use caution with antihypertensive drugs and vasopressor agents due to effects on BP
- Can increase the cardiovascular effects of albuterol

Common side effects: Abdominal pain, constipation, decreased appetite, dry mouth, dysmenorrhea, erectile dysfunction, fatigue, headache, insomnia, nausea, menstrual disorder, tachycardia, urinary hesitation, urinary retention, vomiting

Contraindications: Liver disease, hypersensitivity, eating disorder, pheochromocytoma, angle-closure glaucoma, severe cardiac disorders, within 2 weeks of discontinuing MAOI

Recommended lab tests: LFTs

Overdose: Seizures, dizziness, tremor, hyperactivity, elevated BP/HR; OD rare

Tapering/withdrawal: Gradual taper recommended

Special populations:

Pregnancy: Risk Category C

Lactation: Avoid

Elderly: Lower dose recommended

Hepatic impairment: No dose adjustment necessary in mild to moderate, lower dose recommended in severe

Renal impairment: No dose adjustment necessary

Cardiac impairment: Use caution, contraindicated in structural heart defects

Important notes:
- First nonstimulant approved for ADHD with no abuse potential
- Does not need a physical prescription as it is not a controlled substance
- Monitor growth regularly in children
- May be more effective for inattention than hyperactivity
- Stop if pruritus, dark urine, right-sided abdominal pain, or unexplained flu-like symptoms appear
- Less effective than stimulants for ADHD and it takes a several weeks for maximum effect

Clonidine hydrochloride[1,9,12,16,17,18,24,36,37,38,44,45,48]

Brand name: Catapres, Catapres-TTS

FDA approved for: Hypertension

Other potential uses (off-label): ADHD, aggression, autism, insomnia (caused by stimulants), opioid withdrawal, severe agitation, tic disorder

Medication forms: *Tab* (0.1, 0.2, 0.3 mg); *ER transdermal patch* (0.1, 0.2, 0.3 mg/day)
Dosage:
- ADHD:
  - *IR tab:* 0.05 to 0.1 mg hs initially, can be increased based on tolerance/response to max 0.6 mg divided
  - *ER transdermal patch*: same dose as oral

MOA: Stimulates α-adrenergic receptors in brain, reducing sympathetic outflow from CNS and decreasing peripheral and renal vascular resistance, HR, and BP

Pharmacokinetics: t_{max}=2 hrs, $t_{1/2}$=12.7–13.7 hrs

Warnings:
- Can aggravate depression in patients with history of MDD
- May cause HSR (skin rash, urticaria, angioedema)
- May worsen SA-nodal and AV-nodal block

Drug interactions:
- Do not use with other anticoagulants due to life-threatening bleeding
- Concurrent use with TCAs decreases effect of clonidine
- Potentiates CNS-depressive effects of alcohol, barbiturates, and other CNS depressants
- Can cause sinus bradycardia requiring pacemaker insertion when used with diltiazem or verapamil
- High IV dose with haloperidol can increase QT prolongation or ventricular fibrillation
- Can cause symptoms of orthostatic dysregulation when combined with neuroleptics

Common side effects: Anorexia, confusion, constipation, dizziness, drowsiness, dry mouth, erectile dysfunction, fatigue, hallucinations, headache, hives, hypotension, pruritus, rash, sedation, somnolence, vomiting

Contraindications: Hypersensitivity

Recommended lab tests: BP

Overdose: Apnea, respiratory depression, coma, hypotension

Tapering/withdrawal: Tapering required; abrupt withdrawal can cause rebound hypertension

Important notes:
- Centrally acting α-agonist that lowers BP and HR
- Administer before bedtime to avoid daytime sedation
- Often used with stimulants to reduce side effects, hyperactivity, and hyperkinesis
- Useful option for reducing stimulant-induced insomnia and impulsivity
- Should be avoided in lactation

Kapvay[1,12,14,16,17,18,24,36,37,38,44,45,48]
(ER formulation of clonidine hydrochloride)

FDA approved for: ADHD in children/adolescents (ages 6–17 yrs)
Medication forms: *ER tab* (0.1, 0.2 mg)
Dosage:
- ADHD (ages 6–17 yrs): 0.1 mg qhs initially, can be increased based on tolerance/response to max 0.4 mg/day

Common side effects: Constipation, dizziness, dry mouth, fatigue, headache, insomnia, irritability, somnolence
Tapering/withdrawal: Discontinue by 0.1 mg q3–7days
Important notes:
- Administer before bedtime
- Swallow whole; do not chew/break

Guanfacine[1,12,16,17,18,24,35,36,37,38,44,45,48]
Brand name: Tenex
FDA approved for: ADHD in children/adolescents (ages 6–17 yrs), hypertension
Other potential uses (off-label): Aggression, tic disorder, Tourette syndrome
Medication forms: *Tab* (1, 2 mg)
Dosage:
- ADHD (ages 6–17 yrs): 1 mg qd, can be increased based on tolerance/response to max 4–6 mg/day

MOA: Stimulates α_{2A}-adrenergic receptors, decreasing sympathetic outflow and lowering HR; precise MOA in ADHD unknown
Pharmacokinetics: t_{max}=2.6–5 hrs, $t_{1/2}$=14–17 hrs
Warnings:
- May cause orthostatic hypotension and severe skin allergy
- Use with caution in patients with severe coronary insufficiency, recent MI, or cerebrovascular disease

Drug interactions:
- Avoid with any medication that has antihypertensive effects
- Avoid with other CNS depressants as guanfacine potentiates their effects
- Amitriptyline and amoxapine decrease guanfacine's effect
- Drug metabolism altered by use of CYP450 inducers and inhibitors; dose adjustment possibly required

Common side effects: Abdominal pain, bradycardia, constipation, dizziness, dry mouth, headache, lethargy, sedation, somnolence, weakness
Contraindications: Hypersensitivity
Recommended lab tests: Monitor HR and BP at initiation and with dosage changes
Overdose: Drowsiness, QTc prolongation, hypotension, blurred vision, bradycardia

Tapering/withdrawal: Slow taper recommended; abrupt cessation can cause rebound hypertension

Important notes:

* Can be taken at bedtime if it causes sedation in morning
* Best when taken on an empty stomach; do not take with high-fat meal

Intuniv[1,12,16,17,18,24,35,36,37,38,40,44,45,48]

(ER form of guanfacine)

FDA approved for: ADHD in children/adolescents (ages 6–17 yrs)

Other potential uses (off-label): Aggression, tic disorder, Tourette syndrome

Medication forms: *ER tab* (1, 2, 3, 4 mg)

Dosage:

* ADHD (children/adolescents): 1 mg qd initially, can be increased based on tolerance/response to max 4 mg/day (children ages 6–12 yrs) or max 7 mg/day (adolescents ages 13–17 yrs)

Warnings:

* Use caution in patients with kidney/liver disease, hypersensitivity, or hypertension
* Can cause dizziness, drowsiness, somnolence, bradycardia, hypotension
* May worsen SA-nodal and AV-nodal block

Drug interactions: See guanfacine/Tenex above

Common side effects: Abdominal pain, constipation, dizziness, dry mouth, fatigue, headache, hypotension, insomnia, irritability, lethargy, nausea, somnolence

Important notes:

* No clear study on safety during pregnancy and breastfeeding; use caution
* Can be used in conjunction with stimulants

Bupropion[16,24,44]

(Refer to *Chapter 4: Depressive Disorders and Antidepressants* for further details)

Other potential uses (off-label): ADHD

Dosage:

* ADHD: 150 mg/day initially, can be increased based on tolerance/response to max 450 mg/day (can administer divided or in ER/SR formulations)

TCAs: desipramine, imipramine, nortryptyline[16,24,44]

(Refer to *Chapter 4: Depressive Disorders and Antidepressants* for further details)

TCAs are typically prescribed for ADHD when a patient does not demonstrate improvement with stimulants or other nonstimulants. TCAs are also prescribed if the patient has comorbid depression or anxiety in addition to ADHD.[44,52] Higher doses of desipramine and imipramine are potentially dangerous.

References:

1. Albers, Lawrence J., Rhoda K. Hahn, and Christopher Reist. 2010. *Handbook of Psychiatric Drugs*. 2011 ed. 91–98. Current Clinical Strategies Publishing.

2. Amedra Pharmaceuticals, LLC. 2014. "DEXEDRINE- dextroamphetamine sulfate tablet." US National Library of Medicine: Daily Med. Accessed November 18, 2014. http://dailymed.nlm.nih.gov/dailymed/drugInfo.cfm?setid=9ee6fd99-88ea-4cea-8370-a8945581325f.

3. Amedra Pharmaceuticals, LLC. 2013. "DEXEDRINE SPANSULE- dextroamphetamine sulfate capsule, extended release." US National Library of Medicine: Daily Med. Accessed November 18, 2014. http://dailymed.nlm.nih.gov/dailymed/drugInfo.cfm?setid=a37b6ef9-78b4-4b18-8797-ecb583502500.

4. American Psychiatric Association (APA). 2013a. *Diagnostic and Statistical Manual of Mental Disorders*. 5th ed. (DSM-5®). Washington, DC: American Psychiatric Publishing.

5. American Psychiatric Association (APA). 2013b. "Highlights of Changes from DSM-IV-TR to DSM-5." Accessed. January 13, 2015. http://www.dsm5.org/Documents/changes%20from%20dsm-iv-tr%20to%20dsm-5.pdf.

6. Arnsten, A.F.T. 2006. "Stimulants: therapeutic actions in ADHD." *Neuropsychopharmacology* 31:2376–2383.

7. Barr Laboratories, Inc. 2013. "ADDERALL- dextroamphetamine saccharate, amphetamine aspartate monohydrate, dextroamphetamine sulfate and amphetamine sulfate tablet." US National Library of Medicine: Daily Med. Accessed November 18, 2014. http://dailymed.nlm.nih.gov/dailymed/drugInfo.cfm?setid=24af5ced-ed01-4188-95f0-b6b8e4f70aab.

8. Biederman, J., and S.V. Faraone. 2005. "Attention-deficit hyperactivity disorder." *Lancet* 366:237–248.

9. Boehringer Ingelheim Pharmaceuticals, Inc. 2012. "CATAPRES- clonidine hydrochloride tablet." US National Library of Medicine: Daily Med. Accessed November 24, 2014. http://dailymed.nlm.nih.gov/dailymed/drugInfo.cfm?setid=d7f569dc-6bed-42dc-9bec-940a9e6b090d.

10. Carlson, C. L., L. Tamm, and M. Gaub. 1997. "Gender differences in children with ADHD, ODD, and co-occurring ADHD/ODD identified in a school population." *J Am Acad Child Adolesc Psychiatry* 36(12):1706–1714. doi: 10.1097/00004583-199712000-00019.

11. Centers for Disease Control (CDC). 2014. "Attention-Deficit / Hyperactivity Disorder (ADHD), Data & Statistics." Accessed March 16, 2015. http://www.cdc.gov/ncbddd/adhd/data.html#1.

12. Center Watch. 2015. "FDA Approved Drugs by Therapeutic Area." Accessed February 3, 2015. http://www.centerwatch.com/drug-information/fda-approved-drugs/therapeutic-area/17/psychiatry-psychology.

13. Chavez, B., M.A. Sopko Jr., M.J. Ehret, R.E. Paulino, K.R. Goldberg, K. Angstadt, and G.T. Bogart. 2009. "An update on central nervous system stimulant formulations in children and adolescents with attention-deficit/hyperactivity disorder." *Ann Pharmacother* 43:1084–1095.

14. Concordia Pharmaceuticals, Inc. 2014. "KAPVAY- clonidine hydrochloride tablet, extended release." US National Library of Medicine: Daily Med. Accessed January 8, 2015. http://dailymed. nlm.nih.gov/dailymed/drugInfo.cfm?setid=aa7700e2-ae5d-44c4-a609-76de19c705a7.

15. Eli Lilly and Company. 2015. "STRATTERA- atomoxetine hydrochloride capsule." US National Library of Medicine: Daily Med. Accessed January 8, 2015. http://dailymed.nlm.nih.gov/dailymed/ drugInfo.cfm?setid=309de576-c318-404a-bc15-660c2b1876fb.

16. Elsevier Gold Standard, Inc. 2015. "Clinical Pharmacology." Accessed March 12, 2015. https:// www.clinicalpharmacology.com.

17. Epocrates. 2015. Accessed March 25, 2015. https://online.epocrates.com.

18. Gabbard, Glen O., ed. 2007. *Gabbard's Treatments of Psychiatric Disorders*. 4th ed. 47–72, 263–270. Washington, DC: American Psychiatric Publishing.

19. Golden State Medical Supply. 2013. "METHYLIN- methylphenidate hydrochloride tablet." US National Library of Medicine: Daily Med. Accessed November 20, 2014. http://dailymed.nlm.nih. gov/dailymed/drugInfo.cfm?setid=dc11e45a-016f-44cc-b1b7-b736b8534eb6.

20. Hales, Robert. E., S. Yudofsky, and L. Roberts, eds. 2014. *The American Psychiatric Publishing Textbook of Psychiatry*. 6th ed. 929, 1004. Washington, DC: American Psychiatric Publishing.

21. Janssen Pharmaceuticals, Inc. 2014. "CONCERTA- methylphenidate hydrochloride tablet, extended release." US National Library of Medicine: Daily Med. Accessed November 20, 2014. http:// dailymed.nlm.nih.gov/dailymed/drugInfo.cfm?setid=1a88218c-5b18-4220-8f56-526de1a276cd.

22. Kessler, R.C., L. Adler, R. Barkley, J. Biederman, C.K. Conners, O. Demler, S.V. Faraone, L.L. Greenhill, M.J. Howes, K. Secnik, T. Spencer, T.B. Ustun, E.E. Walters, and A.M. Zaslavsky. 2006. "The prevalence and correlates of adult ADHD in the United States: results from the National Comorbidity Survey Replication." *Am J Psychiatry* 163(4):716–723. doi: 10.1176/ ajp.2006.163.4.716.

23. Kolar, Susan, Amanda Keller, Maria Golfinopoulos, Lucy Cumyn, Cassidy Syer, and Lily Hechtman. 2008. "Treatment of adults with attention-deficit/hyperactivity disorder." *Neuropsychiatric Disease and Treatment* 4(2):389–403.

24. Medscape: Drugs & Diseases. 2015. "Psychiatrics." Accessed February 3, 2015. http://reference.med-scape.com/drugs/psychiatrics.

25. Medscape. 2015. "Psychiatry and Mental Health." Accessed March 12, 2015. http://www.medscape. com/psychiatry.

26. Mosby Drug Database Browser. 2014. "Ritalin." *PSNI*. Accessed January 14, 2015. http://psni.cc/ SNAPDrugInfo/DrugInfo.aspx?ID=391&Name=Ritalin.

27. National Institute of Mental Health (NIMH). 2014. "Attention Deficit Hyperactivity Disorder (ADHD)." Accessed February 6, 2012. http://www.nimh.nih.gov/health/topics/attention-deficit-hyperactivity-disorder-adhd/index.shtml.

28. NextWave Pharmaceuticals, Inc. 2014. "QUILLIVANT XR- methylphenidate hydrochloride powder, for suspension." US National Library of Medicine: Daily Med. Accessed November

20, 2014. http://dailymed.nlm.nih.gov/dailymed/drugInfo.cfm?setid=e0157005-6e3e-4763-b910-9eb0937608c9.

29. Novartis Pharmaceuticals Corporation. 2013. "FOCALIN- dexmethylphenidate hydrochloride tablet." US National Library of Medicine: Daily Med. Accessed November 20, 2014. http://dailymed.nlm.nih.gov/dailymed/drugInfo.cfm?setid=7c552f11-e24a-4d9b-bb8d-be10c928eca8.

30. Novartis Pharmaceuticals Corporation. 2013. "FOCALIN XR- dexmethylphenidate hydrochloride capsule, extended release." US National Library of Medicine: Daily Med. Accessed November 20, 2014. http://dailymed.nlm.nih.gov/dailymed/drugInfo.cfm?setid=1a1da905-42a0-4748-9c39-67eca45deccc.

31. Novartis Pharmaceuticals Corporation. 2013. "RITALIN LA- methylphenidate hydrochloride capsule, extended release." US National Library of Medicine: Daily Med. Accessed November 20, 2014. http://dailymed.nlm.nih.gov/dailymed/drugInfo.cfm?setid=effd952d-ac94-47bb-b107-589a4934dcca.

32. Novartis Pharmaceuticals Corporation. 2013. "RITALIN- methylphenidate hydrochloride tablet." US National Library of Medicine: Daily Med. Accessed November 20, 2014. http://dailymed.nlm.nih.gov/dailymed/drugInfo.cfm?setid=c0bf0835-6a2f-4067-a158-8b86c4b0668a.

33. Noven Therapeutics, LLC. 2014. "DAYTRANA - methylphenidate patch." US National Library of Medicine: Daily Med. Accessed November 20, 2014. http://dailymed.nlm.nih.gov/dailymed/drugInfo.cfm?setid=2c312c31-3198-4775-91ab-294e0b4b9e7f.

34. Preston, John D., and James Johnson. 2011. *Clinical Psychopharmacology Made Ridiculously Simple*. 7th ed. 1–79. Miami: MedMaster Inc.

35. Promius Pharma, LLC. 2013. "TENEX - guanfacine hydrochloride tablet." US National Library of Medicine: Daily Med. Accessed November 24, 2014. http://dailymed.nlm.nih.gov/dailymed/drugInfo.cfm?setid=886e050c-dd22-4f35-ac3b-243f091125c3.

36. RxList. 2015. "Drugs A-Z List." Accessed March 25, 2015. http://www.rxlist.com/drugs/alpha_a.htm.

37. Schatzberg, A.F., and C.B. Nemeroff, eds. 2009. *The American Psychiatric Publishing Textbook of Psychopharmacology*. 4th ed. 843–860. Washington, DC: American Psychiatric Publishing.

38. Schatzberg, A.F., Jonathan O. Cole, and Charles DeBattista. 2010. *Manual of Clinical Psychopharmacology*. 7th ed. 467–488. Washington, DC: American Psychiatric Publishing.

39. Shire, PLC. 2013. "ADDERALL XR- dextroamphetamine sulfate, dextroamphetamine saccharate, amphetamine aspartate monohydrate and amphetamine sulfate capsule, extended release." US National Library of Medicine: Daily Med. Accessed November 18, 2014. http://dailymed.nlm.nih.gov/dailymed/drugInfo.cfm?setid=aff45863-ffe1-4d4f-8acf-c7081512a6c0.

40. Shire PLC. 2014. "INTUNIV- guanfacine hydrochloride tablet, extended release." US National Library of Medicine: Daily Med. Accessed January 8, 2015. http://dailymed.nlm.nih.gov/dailymed/drugInfo.cfm?setid=b972af81-3a37-40be-9fe1-3ddf59852528.

41. Shire, PLC. 2014. "VYVANSE- lisdexamfetamine dimesylate capsule." US National Library of Medicine: Daily Med. Accessed January 6, 2015. http://dailymed.nlm.nih.gov/dailymed/drugInfo.cfm?setid=704e4378-ca83-445c-8b45-3cfa51c1ecad.

42. Soreff, S. 2015. "Attention Deficit Hyperactivity Disorder" Accessed January 13, 2015. emedicine.mescape.com/article/289350-overview.

43. Stahl, S.M. 2008. *Essential Psychopharmacology: Neuroscientific Basis and Practical Applications.* 3rd ed. 471–502. New York: Cambridge Press.

44. Stahl, S.M. 2011. *Essential Psychopharmacology: the Prescriber's Guide.* 4th ed. 41–46, 35–40, 65–69, 123–127, 359–363, 365–371. Cambridge: Cambridge University Press.

45. Truven Health Analytics. 2015. *Micromedex 2.0.* Accessed March 20, 2015. http://www.micromedexsolutions.com/home/dispatch.

46. Unither Manufacturing, LLC. 2013. "METADATE CD- methylphenidate hydrochloride capsule, extended release." US National Library of Medicine: Daily Med. Accessed November 20, 2014. http://dailymed.nlm.nih.gov/dailymed/drugInfo.cfm?setid=a6aedc40-5725-4bd3-9037-033746e8599e.

47. Unither Manufacturing, LLC. 2014. "METADATE ER- methylphenidate hydrochloride tablet, extended release." US National Library of Medicine: Daily Med. Accessed November 20, 2014. http://dailymed.nlm.nih.gov/dailymed/drugInfo.cfm?setid=739bbd64-d9e1-4771-967b-a2cd08f4eaf5.

48. UpToDate. 2015. Accessed March 12, 2015. http://www.uptodate.com/home.

49. US Food & Drug Administration (FDA). 2005. "Amphetamines have a high potential for abuse." Accessed January 14, 2015. http://www.fda.gov/ohrms/dockets/ac/06/briefing/2006-4210b_05_06_MixedSaltFDAlabel.pdf.

50. US National Library of Medicine. 2015. "Drugs and Lactation Database (LactMed)." Accessed February 3, 2015. http://toxnet.nlm.nih.gov/newtoxnet/lactmed.htm.

51. US National Library of Medicine. 2015. "Toxicology Data Network." Accessed March 17, 2015. http://toxnet.nlm.nih.gov.

52. Waxmonsky, J. G. 2005. "Nonstimulant therapies for attention-deficit hyperactivity disorder (ADHD) in children and adults." *Essent Psychopharmacol* 6(5):262–276.

53. Wegmann, J. 2008. *Psychopharmacology: Straight Talk on Mental Health Medications.* 125–134. Eau Claire: Pesi, LLC.

Chapter 8
Psychotic Disorders And Antipsychotics

Psychosis refers to a gross impairment of thinking and perception causing a loss of touch with reality. Psychotic disorders include all mental disorders with psychosis as the predominant symptom. Specific symptoms of psychosis include paranoia, delusion, disorganization, hallucination, and thought disorder.[5] The diagnosis is mostly clinical and requires thorough evaluation of a patient's current and past symptoms, longitudinal course, and family history.[20]

Symptoms of Psychosis[18,23,44,56]
Positive symptoms: Auditory hallucinations, delusions, disorganized speech/behavior
Negative symptoms: Decreased emotional range, poverty of speech, social isolation, and loss of interest, inertia, and drive
Cognitive symptoms: Impaired memory/attention, decline in interpersonal skills
Mood symptoms: Depression, hypomania, mania

DSM-5 Diagnostic Types[5]
- Delusional disorder
- Brief psychotic disorder
- Schizophreniform disorder
- Schizophrenia
- Schizoaffective disorder
- Substance/medication-induced psychotic disorder
- Psychotic disorder due to another medical condition
- Schizophrenia spectrum and other psychotic disorders

Management
Management of psychotic disorders requires a combination of pharmacotherapy and psychosocial interventions. A variety of psychosocial treatments can enable a patient to acquire better social and vocational skills and to manage residual psychotic symptoms.[43,44] These psychosocial interventions include[14,15,23,43,44]:

- Individual/group therapy
- Psycho-education
- Cognitive behavioral therapy (CBT)
- Social skills training
- Family intervention
- Cognitive remediation
- Arts therapy
- Adherence therapy

Long-term management of psychotic disorders requires the integration of medical, psychological, and psychosocial therapies by a multidisciplinary team.[23,43] With proper treatment, psychosocial intervention, and family support, many people with psychotic disorders can live independent and productive lives.

Prevention: Early detection and treatment of the first episode of psychosis may improve the long-term prognosis of psychotic disorders.[35,43] Early stage psychosocial interventions such as CBT and medication may prevent full-blown psychosis.[43]

Important notes[3,14,16,19,20,38,44,47,48,56]:

- Schizophrenia is a chronic and relapsing disorder; for long-term stabilization, medication should be continued even if symptoms are not apparent.[43,44]
- Full recovery from schizophrenia is rare; symptoms usually follow a waxing/waning course.[23]
- Patients with schizophrenia have a 5–10% lifetime risk of suicide.[43]
- Poor prognosis is associated with early onset of disease and family history of schizophrenia.[23]
- Inform patients of the side effects of antipsychotic medications to decrease likelihood of noncompliance.[38]
- Stimulant drugs (e.g., amphetamines, levodopa) should be avoided, as they can precipitate psychosis.
- Antipsychotics often produce emotional blunting, apathy, or Parkinsonian symptoms, which may be misdiagnosed as negative symptoms.[38,44]
- Antipsychotics can reduce the positive symptoms of psychosis in 7–14 days, but they do not affect negative symptoms or cognitive dysfunction.
- Typical antipsychotics are associated with a higher risk of extrapyramidal symptoms (EPS) than second generation antipsychotic (SGA) drugs; however, SGA's have higher risk of metabolic syndrome.[38,44,56]
- For noncompliance, long-acting depot preparations of antipsychotics may reduce the risk of relapse.

Black Box Warning Regarding Antipsychotic Use in the Elderly

This warning applies to all antipsychotics and includes the following statement:

Elderly patients with dementia-related psychosis treated with atypical antipsychotic drugs are at an increased risk of death compared with placebo. Although the causes of death in clinical trials were varied, most of the deaths appeared to be either cardiovascular (e.g., heart failure, sudden death) or infectious (e.g., pneumonia) in nature. Observational studies suggest that antipsychotic drugs may increase mortality. It is unclear from the observational studies to what extent these mortality findings may be attributed to the antipsychotic drug as opposed to patient characteristics.[5]

Medications

Atypical Antipsychotics (Second Generation)
Class Profile[14,15,23,38,43,44,46,56]
Overview: Atypical antipsychotics act on different receptors in the brain's dopamine pathways and are less likely to cause EPS than typical antipsychotics. Although they appear safer than typicals, atypical antipsychotics can involve severe side effects (e.g., diabetes mellitus, metabolic syndrome, weight gain, increased stroke risk, blood clots, and sudden cardiac death).[31] Atypical antipsychotics include[23,47]:

- Aripiprazole
- Asenapine
- Clozapine
- Iloperidone
- Lurasidone
- Olanzapine
- Paliperidone
- Quetiapine
- Risperidone
- Ziprasidone

Warnings:
- **Black box warning:** Increased risk of death in elderly patients with dementia-related psychosis
- May alter blood glucose levels and cause weight gain and other metabolic changes
- Can cause TD, NMS, and EPS and increase risk of cognitive/motor impairment
- Can cause orthostatic hypotension, syncope, QT prolongation, and lower the seizure threshold; use caution in patients with cerebrovascular/cardiovascular disorders
- May cause esophageal dysmotility and lead to aspiration pneumonia
- Associated with blood dyscrasias (leukopenia, neutropenia, agranulocytosis), hyperprolactinemia, and impaired body temperature regulation
- May increase risk of suicide

Drug interactions:
- Can potentiate the effects of certain antihypertensive drugs
- Use caution with other CNS-active drugs or alcohol
- SSRIs can increase drug levels; use with TCAs can increase both drug levels
- CYP450 inducers decrease plasma levels; CYP450 inhibitors increase plasma levels
- Decreased drug levels with carbamazepine and nicotine
- Can decrease efficacy of dopamine agonists
- Absorption decreased by antacids
- Increased sedation and hypotension with meperidine
- Use with beta-blockers can increase both drug levels increasing risk of hypotension

Class side effects: Abdominal pain, akathisia, anxiety, asthenia, blurred vision, constipation, dizziness, drowsiness, dyskinesia, EPS, fatigue, headache, hypersalivation, hypotension, increased appetite, indigestion, insomnia, myalgia, nasal congestion, orthostatic hypotension, Parkinsonism, rash, restlessness, sedation, sexual dysfunction, somnolence, tachycardia, tremor, urinary incontinence, vertigo, vomiting, weight gain.

Metabolic syndrome (MS): MS refers to the cluster of risk factors leading to cardiac and metabolic diseases. Patients should be fully assessed, informed about, and monitored for metabolic syndrome during treatment.[40] MS diagnosis includes three or more of the following[44]:

- Personal/family history of obesity, diabetes, heart disease, high cholesterol, or high BP
- Large weight and height ratio (BMI>25)
- Large waist circumference (>40 inches in males; >35 inches in females)
- Increased BP (>130/85)
- Fasting blood glucose levels (>110)
- Fasting cholesterol levels (HDL <40; total >200)
- Fasting triglyceride levels (>175)

Guidelines for monitoring metabolic syndrome [4,8,44]

The following tests should be performed at the designated time frame to monitor for risk factors and signs of metabolic syndrome during treatment with atypical antipsychotics:

- *Baseline:* Personal/family history, weight (BMI), waist circumference, BP, fasting plasma glucose, fasting lipid profile
- *4 weeks:* Weight (BMI)
- *8 weeks:* Weight (BMI)
- *12 weeks:* Weight (BMI), BP, fasting plasma glucose, fasting lipid profile
- *Quarterly:* Weight (BMI)
- *Annually:* Personal/family history, waist circumference, BP, fasting plasma glucose
- *Every 5 years*: Fasting lipid profile

Individual Drug Profiles

Aripiprazole[2,9,11,12,14,22,23,34,39,43,44,47,50,51,54]

Brand name: Abilify, Abilify Discmelt, Abilify Maintena

FDA approved for: Schizophrenia (acute and maintenance), acute treatment and maintenance of mania or mixed episodes of bipolar I disorder (as monotherapy or as adjunct to lithium/valproate), acute treatment of agitation associated with schizophrenia or bipolar I disorder (IM), MDD (adjunct), autism-related irritability

Other potential uses (off-label): Bipolar depression, BPD, drug-induced hyperprolactinemia, schizoaffective disorder

Medication forms: *Tab* (2, 5, 10, 15, 20, 30 mg); *ODT* (10, 15 mg); *oral sol* (1 mg/ml); *injectable* (9.75 mg/1.3 ml [7.5mg/ml]); *ER injectable* (300, 400 mg/vial)

Dosage:

- Schizophrenia:
    - *Oral:* 10–15 mg po qd initially, can be increased based on tolerance/response to max 30 mg/day

- *ER injection:*
  - Establish tolerability with oral aripiprazole
  - Initial and maintenance dose: 400 mg IM once monthly, give 10–20 mg oral aripiprazole or another antipsychotic after first injection and continue for 14 consecutive days
- Bipolar disorder/schizophrenia agitation:
  - 9.75 mg IM initially (range 5.25–15 mg), second dose may be required, max 30 mg/day
  - For ongoing therapy, replace injection with oral aripiprazole 10–30 mg/day as soon as possible
- Bipolar I disorder:
  - *Adjunctive to lithium/valproate:* 10–15 mg po qd initially, can be increased based on tolerance/response to max 30 mg/day (target 15 mg qd)
  - *Monotherapy, manic or mixed episodes:* 15 mg po qd initially, can be increased based on tolerance/response to max 30 mg/day
- MDD (adjunctive to antidepressants): 2–5 mg po qd initially, can be increased based on tolerance/response to max 15 mg/day
- Autism (ages 6–17 yrs): 2 mg/day po initially, can be increased based on tolerance/response to max 15 mg/day

MOA: Partial agonist at D_2 and 5-HT_{1A} receptors, antagonist at 5-HT_{2A} receptors

Pharmacokinetics: t_{max}=3–5 hrs, $t_{1/2}$=75 hrs

Warnings:
- Similar to *Atypical Class Profile*
- **Black box warnings:**
  - Increased risk of death in elderly patients with dementia-related psychosis
  - Increased risk of suicidal thoughts and behavior with antidepressant use in children, adolescents, and young adults under the age of 24 years; closely monitor patients of all ages for emerging suicidal thoughts and behaviors

Drug interactions:
- Similar to *Atypical Class Profile*
- Plasma levels increased when used with strong CYP3A4 (e.g., ketoconazole) and CYP2D6 inhibitors
- Plasma levels decreased with CYP3A4 inducers (e.g., carbamazepine)

Common side effects: Agitation, akathisia, anxiety, blurred vision, constipation, dizziness, EPS, fatigue, headache, indigestion, insomnia, lightheadedness, nausea, restlessness, sedation, tremor, vomiting

Contraindications: Hypersensitivity

Recommended lab tests: Metabolic screening/monitoring (BMI, lipid panel, blood glucose, LFT)

Overdose: Hypotension, NMS, coma; OD rare

Tapering/withdrawal: Slow taper recommended
Special populations:
Pregnancy: Risk Category C
Lactation: Avoid
Elderly: Lower dose recommended
Hepatic impairment: No dose adjustment necessary
Renal impairment: No dose adjustment necessary
Important notes[44]:
- Less weight gain and sedation than other antipsychotics
- Does not increase prolactin levels or prolong QT interval; in fact, it may decrease prolactin levels
- Can be used as adjunct to SSRIs/SNRIs for depression
- Sedation and EPS are more problematic in children

Asenapine[2,9,11,12,13,14,15,22,23,39,43,44,47,50,51,54]
Brand name: Saphris
FDA approved for: Schizophrenia (acute and maintenance), acute mania or mixed episodes associated with bipolar I disorder (as monotherapy or in combination with lithium/valproate)
Other potential uses (off-label): Agitation, bipolar depression
Medication forms: *Tab* (5, 10 mg for SL administration)
Dosage:
- Schizophrenia: 5 mg bid initially, can be increased based on tolerance/response to max 10 mg bid
- Bipolar disorder (manic or mixed):
  - *Monotherapy:* 5 mg bid initially, can be increased based on tolerance/response to max 10 mg bid
  - *Combination therapy with lithium/valproate:* 5 mg bid initially, can be increased based on tolerance/response to max 10 mg bid
MOA: Combination of antagonist activity at D_2 and $5-HT_{2A}$ receptors
Pharmacokinetics: t_{max}=0.5–1.5 hrs, $t_{1/2}$=24 hrs
Warnings:
- Similar to *Atypical Class Profile*
- **Black box warning:** Increased risk of death in elderly patients with dementia-related psychosis
- May cause type I HSR including angioedema and anaphylactic reactions, even after first dose
- May prolong QTc interval; avoid in patients with electrolyte derangement (e.g., hypokalemia, hypomagnesemia)

Drug interactions:
- Similar to *Atypical Class Profile*
- Raises levels of paroxetine by 50% when used in combination
- Do not use with other drugs which can cause QT prolongation

Common side effects: Akathisia, dizziness, EPS, headache, insomnia, oral hypoesthesia, restlessness, somnolence, weight gain

Contraindications: Hypersensitivity, severe hepatic impairment

Recommended lab tests: Metabolic monitoring/screening (BMI, lipid panel, blood glucose, LFT)

Overdose: Agitation, confusion, hyperglycemia

Tapering/withdrawal: Slow taper recommended

Special populations:

Pregnancy: Risk Category C

Lactation: Avoid

Elderly: No dose adjustment necessary

Hepatic impairment: No dose adjustment necessary in mild to moderate, avoid in severe

Renal impairment: No dose adjustment necessary

Important notes:
- Patients complain of oral hypoesthesia and taste problems
- Some patients cannot tolerate morning dose due to sedation

Clozapine[2,9,11,12,14,22,23,32,39,43,44,47,50,51,54]

Brand name: Clozaril, FazaClo ODT, Versacloz

FDA approved for: Treatment-resistant schizophrenia, recurrent suicidal behavior in schizophrenia/schizoaffective disorder

Other potential uses (off-label): Agitation, suicide prevention, treatment-resistant bipolar disorder, tremors

Medication forms: *Tab* (25, 50, 100, 200 mg); *oral suspension* (50mg/ml); *ODT* (12.5, 25, 100, 150 mg)

Dosage:
- Schizophrenia: 12.5 mg qd–bid initially, can be increased based on tolerance/response to target 300–450 mg/day divided, may require 600–900 mg/day for acceptable response

MOA: Antagonizes D_2 and $5\text{-}HT_{2A}$ receptors; also interferes with dopamine binding moderately at D_4 and weakly at D_1, D_3, and D_5 receptors

Pharmacokinetics: t_{max}=2.2–2.5 hrs, $t_{1/2}$=12 hrs

Warnings:
- Similar to *Atypical Class Profile*
- **Black box warnings:**

- Increased risk of death in elderly patients with dementia-related psychosis
- Agranulocytosis: drug available only by enrollment in restricted programs in the National Registry
- Orthostatic hypotension, bradycardia, syncope, cardiac arrest: use caution with cardiovascular/cerebrovascular disease or with conditions predisposing to hypotension
- Seizures: use caution with history of seizures or other predisposing risk factors for seizures
- Myocarditis, cardiomyopathy: potentially fatal; if suspected, discontinue and obtain cardiac evaluation
- May cause eosinophilia, pulmonary embolism, fever, and anticholinergic toxicity

Drug interactions:
- Similar to *Atypical Class Profile*
- Use caution with carbamazepine due to high risk of hematological adverse events
- Contraindicated with QT-prolonging agents (ziprasidone, aripiprazole, risperidone, olanzapine, mesoridazine, pimozide, or thioridazine) due to risk of QT syndrome
- Avoid with agents that cause bone marrow suppression
- Use with CYP1A2, CYP2D6, and CYP3A4 inhibitors raises clozapine plasma levels; inducers of CYP1A2 and CYP3A4 decrease levels

Common side effects: Constipation, dizziness, dry mouth, hypersalivation, hypotension, sedation, sweating, tachycardia, vertigo, visual disturbances, weight gain

Contraindications:
- Hypersensitivity
- History of clozapine-induced agranulocytosis or severe granulocytopenia
- Concurrent use with QT-prolonging agents, carbamazepine, and epinephrine

Recommended lab tests: Metabolic screening/monitoring (BMI, lipid panel, blood glucose, LFT), EKG, CBC (before treatment, weekly for 6 months, biweekly for months 6–12, every 4 weeks thereafter)
- Suspend treatment immediately if ANC <1,000/mm^3 and WBC <2,000/mm^3; treatment may resume once ANC >2,000/mm^3 and WBC >3,500/mm^3; discontinue if ANC <500/mm^3

Overdose: Delirium, seizures, coma, hyperthermia, severe hypotension

Tapering/withdrawal: Slow taper recommended

Special populations:

Pregnancy: Risk Category B

Lactation: Avoid

Elderly: Cautious dose selection recommended

Hepatic impairment: No dose adjustment necessary in mild to moderate, use caution in severe

Renal impairment: No dose adjustment necessary in mild to moderate, lower dose recommended in severe

Important notes:

- Only antipsychotic medication which does not cause any EPS or TD
- One of only two medications indicated to reduce suicidal behavior and impulsivity
- Greater weight gain and risk of seizures compared to other antipsychotics
- Often only used for psychosis after three failed attempts with other antipsychotics

Iloperidone[2,9,11,12,14,22,23,33,39,43,44,47,50,51,54]

Brand name: Fanapt, Fanapt titration pack

FDA approved for: Schizophrenia

Other potential uses (off-label): Agitation

Medication forms: *Tab* (1, 2, 4, 6, 8, 10, 12 mg)

Dosage:

- Schizophrenia: 1 mg bid on day 1, 2 mg bid on day 2, can be increased based on tolerance/response to effective dose of 6–12 mg bid (max 24 mg/day)

MOA: Antagonist at D_2 receptors and 5-HT_2 receptors

Pharmacokinetics: t_{max}=2–4 hrs, $t_{1/2}$=18–33 hrs

Warnings:

- Similar to *Atypical Class Profile*
- Avoid use in patients with abnormal LFTs
- May cause priapism

Drug interactions:

- Similar to *Atypical Class Profile*
- **Black box warning:** Increased risk of death in elderly patients with dementia-related psychosis
- Avoid use with drugs that prolong QTc (e.g., ziprasidone, chlorpromazine, thioridazine, quinidine, procainamide, amiodarone, sotalol, moxifloxacin)
- Reduce dose in patients co-administered a strong CYP2D6 or CYP3A4 inhibitors

Common side effects: Akathisia, dizziness, dry mouth, fatigue, nasal congestion, nausea, orthostatic hypotension, somnolence, tachycardia, tremor, urinary incontinence, URTI, weight gain, weight loss

Contraindications: Hypersensitivity, concurrent use with drugs that prolong the QT interval

Recommended lab tests: Metabolic screening/monitoring (BMI, lipid panel, blood glucose, LFT), AIMS

Overdose: Drowsiness, severe EPS, torsades de pointes; OD rare

Tapering/withdrawal: Slow taper recommended
Special populations:
Pregnancy: Risk Category C
Lactation: Avoid
Elderly: Lower dose recommended
Hepatic impairment: No dose adjustment necessary in mild, use caution in moderate, avoid in severe
Renal impairment: No dose adjustment necessary
Important notes:
- Due to possible arrhythmias and sudden death associated with QTc prolongation, consider other treatment options before prescribing
- Slow dose titration required due to risk of hypotension

Lurasidone[2,7,9,11,12,14,22,23,39,43,44,47,50,51,54]
Brand name: Latuda
FDA approved for: Schizophrenia, depressive episodes associated with bipolar I disorder
Other potential uses (off-label): Agitation, bipolar disorder, depression
Medication forms: *Tab* (20, 40, 60, 80, 120 mg)
Dosage:
- Schizophrenia: 40 mg/day initially with food, can be increased based on tolerance/response to max 160 mg/day
- Bipolar depression: 20 mg/day initially with food, can be increased based on tolerance/response to max 120 mg/day
MOA: Antagonist at D_2 and 5-HT_{2A} receptors, moderate antagonistic activity at α_{2C}- and α_{2A}-adrenergic receptors, partial agonist at 5-HT_{1A} receptors
Pharmacokinetics: t_{max}=1–3 hrs, $t_{1/2}$=18 hrs
Warnings:
- Similar to *Atypical Class Profile*
- **Black box warning:**
  - Increased risk of death in elderly patients with dementia-related psychosis
  - Increased risk of suicidal thoughts and behavior with antidepressant use in children, adolescents, and young adults under the age of 24 years; closely monitor patients of all ages for emerging suicidal thoughts and behaviors
Drug interactions:
- Similar to *Atypical Class Profile*
- Inhibitors of CYP3A4 increase plasma levels while inducers of CYP3A4 decrease levels
Common side effects: Akathisia, agitation, nausea, Parkinsonism, somnolence

Contraindications:

- Hypersensitivity
- History of hematological disease
- Concurrent use with strong CYP3A4 inhibitors (e.g., ketoconazole) or with strong CYP3A4 inducers (e.g., carbamazepine, rifampin)

Lab test recommended: Metabolic screening/monitoring (BMI, lipid panel, blood glucose, LFT), AIMS

Overdose: Rare, even at high doses

Tapering/withdrawal: Slow taper recommended

Special populations:

Pregnancy: Risk Category B

Lactation: Avoid

Elderly: Use caution

Hepatic impairment: No dose adjustment necessary in mild to moderate, max 40 mg/day in severe

Renal impairment: No dose adjustment necessary in mild to moderate, max 40 mg/day in severe

Important notes[44]:

- Good metabolic profile (lower weight gain) compared to other atypicals
- Only atypical not associated with QTc prolongation
- Only atypical with Category B warning for pregnancy
- Use with food increases the absorption rate by 2–3x

Olanzapine[2,9,10,11,12,14,22,23,39,43,44,47,50,51,53,54]

Brand name: Zyprexa, Zyprexa Relprevv, Zyprexa Zydis

FDA approved for: Schizophrenia, acute agitation associated with schizophrenia and bipolar I mania (IM), acute treatment and maintenance of mania or mixed episodes of bipolar I disorder (as monotherapy or as adjunct to lithium/valproate) bipolar depression (in combination with fluoxetine), treatment-resistant depression (in combination with fluoxetine)

Other potential uses (off-label): Anorexia, anxiety disorders, cluster headaches, delirium, dementia, MDD with psychosis, OCD, PTSD

Medication forms: *Tab* (2.5, 5, 7.5, 10, 15, 20 mg); *ODT* (5, 10, 15, 20 mg); *IM sol powder* (10 mg/vial); *ER injectable* (210, 300, 405 mg/vial)

Dosage:

- Schizophrenia: 5–10 mg/day initially, can be increased based on tolerance/response to max 20 mg/day
- Schizophrenia/bipolar-related agitation: 10 mg IM (short-acting), consider 5–7.5 mg for geriatric, max 30 mg/day

- Bipolar mania:
  - *Monotherapy:* 10–15 mg/day po initially, can be increased based on tolerance/response to max 20 mg/day
  - *Adjunct to lithium/valproate:* 10 mg/day po initially, can be increased based on tolerance/response to max 20 mg/day
- Treatment-resistant depression, depression associated with bipolar I disorder (*see package insert for Symbax when used in combination with fluoxetine*): 25 mg fluoxetine/6 mg olanzapine po each evening, can be increased based on tolerance/response to max 75 mg/18 mg per day

MOA: Blocks D_1, D_2, D_3, D_4, 5-HT_{2A}, 5-HT_{2C}, H_1, and α_1 adrenergic receptors

Pharmacokinetics: t_{max}=6 hrs, $t_{1/2}$=21–54 hrs

Warnings:

- Similar to *Atypical Class Profile*
- **Black box warning:**
  - Increased risk of death in elderly patients with dementia-related psychosis
  - Intramuscular Post-Injection Delirium/Sedation Syndrome: patients are required to receive the Zyprexa Relprevv injection at an REMS-certified health care facility, to be monitored at the facility for at least 3 hours post-injection, and to be accompanied home from the facility

Drug interactions:

- Similar to *Atypical Class Profile*
- Avoid use with drugs that prolong QTc interval (e.g., mesoridazine, pimozide, thioridazine, or ziprasidone)
- Inducers of CYP1A2 can increase clearance (decrease plasma levels); inhibitors of CYP1A2 can decrease clearance (increase plasma levels)
- Use with diazepam or alcohol may potentiate orthostatic hypotension
- Use with ritonavir may reduce olanzapine serum concentrations by approximately 50%
- IM use with lorazepam (IM) can increase somnolence

Common side effects: Akathisia, amnesia, asthenia, back pain, constipation, dizziness, dry mouth, hypertriglyceridemia, increased appetite, increased salivation, indigestion, insomnia, orthostatic hypotension, paresthesia, peripheral edema, personality disorder, somnolence, speech disorder, tremor, weakness, weight gain

Contraindications: None listed by manufacturer

Recommended lab tests: Metabolic screening/monitoring (BMI, lipid panel, blood glucose, LFT), AIMS, neurologic function, serum cholesterol profile

Overdose: Seizures, delirium, coma, respiratory depression; OD rare

Tapering/withdrawal: Slow tapering/cross tapering recommended

Special populations:

Pregnancy: Risk Category C

Lactation: Use caution

Elderly: Lower dose recommended initially (5 mg)

Hepatic impairment: No dose adjustment necessary in mild to moderate, lower dose recommended in severe

Renal impairment: No dose adjustment necessary

Important notes:

- Performed better than most others in Clinical Antipsychotic Trials of Intervention Effectiveness (CATIE)
- Strong mood stabilizing and antipsychotic properties
- Smokers who are on this medications may need a higher dose
- Avoid use of IM formulation with parenteral benzodiazepines
- Weight gain is the major side effect of this medication

Paliperidone[2,9,11,12,14,17,22,23,39,43,44,47,50,51,54]

Brand name: Invega, Invega Sustenna

FDA approved for: Schizophrenia, schizoaffective disorder

Other potential uses (off-label): Agitation, bipolar disorder

Medication forms: *ER tab* (1.5, 3, 6, 9, 12 mg); *IM suspension* (39, 78, 117, 156, 234 mg)

Dosage:

- Schizophrenia and schizoaffective disorder:
    - *IM:* 234 mg in deltoid on day 1, then 156 mg 1 week later; use 117 mg monthly for maintenance (monthly range 39–234 mg for schizophrenia, 78–234 for schizoaffective disorder)
    - *Oral:* 6 mg qam, can be increased based on tolerance/response to max 12 mg/day

MOA: Antagonist of D_2, 5-HT_{2A}, H_1 and α_1- and α_2-adrenergic receptors

Pharmacokinetics: t_{max}=24 hrs, $t_{1/2}$=23 hrs

Warnings:

- Similar to *Atypical Class Profile*
- **Black box warning:** Increased risk of death in elderly patients with dementia-related psychosis
- Avoid use in patients with GI problems (e.g., small intestine IBD, short bowel syndrome) due to risk of GI obstruction
- May cause priapism and antiemetic effect

Drug interactions:

- Similar to *Atypical Class Profile*
- Can cause paradoxical epinephrine reversal if used with epinephrine
- Can cause QTc prolongation with other QTc agents (e.g., mesoridazine, pimozide, thioridazine, ziprasidone)

- Risk of additive effect with drugs causing orthostatic hypertension
- Use with strong CYP3A4/P-glycoprotein (P-gp) inducers (e.g., carbamazepine) may require dosage increase; on discontinuation of strong inducer, decrease paliperidone dosage
- Co-administration of divalproex sodium increases levels by approximately 50%

Common side effects: Akathisia, blurred vision, constipation, EPS, headache, indigestion, insomnia, nasal inflammation, Parkinsonism, restlessness, sexual dysfunction, somnolence, tachycardia, vomiting, weight gain

Contraindications: Hypersensitivity (including to risperidone products)

Recommended lab tests: Metabolic screening/monitoring (BMI, lipid panel, blood glucose, LFT), AIMS

Overdose: Agitation, tachycardia, and hypertension; OD rare

Tapering/withdrawal: Slow taper recommended

Special populations:

Pregnancy: Risk Category C

Lactation: Avoid

Elderly: Lower dose recommended

Hepatic impairment: No dose adjustment necessary in mild to moderate; use caution in severe

Renal impairment: Max 6 mg/day in mild to moderate; max 3 mg/day in severe

Important notes:

- Greater chance of prolonged QTc interval compared to other antipsychotics
- Due to high cost, IM Sustenna is not the first choice among IM depot medications

Quetiapine[2,6,9,11,12,14,22,23,39,43,44,47,50,51,54]

Brand name: Seroquel, Seroquel XR

FDA approved for: Schizophrenia (acute and maintenance), acute mania or mixed episodes associated with bipolar I disorder (as monotherapy or in combination with lithium/valproate), maintenance of bipolar I disorder (adjunctive to lithium/valproate) bipolar depression, adjunctive for the treatment of MDD

Other potential uses (off-label): Agitation, anxiety, BPD, insomnia, delirium, OCD, Parkinson's disease, PTSD

Medication forms: *Tab* (25, 50, 100, 200, 300, 400 mg); *XR tab* (50, 150, 200, 300, 400 mg)

Dosage:

- Schizophrenia:
  - *IR:* 25 mg bid initially, can be increased based on tolerance/response to max 750 mg/day
  - *XR:* 300 mg/day initially, can be increased based on tolerance/response to max 800 mg (usual range 150–750 mg/day)

- *Maintenance (monotherapy):* 400–800 mg/day
- Bipolar I disorder, mania (as monotherapy or as adjunct to lithium/valproate):
  - *IR:* 50 mg bid initially, can be increased based on tolerance/response to max 800 mg/day (usual range 400–800 mg/day)
  - *XR:* 300 mg qd initially, can be increased based on tolerance/response to max 800 mg/day
  - *Maintenance therapy (IR or ER):* 400–800 mg/day, max 800 mg/day
- Bipolar I disorder, depressive episodes associated with bipolar I or II disorder
  - *IR:* 50 mg qd hs initially, can be increased based on tolerance/response to max 300 mg/day
  - *XR:* 50 mg qd hs initially, can be increased based on tolerance/response to max 300 mg/day
- Adjunctive for the treatment of MDD
  - *XR:* 50 mg qd hs initially, can be increased based on tolerance/response to max 300 mg/day

MOA: Antagonist at 5-HT_{1A}, 5-HT_2, D_1, D_2, H_1, α_1- and α_2-adrenergic receptors

Pharmacokinetics: t_{max}=1.5 hrs (IR)/6 hrs (XR), $t_{1/2}$=6–12 hrs

Warnings:

- Similar to *Atypical Class Profile*
- **Black box warning:**
  - Increased risk of death in elderly patients with dementia-related psychosis
  - Increased risk of suicidal thoughts and behavior in children, adolescents and young adults taking antidepressants; not approved for patients under 10 years of age. Monitor patients closely for clinical worsening and emergence of suicidal thoughts and behaviors.
- Can cause cataracts

Drug interactions:

- Similar to *Atypical Class Profile*
- With strong CYP3A4 inhibitors, reduce quetiapine dose to one sixth
- With strong CYP3A4 inducers, increase quetiapine dose up to 5 fold
- Reduce quetiapine dose by 5 fold within 7–14 days of discontinuation of strong CYP3A4 inducers
- Can reduce oral clearance of lorazepam

Common side effects: Asthenia, constipation, dizziness, dry mouth, fatigue, headache, increased appetite, indigestion, orthostatic hypertension, pharyngitis, somnolence, tachycardia, vomiting, weight gain

Contraindications: Hypersensitivity

Recommended lab tests: Metabolic monitoring/screening (BMI, lipid panel, blood glucose, LFT), AIMS

Overdose: CNS depression, seizures, tachycardia; OD rare
Tapering/withdrawal: Slow taper recommended
Special populations:
Pregnancy: Risk Category C
Lactation: Avoid
Elderly: Lower dose recommended
Hepatic impairment: No dose adjustment necessary in mild to moderate, lower dose in severe
Renal impairment: No dose adjustment necessary
Important notes:
- Preferred in patients with Parkinson's disease who develop psychosis
- Only antipsychotic approved for monotherapy to treat depressive episodes in bipolar I and II disorders
- Promising for schizoaffective disorder
- Used frequently off-label for insomnia

Risperidone[2,9,11,12,14,18,22,23,39,43,44,47,50,51,54]
Brand name: Risperdal, Risperdal Consta, Risperdal M-TAB
FDA approved for: Schizophrenia (acute and maintenance), acute mania or mixed episodes of bipolar I disorder (as monotherapy or as adjunct to lithium/valproate), bipolar 1 disorder maintenance (IM, in monotherapy or as adjunct to lithium/valproate), autism-related irritability
Other potential uses (off-label): Agitation, anxiety associated with drug withdrawal, OCD, oppositional defiant disorder, psychotic depression, PTSD, Tourette syndrome
Medication forms: *Tab* (0.25, 0.5, 1, 2, 3, 4 mg); *oral sol* (1 mg/ml [30 ml bottle]); *ODT* (0.25, 0.5, 1, 2, 3, 4 mg); *long-acting IM* (12.5, 25, 37.5, 50 mg)
Dosage:
- Schizophrenia:
  - *Oral:* 2 mg daily in 1–2 divided doses, can be increased based on tolerance/response to 4–8 mg daily, max 16 mg/day
  - *IM* (Risperdal Consta)*:* 25–50 mg in deltoid/gluteal muscle every 2 weeks
- Bipolar 1 mania: 2–3 mg po qd initially, range 1–6 mg daily
- Bipolar 1 maintenance: 25 mg IM in deltoid/gluteal muscle every 2 weeks initially, max 50 mg every 2 weeks
- Irritability associated with autistic spectrum disorder in children:
  - *5–16 years (weight <20 kg):* 0.25 mg/day po initially, can be increased based on tolerance/response to target 0.5 mg/day, max 3 mg/day
  - *5–16 yrs (weight ≥20 kg):* 0.5 mg/day po initially, can be increased based on tolerance/response to target 1 mg/day, max 3 mg/day

MOA: Antagonist at D_2, 5-HT_{2A}, H_1, a_1- and a_2-adrenergic receptors

Pharmacokinetics: t_{max}=1 hr (oral)/29–31 days (IM), $t_{1/2}$=3–20 hrs (oral)/2.6–9 days (IM)

Warnings:
- Similar to *Atypical Class Profile*
- **Black box warning:** Increased risk of death in elderly patients with dementia-related psychosis
- Has propensity to cause stroke in elderly people

Drug interactions:
- Similar to *Atypical Class Profile*
- CYP2D6 inhibitors (e.g., fluoxetine, paroxetine) and inducers (e.g., carbamazepine) can elevate or lower serum concentrations, respectively
- Avoid use with amoxapine, mesoridazine, pimozide, thioridazine, ziprasidone or other QT-prolonging drugs due to risk of additive QT prolongation
- Use with clozapine can increase levels
- Increased mortality rates with furosemide in elderly patients

Common side effects: Akathisia, anxiety, blurred vision, constipation, cough, dizziness, drooling, dry mouth, fatigue, headache, increased appetite, indigestion, insomnia, nasopharyngitis, nausea, Parkinsonism, rash, restlessness, sedation, sexual dysfunction, tremor, abdominal pain, urinary incontinence, URTI, vomiting, weight gain

Contraindications: Hypersensitivity

Recommended lab tests: Metabolic screening/monitoring (BMI, lipid panel, blood glucose, LFT), AIMS

Overdose: QTc prolongation, respiratory depression, seizure, NMS, coma; OD rare

Tapering/withdrawal: Slow taper recommended

Special populations:

Pregnancy: Risk Category C

Lactation: Avoid

Elderly: Initiate at 0.5 mg po bid and gradually titrate up to 2 mg

Hepatic impairment: No dose adjustment necessary in mild to moderate, 1 mg bid recommended in severe

Renal impairment: 0.5–1.5 mg/day

Important notes:
- Notorious among antipsychotics for causing hyperprolactinemia, which can cause galactorrhea and gynecomastia, particularly in youth
- Most common atypical antipsychotic for children/adolescents
- Associated with increased EPS in African-American males
- Risperdal Consta is very expensive, making it a difficult choice compared to typical IM medications

Ziprasidone[2,9,11,12,14,22,23,36,39,43,44,47,50,51,54]

Brand name: Geodon

FDA approved for: Schizophrenia (acute and maintenance), acute treatment of agitation associated with schizophrenia (IM), acute mania and mixed episodes of bipolar I, bipolar I maintenance (as adjunct to lithium/valproate)

Other potential uses (off-label): Agitation, bipolar disorder, schizoaffaffective disorder, Tourette syndrome

Medication forms: *Cap* (20, 40, 60, 80 mg); *injectable* (20 mg/ml)

Dosage:
- Schizophrenia: 20 mg po bid with food initially, can be increased based on tolerance/response to max 80 mg bid
- Acute agitation with schizophrenia:
  - IM: 10 mg q2hr or 20 mg q4hr, max 40 mg/day
  - Oral: 40 mg bid initially, max 120–160 mg/day
- Bipolar I disorder: 40 mg po bid initially, can be increased based on tolerance/response to max 120–160 mg/day

MOA: Antagonist at α_1-adrenergic, D_2, 5-HT$_{2A}$, and other dopamine and serotonin receptors; also has moderate affinity for H_1 receptors

Pharmacokinetics: t_{max}=6–8 hrs, $t_{1/2}$=7 hrs

Warnings:
- Similar to *Atypical Class Profile*
- **Black box warning:** Increased risk of death in elderly patients with dementia-related psychosis
- May cause drug reaction with eosinophilia and systemic symptoms (DRESS) and rash
- Discontinue if QTc interval >500 msec

Drug interactions:
- Similar to *Atypical Class Profile*
- Can enhance QTc-prolongation ability of other drugs; concomitant use with drugs that prolong QT interval is contraindicated

Common side effects: Abnormal vision, akathisia, asthenia, constipation, diarrhea, dizziness, EPS, headache, indigestion, lightheadedness, nausea, rash, somnolence, vomiting, weight gain

Contraindications:
- Hypersensitivity
- Congenital long QTc syndrome, recent MI, CHF, uncompensated heart failure, history of prolonged QTc or arrhythmia
- Patients taking pimozide, thioridazine, moxifloxacin, sparfloxacin, or other drugs which prolong the QT interval

Recommended lab tests: Metabolic screening/monitoring (BMI, lipid panel, blood glucose, LFT), AIMS, baseline ECG when cardiac risk factors are present

Overdose: Hypotension, hypertension, tachycardia, prolonged QRS and QTc intervals, torsades de pointes; OD rare

Tapering/withdrawal: Slow taper recommended

Special populations:

Pregnancy: Risk Category C

Lactation: Avoid

Elderly: Lower dose with slow titration recommended

Hepatic impairment: No dose adjustment necessary

Renal impairment: No dose adjustment necessary in mild to moderate; 20–80 mg/day max in severe, use caution with IM doses

Cardiac impairment: Contraindicated in QTc prolongation

Important notes:

- Considered to be a weight-neutral atypical antipsychotic
- Causes greater QTc prolongation than other antipsychotics
- QTc prolongation has been a major cause of physician anxiety when prescribing this medication
- Absorption increased up to 100% with food

Typical Antipsychotics (First Generation)

Class Profile[14,15,23,38,43,44,46,56]

Overview: Typical or first-generation antipsychotic medications (FGAs), also known as neuroleptics or conventional antipsychotics, are used to treat psychosis and other conditions like acute mania and agitation. Since FGAs are considerably less expensive than and as effective as newer antipsychotics, they are a valuable treatment option for psychotic disorders. The primary FGAs used include:

- *Low potency:* Chlorpromazine, mesoridazine, thrioridazine
- *High potency:* Fluphenazine, flupentixol, haloperidol, loxapine, molindone, perphenazine, pimozide, thiothixene, trifluperazine

Warnings:

- **Black box warning:** Increased risk of death in elderly patients with dementia-related psychosis
- Can cause TD, NMS, EPS, and orthostatic hypotension
- Use caution in cerebrovascular/cardiovascular disorders and respiratory impairment
- Associated with blood dyscrasias (leukopenia, neutropenia, agranulocytosis), hyperprolactinemia, and impaired body temperature regulation
- Can impair mental/physical abilities and lower seizure threshold

Drug interaction:

- Increased sedation with CNS depressants; avoid with alcohol, other CNS depressants
- Levels decreased with carbamazepine and nicotine

- Levels increased with SSRIs; use with TCAs can increase both drug levels
- Increased sedation and hypotension with meperidine
- Use with beta-blockers can increase both drug levels, increasing risk of hypotension
- Use caution with anticholinergic agents and organophosphates
- Diminishes effects of oral anticoagulants
- Can produce α-adrenergic blockade

Class side effects: Akathisia, blurred vision, breast engorgement, confusion, constipation, decreased sweating, drowsiness, dry mouth, dystonia, EPS, galactorrhea, impotence, insomnia, lactation, orthostatic hypotension, Parkinsonism, rash, restlessness, salivation, TD, visual disturbances, weight gain.

Recommended lab tests: BMI during treatment, AIMS; evaluate for pre-diabetes, diabetes, and dyslipidemia if weight gain >5%.

Overdose: Severe CNS depression or coma, pulmonary edema, NMS, agitation, seizures, hypotension, cardiac arrest, and sudden death.

Tapering/withdrawal: Slow titration and cross titration recommended.

Individual Drug Profiles

Chlorpromazine[2,9,11,12,14,22,23,39,41,43,44,47,50,51,54]

Brand name: Thorazine

FDA approved for: Schizophrenia, other psychotic disorders, manifestations of manic-depressive illness, severe behavioral problem in children (ages 1–12 yrs), tetanus (adjunct), intractable hiccups, nausea/vomiting, acute intermittent porphyria, restlessness and apprehension before surgery

Other potential uses (off-label): Agitation, dementia, insomnia, migraines

Medication forms: *Tab* (10, 25, 50, 100, 200 mg); *injectable* (25 mg/ml)

Dosage:
- Schizophrenia, psychotic disorders:
  - *Oral:* 30–75 mg/day divided bid–tid initially, maintenance 200 mg/day
  - *IV/IM:* 25–50 mg initially, followed prn 25–50 mg after 1–4 hours, can be increased based on tolerance/response to max 400 mg q4–6hr (usual dosage 300–800 mg/day)

MOA: Antagonist at D_1 and D_2 and $α_1$-adrenergic receptors

Pharmacokinetics: t_{max}=2.8 hrs (oral), $t_{1/2}$=6 hrs

Warnings:
- Similar to *Typical Class Profile*
- **Black box warning**: Increased risk of death in elderly patients with dementia-related psychosis

Drug interactions:
- Similar to *Typical Class Profile*
- Use with lithium increases risk of encephalopathic syndrome

- Use with thiazide potentiates orthostatic hypotension
- Can increase valproic acid levels and decrease the effect of guanethidine

Common side effects: Akathisia, anticholinergic effects, dizziness, drowsiness, dry mouth, EPS, hypotension, pigmentary retinopathy, sedation, photosensitivity to sunlight

Contraindications: Coma, hypersensitivity to chlorpromazine or any phenothiazine, use with CNS depressants (alcohol, barbiturates, narcotics, etc.)

Special populations:

Pregnancy: Risk Category C

Lactation: Avoid

Elderly: Lower dose recommended

Hepatic impairment: Use caution

Renal impairment: No dose adjustment necessary

Important notes:

- Used widely for treating nausea and hiccups

Fluphenazine[2,9,11,12,14,22,23,26,39,43,44,47,50,51,54]

Brand name: Prolixin, Rho-Fluphenazine

FDA approved for: Psychotic disorders, behavioral complications in patients with mental retardation

Other potential uses (off-label): Agitation, dementia

Medication forms: *Tab* (1, 2.5, 5, 10 mg); *elixir* (2.5 mg/5 ml); *oral conc* (5mg/ml); *injectable sol* (0.5 mg/ml fluphenazine hydrochloride or 25 mg/ml fluphenazine decanoate)

Dosage:

- Schizophrenia:
  - *Oral:* 2.5–10 mg/day divided tid–qid, can be increased based on tolerance/response to max 40 mg/day (maintenance 1–5 mg/day)
  - *IM*: 12.5–25 mg (25 mg/ml) IM/SC every 2–4 weeks

MOA: Selectively antagonizes D_2 receptors

Pharmacokinetics: t_{max}=2.8 hrs (oral)/1 day (decanoate), $t_{1/2}$=10–20 hrs (oral)/14–26 days (decanoate)

Warnings:

- Similar to *Typical Class Profile*
- **Black box warning:** Increased risk of death in elderly patients with dementia-related psychosis
- May cause liver damage, pigmented retinopathy, lenticular and corneal dyskinesia with prolonged therapy

Drug interactions: Similar to *Typical Class Profile*

Common side effects: Blurred vision, constipation, drowsiness, dry mouth, dystonia, EPS, NMS, orthostatic hypotension, TD, pseudo-Parkinsonism

Contraindications: Hypersensitivity, severe CNS depression, coma, brain damage, hepatic disease, blood dyscrasias

Special populations:

Pregnancy: Risk Category C

Lactation: Avoid

Elderly: Use caution and lower dose

Hepatic impairment: Avoid

Renal impairment: Use caution

Important notes:

- Used primarily patients who require depot therapy with long-lasting injection
- Side effect profile similar to haloperidol
- Sudden discontinuation may cause severe GI symptoms
- Prolixin available in long-acting forms (IM) for dosing on two-week or monthly basis; particularly helpful for noncompliant psychotic patients

Flupentixol[22,47,50,51]

Brand name: Depixol, Fluanxol

FDA approved for: None (used in many countries as IM injection for non- compliant schizophrenic patients.)

Other potential uses (off-label): Anxiety

Medication forms: None available in US

Dosage:

- Oral: 3-9 mg/day initially divided, max 18 mg/day
- IM: 40–120 mg every 1–4 weeks

MOA: Antagonizes D_2 and/or $5\text{-}HT_{2A}$ receptors

Common side effects: Amenorrhea, agitation, galactorrhea, EPS, insomnia, Parkinsonism, restlessness, sedation, TD, weight gain

Haloperidol[2,9,11,12,14,22,23,27,39,43,44,47,50,51,54]

Brand name: Haldol, Haldol Decanoate

FDA approved for: Schizophrenia, Tourette syndrome, severe behavior problems in children with combative and explosive hyper-excitability, short-term treatment of hyperactive children showing excessive motor activity with accompanying conduct disorder, schizophrenia requiring prolonged therapy (IM decanoate)

Other potential uses (off-label): Agitation, autism, chronic hiccups, delirium, dementia, mania

Medication forms: *Tab* (0.5, 1, 2, 5, 10, 20 mg)*; oral conc* (2 mg/ml)*; injectable lactate sol* (5 mg/ml)*; injectable decanoate sol* (50, 100 mg/ml)

Dosage:
- Schizophrenia, psychosis:
  - *Oral:* 0.5–5 mg bid–tid, max 30 mg/day
  - *IM (as lactate):* 2–5 mg every 4–8 hours prn, max 8–10 mg
  - *IM (as decanoate):* 10–20x daily oral dose q4-week intervals initially, maintenance 10–15x initial oral dose
- Tourette disorder: 0.5 mg/day po bid–tid initially, max 0.15 mg/kg/day
- Acute agitation in children ages >12 yrs:
  - *Oral:* 0.5–3 mg po initially, repeated 1 hr prn

    or
  - *IM:* 2–5 mg initally, repeated 1 hr prn

MOA: Blocks postsynaptic D_2 receptors in mesolimbic system and blocks D_2 somatodendritic autoreceptors

Pharmacokinetics: t_{max}=20 min (IM)/2–6 hrs (oral)/6 days (decanoate), $t_{1/2}$=18 hrs (oral)/3 weeks (decanoate)

Warnings:
- Similar to *Typical Class Profile*
- **Black box warning**: Increased risk of death in elderly patients with dementia-related psychosis
- May cause hyperpyrexia, heat stroke, and bronchopneumonia
- Use caution with QT prolongation

Drug interactions:
- Similar to *Typical Class Profile*
- Counteracts increased action of norepinephrine and dopamine in narcolepsy
- Antagonizes effects of epinephrine
- Can cause QTc interval prolongation when used with amiodarone or other drugs which prolong the QT interval
- Can cause encephalopathic syndrome with lithium

Common side effects: Blurred vision, drowsiness, dry mouth, dystonia, hallucinations, impotence, insomnia, TD, visual disturbances

Contraindications: Coma, CNS depression, Parkinson's disease, hypersensitivity

Recommended lab tests: CBC, prolactin, lipids

Special populations:

Pregnancy: Risk Category C

Lactation: Use caution

Elderly: Lower dose recommended

Hepatic impairment: Use caution

Renal impairment: No dose adjustment necessary

Important notes:
- IM formulation allows dosage on two-week or monthly basis; particularly helpful for noncompliant psychotic patients

Loxapine[2,9,11,12,14,22,23,28,39,43,44,47,50,51,54]

Brand name: Loxitane, Adasuve

FDA approved for: Schizophrenia (acute and maintenance), agitation associated with bipolar disorder/schizophrenia

Other potential uses (off-label): Bipolar disorder, insomnia

Medication forms: *Cap* (5, 10, 25, 50 mg); *powder for oral inhalation* (10 mg/single-use inhaler)

Dosage:
- Schizophrenia: 10 mg po bid initially, can be increased based on tolerance/response to max 250 mg/day (maintenance 60–100 mg/day divided bid–tid)
- Schizophrenia and bipolar I agitation: 10 mg inhaled po once within a 24-hr period, must be administered by a healthcare professional

MOA: Blocks D_1, D_2, D_3, D_4, and 5-HT$_{2A}$ receptors

Pharmacokinetics: t_{max}=1.13 min (oral inhalation), $t_{1/2}$=7.6 hrs

Warnings:
- Similar to *Typical Class Profile*
- **Black box warning:**
  - Increased risk of death in elderly patients with dementia-related psychosis
  - *Inhalation, Oral (Powder), Bronchospasm:* Can cause bronchospasm that has the potential to lead to respiratory distress/arrest; monitor for signs and symptoms of bronchospasm following treatment. Because of the risk of bronchospasm, loxapine powder for oral inhalation is available only through a restricted program under a Risk Evaluation and Mitigation Strategy (REMS) called the Adasuve ™ REMS.
- Use caution in patients with glaucoma and urinary retention
- Antiemetic effects may mask the toxicity of other drugs and may hide the presence of a brain tumor or intestinal obstruction

Drug interactions:
- Similar to *Typical Class Profile*
- Risk of respiratory depression, stupor, and hypotension with lorazepam
- Antagonizes effects of epinephrine

Common side effects: Akathisia, confusion, constipation, drowsiness, dry mouth, EPS, nasal congestion, orthostatic hypotension, Parkinson's symptoms, rash, urinary retention, weight gain

Contraindications: Asthma, COPD, coma, use of CNS depressants (alcohol, barbiturates, narcotics, etc.), hypersensitivity to loxapine or amoxapine

Special populations:

Pregnancy: Risk Category C

Lactation: Avoid

Elderly: Lower dose recommended

Hepatic impairment: Lower dose recommended for oral form, no dose adjustment required for inhalation form

Renal impairment: No dose adjustment necessary

Important notes:

- Striking similarities to clozapine
- Inhaled loxapine is an innovative and rapid option for agitation

Mesoridazine[2,9,11,12,14,22,23,39,43,44,47,50,51]

Brand name: Serentil, Lidanil

FDA approved for: None (discontinued in US; previously approved for management of schizophrenic patients unresponsive to other antipsychotics)

Other potential uses (off-label): None

Medication forms: *Tab* (10, 25, 50, 100 mg); *injectable* (25 mg/ml); *conc* (25 mg/ml)

Dosage:

- Oral: 100–400 mg/day
- Injection: 25–200 mg/day

Warnings: Similar to *Typical Class Profile*

Drug interactions:

- Similar to *Typical Class Profile*
- May cause serious cardiotoxicity if used with other drugs that prolong QTc

Common side effects: Constipation, dry mouth, EPS, sexual dysfunction, pigmentary retinopathy

Important notes:

- Rarely ever used due to QTc effect

Molindone[2,9,11,12,14,22,23,39,43,44,47,50,51,54]

Brand name: Moban

FDA approved for: Schizophrenia

Other potential uses (off-label): Bipolar disorders

Medication forms: *Tab* (5, 10, 25, 50, 100 mg); *cap* (5, 10, 25 mg); *conc* (20 mg/ml)

Dosage:

- Schizophrenia: 50–75 mg/day divided, max 225 mg/day

Warnings:

- Similar to *Typical Class Profile*
- **Black box warning**: Increased risk of death in elderly patients with dementia-related psychosis

Drug interactions:

- Similar to *Typical Class Profile*

- Can interfere with calcium sulfate, phenytoin sodium, and tetracycline

Common side effects: Decreased sweating, difficult urination, drowsiness, dry mouth, EPS, headache, nausea

Contraindications: Hypersensitivity, coma, CNS depression

Special populations:

Pregnancy: Risk Category C

Lactation: Avoid

Elderly: Lower dose recommended

Hepatic impairment: Use caution

Renal impairment: No dose adjustment necessary

Important notes:

- Associated with lower weight gain but higher EPS

Perphenazine[2,9,11,12,14,22,23,39,43,44,42,47,50,51,54]

Brand name: Trilafon

FDA approved for: Schizophrenia, nausea and vomiting

Other potential uses (off-label): Agitation

Medication forms: *Tab* (2, 4, 8, 16 mg)

Dosage:

- Schizophrenia: 4–8 mg bid, can be increased based on tolerance/response to max 24 mg

MOA: Blocks postsynaptic mesolimbic dopaminergic and α-adrenergic receptors

Pharmacokinetics: t_{max}=1–3 hrs, $t_{1/2}$=9–12 hrs

Warnings:

- Similar to *Typical Class Profile*
- **Black box warning**: Increased risk of death in elderly patients with dementia-related psychosis
- Use caution with depression and renal impairment
- May cause photosensitivity
- Antiemetic effects may mask the toxicity of other drugs and may hide presence of a brain tumor or intestinal obstruction

Drug interactions:

- Similar to *Typical Class Profile*
- Additive anticholinergic reaction with atropine
- Increased levels with cytochrome CYP2D6 inhibitors
- Reduce doses of anesthetics and CNS depressants in surgical candidates

Common side effects: Blurred vision, breast engorgement, constipation, drowsiness, dry mouth, EPS, lactation, motor restlessness, orthostatic hypotension, salivation

Contraindications: Bone marrow suppression, coma, hypersensitivity, concurrent use with CNS depressants or antihistamines, blood dyscrasias, liver damage, subcortical damage

Special populations:

Pregnancy: Risk Category C

Lactation: Use caution

Elderly: Lower dose recommended

Hepatic impairment: No dose adjustment necessary in mild to moderate, use caution in severe

Renal impairment: No dose adjustment necessary

Important notes:

- Effective for positive symptoms of schizophrenia; less effective for negative symptoms
- May have less weight gain compared to others in this class

Pimozide[2,9,11,12,14,22,23,39,43,44,47,49,50,51,54]

Brand name: Orap

FDA approved for: Tourette syndrome

Other potential uses (off-label): Chronic schizophrenia, delusional paristosis

Medication forms: *Tab* (1, 2 mg)

Dosage:

- Chronic schizophrenia: 1–2 mg qd initially, can be increased based on tolerance/response to max 10 mg/day

MOA: Potent centrally acting D-receptor antagonist

Pharmacokinetics: t_{max}=6–8 hrs, $t_{1/2}$=55–66 hrs

Warnings:

- Similar to *Typical Class Profile*
- **Black box warning:** Increased risk of death in elderly patients with dementia-related psychosis
- Use caution with history of seizure, EEG abnormalities, severe hepatic/renal impairment
- Associated with sudden death, QTc prolongation, pituitary tumors

Drug interactions:

- Similar to *Typical Class Profile*
- Can cause bradycardia with fluoxetine
- Avoid combination with drugs that cause QTc prolongation
- Avoid with strong CYP3A4 inhibitors (e.g., azole antifungals)

Common side effects: Abnormal heart rhythm, adverse behavior effects, akinesia, constipation, drowsiness, dry mouth, EPS, gingival hyperplasia, hypotension, impotence, NMS, Parkinson symptoms, rash, sedation, visual disturbances

Contraindications:

- Hypersensitivity
- Comatose state, CNS depression
- Congenital long QTc syndrome or use with QTc prolonging drugs
- Simple tics and tics caused by pemoline, methylphenidate, amphetamines
- Hypokalemia, hypomagnesaemia
- Use with macrolide antibiotics (QTc syndrome) and azole antifungals
- Use with citalopram, escitalopram, sertraline, CYP2D6 inhibitors, nefazodone, zileuton, or other protease inhibitors

Special populations:

Pregnancy: Risk Category C
Lactation: Avoid
Elderly: Lower dose recommended
Hepatic impairment: No data available
Renal impairment: No data available

Important notes:

- Rarely used due to cardiovascular risk

Thioridazine[2,9,11,12,14,22,23,25,39,43,44,47,50,51,54]

Brand name: Mellaril

FDA approved for: None (no longer approved due to potential cardiotoxicity and retinopathy; previously approved for schizophrenia not responsive to other antipsychotics)

Other potential uses (off-label): Agitation, psychotic depression

Medication forms: *Tab* (10, 15, 25, 50, 100, 150, 200 mg); *liq* (30, 100 mg/ml [120 ml bottle]); *suspension* (5 mg/ml, 20 mg/ml, 25 mg/5 ml)

Dosage:

- Schizophrenia: 50–100 mg tid initially, can be increased based on tolerance/response to max 800 mg/day divided
- Depressive disorders: 25 mg qid, can be increased based on tolerance/response to max 200 mg/day

MOA: Blocks postsynaptic mesolimbic dopaminergic and α-adrenergic receptors and also has calcium antagonist effect

Pharmacokinetics: t_{max}=2–4 hrs, $t_{1/2}$=21–24 hrs

Warnings:

- Similar to *Typical Class Profile*
- **Black box warning:**
    - Increased risk of death in elderly patients with dementia-related psychosis
    - Has been shown to prolong the QTc interval in a dose related manner, which has been associated with torsades de pointes-type arrhythmias and sudden

    death; should be reserved for use in the treatment of schizophrenic patients who fail to show an acceptable response to adequate courses of treatment with other antipsychotic drugs

- Associated with pigmentary retinopathy

Drug interactions:
- Similar to *Typical Class Profile*
- Levels increased with fluvoxamine, pindolol
- Avoid use with drugs that prolong QTc interval
- Avoid use with CYP2D6 inhibitors (e.g., fluoxetine, sertraline, paroxetine) due to increased plasma levels

Common side effects: Blurred vision, constipation, drowsiness, dry mouth, ejaculation disorder, EPS, galactorrhea, restlessness

Contraindications:
- Hypersensitivity
- CNS depression, comatose state
- History of QTc prolongation or use with drugs that can prolong the QTc interval
- Circulatory collapse, recent acute MI, severe hypertension/hypotension, history of cardiac arrhythmia
- Presence of blood dyscrasias
- Use with CYP2D6 inhibitors

Special populations:
Pregnancy: Risk Category C
Lactation: Avoid
Elderly: Lower dose recommended
Hepatic impairment: Lower dose recommended
Renal impairment: No dose adjustment necessary

Thiothixene[2,9,11,12,14,22,23,37,39,43,44,47,50,51,54]
Brand name: Navane
FDA approved for: Schizophrenia
Other potential uses (off-label): Agitation
Medication forms: *Cap* (1, 2, 5, 10, 20 mg); *conc* (5 mg/ml [120 ml bottle])
Dosage:
- Schizophrenia:
  - *Cap:* 2–5 mg/day initially, increase to target 15– 30 mg/day, max 60 mg/day
  - *Conc:* 2–3 mg tid, max 60 mg/day

MOA: Postsynaptic blockade of CNS D-receptors and ⊠-adrenergic blocking activity
Pharmacokinetics: t_{max}=1–2 hrs, $t_{1/2}$=34 hrs

Warnings:
- Similar to *Typical Class Profile*
- **Black box warning**: Increased risk of death in elderly patients with dementia-related psychosis
- Monitor for retinopathy and lenticular pigmentation
- Antiemetic effects may mask the toxicity of other drugs and may hide the presence of a brain tumor or intestinal obstruction

Drug interactions:
- Similar to *Typical Class Profile*
- Paradoxical effect with vasopressor agents
- Increased clearance with carbamazepine

Common side effects: Anticholinergic effects, breast engorgement, decreased sweating, drowsiness, dry mouth, dystonia, EPS, increased appetite, orthostatic hypotension, photosensitivity, restlessness, TD, weight gain

Contraindications: Hypersensitivity

Special populations:

Pregnancy: Risk Category C

Lactation: Avoid

Elderly: Lower dose recommended

Hepatic/Renal impairment: Use caution

Trifluoperazine[2,9,11,12,14,22,23,29,39,43,44,47,50,51,54]

Brand name: Stelazine

FDA approved for: Schizophrenia, nonpsychotic anxiety

Other potential uses (off-label): Agitation, bipolar disorder

Medication forms: *Tab* (1, 2, 5, 10 mg); *IM sol* (2 mg/ml)

Dosage:
- Schizophrenia:
  - *Outpatient:* 1–2 mg bid
  - *Inpatient:* maintenance 15–20 mg, max 40mg/day
- Non-psychotic anxiety: 1–2 mg bid, can be increased based on tolerance/response to max 6 mg/day for max 12 weeks

MOA: Blocks postsynaptic mesolimbic dopaminergic and ☒-adrenergic receptors

Warnings:
- Similar to *Typical Class Profile*
- **Black box warning:** Increased risk of death in elderly patients with dementia-related psychosis

- May cause encephalopathic syndrome with lithium, jaundice (cholestatic), pigmented retinopathy, thrombocytopenia and anemia
- Use caution in patients with angina
- Antiemetic action may mask toxic signs of overdose of other medications and may hide the presence of a brain tumor or intestinal obstruction

Drug interactions:
- Similar to *Typical Class Profile*
- Counteracts antihypertensive effects of guanethidine
- Use with thiazide diuretics can accentuate orthostatic hypotension

Common side effects: Blurred vision, dizziness, drowsiness, dry mouth, dystonia, EPS, insomnia, motor restlessness

Contraindications: CNS depression, comatose state, blood dyscrasias, hypersensitivity, bone marrow suppression, preexisting liver damage

Special populations:
Pregnancy: Risk Category C
Lactation: Use caution
Elderly: Lower dose recommended
Hepatic impairment: Contraindicated
Renal impairment: No dose adjustment necessary

Important notes:
- Caution in patients exposed to excessive heat

References:

1. Abou-Setta, Ahmed M., Shima S. Mousavi, Carol Spooner, Janine R. Schouten, Dion Pasichnyk, Susan Armijo-Olivo, Amy Beaith, Jennifer C. Seida, Serdar Dursun, Amanda S. Newton, and Lisa Hartling. 2012. "Comparative Effectiveness Reviews, No. 63." In *First-Generation Versus Second-Generation Antipsychotics in Adults: Comparative Effectiveness*. US Agency for Healthcare Research and Quality.

2. Albers, Lawrence J., Rhoda K. Hahn, and Christopher Reist. 2010. *Handbook of Psychiatric Drugs*. 2011 ed. 39–59. Current Clinical Strategies Publishing.

3. Alvarez-Jimenez, M., A. Priede, S. E. Hetrick, S. Bendall, E. Killackey, A. G. Parker, P. D. McGorry, and J. F. Gleeson. 2012. "Risk factors for relapse following treatment for first episode psychosis: a systematic review and meta-analysis of longitudinal studies." *Schizophr Res* 139(1-3):116–128. doi: 10.1016/j.schres.2012.05.007.

4. American Heart Association (AHA). 2005. "Diagnosis and Management of the Metabolic Syndrome." *Circulation*. 112(17):2735–2752. Accessed February 3, 2015. http://circ.ahajournals.org/content/112/17/2735/T1.expansion.html.

5. American Psychiatric Association (APA). 2013. *Diagnostic and Statistical Manual of Mental Disorders*. 5th ed. (DSM-5). Washington, DC: American Psychiatric Publishing.

6. AstraZeneca Pharmaceuticals LP. 2013. "SEROQUEL- quetiapine fumarate tablet, film coated." US National Library of Medicine: Daily Med. Accessed December 11, 2014. http://dailymed.nlm.nih. gov/dailymed/drugInfo.cfm?setid=0584dda8-bc3c-48fe-1a90-79608f78e8a0.

7. Bushu Pharmaceutical, LTD. 2014. "LATUDA- lurasidone hydrochloride tablet, film coated." US National Library of Medicine: Daily Med. Accessed December 11, 2014. http://dailymed.nlm.nih. gov/dailymed/drugInfo.cfm?setid=88a244d1-eddb-499c-bee2-e1f49056e78f.

8. Center for Quality Assessment and Improvement in Mental Health (CQAIMH). 2015. "Metabolic Monitoring." Accessed January 14, 2015. http://www.cqaimh.org/pdf/tool_metabolic.pdf.

9. Center Watch. 2015. "FDA Approved Drugs by Therapeutic Area." Accessed February 3, 2015. http://www.centerwatch.com/drug-information/fda-approved-drugs/therapeutic-area/17/ psychiatry-psychology.

10. Eli Lilly and Company. 2014. "ZYPREXA - olanzapine tablet." US National Library of Medicine: Daily Med. Accessed January 8, 2015. http://dailymed.nlm.nih.gov/dailymed/drugInfo. cfm?setid=d5051fbc-846b-4946-82df-341fb1216341.

11. Elsevier Gold Standard, Inc. 2015. "Clinical Pharmacology." Accessed March 12, 2015. https:// www.clinicalpharmacology.com.

12. Epocrates. 2015. Accessed March 25, 2015. https://online.epocrates.com.

13. Forest Laboratories, Inc. 2014. "SAPHRIS- asenapine maleate tablet." US National Library of Medicine: Daily Med. Accessed December 11, 2014. http://dailymed.nlm.nih.gov/dailymed/drugInfo.cfm?setid=5429f134-839f-4ffc-9944-55f51238def8.

14. Gabbard, Glen O., ed. 2007. *Gabbard's Treatments of Psychiatric Disorders*. 4th ed. 323–380. Washington, DC: American Psychiatric Publishing.

15. Hales, Robert. E., S. Yudofsky, and L. Roberts, eds. 2014. *The American Psychiatric Publishing Textbook of Psychiatry*. 6th ed. 273–310, 929–1004. Washington, DC: American Psychiatric Publishing.

16. Hor, Kahyee, and Mark Taylor. 2010. "Suicide and schizophrenia: a systematic review of rates and risk factors." *Journal of Psychopharmacology* 24(4 supplement):81–90. doi: 10.1177/1359786810385490.

17. Janssen Pharmaceuticals, Inc. 2014. "INVEGA- paliperidone tablet, extended release." US National Library of Medicine: Daily Med. Accessed December 11, 2014. http://dailymed.nlm.nih.gov/dailymed/drugInfo.cfm?setid=7b8e5b26-b9e4-4704-921b-3c3c0d159916.

18. Janssen Pharmaceuticals, Inc. 2014. "RISPERDAL- risperidone tablet." US National Library of Medicine: Daily Med. Accessed December 11, 2014. http://dailymed.nlm.nih.gov/dailymed/drugInfo.cfm?setid=7e117c7e-02fc-4343-92a1-230061dfc5e0.

19. Kosten, Thomas R., and Douglas M. Ziedonis. 1997. "Substance Abuse and Schizophrenia: Editors' Introduction." *Schizophrenia Bulletin* 23(2):181–186. doi: 10.1093/schbul/23.2.181.

20. Lehman, A.F., J.A. Lieberman, L.B. Dixon, T.H. McGlashan, A.L. Miller, D.O. Perkins, and J. Kreyenbuhl. 2004. "Practice guideline for the treatment of patients with schizophrenia, second edition." American Psychiatric Association Steering Committee on Practice Guidelines. *Am J Psychiatry* 161(2 suppl):1–56.

21. Lieberman, J.A., T.S. Stroup, J.P. McEvoy, M.S. Swartz, Robert A. Rosenheck, Diana O. Perkins, Richard S.E. Keefe, Sonia M. Davis, Clarence E. Davis, Barry D. Lebowitz, Joanne Severe, and John K. Hsiao. 2005. "Effectiveness of antipsychotic drugs in patients with chronic schizophrenia." *N Engl J Med* 353(12):1209–1223.

22. Medscape: Drugs & Diseases. 2015. "Psychiatrics." Accessed February 3, 2015. http://reference.medscape.com/drugs/psychiatrics.

23. Medscape. 2015. "Schizophrenia." Accessed March 12, 2015. http://emedicine.medscape.com/article/288259-overview.

24. Meeks, Thomas W., and Dilip V. Jeste. 2008. "Beyond the Black Box: What is The Role for Antipsychotics in Dementia?" *Current Psychiatry* 7(6):50–65.

25. Mutual Pharmaceutical. 2014. "THIORIDAZINE HYDROCHLORIDE- thioridazine hydrochloridetablet,filmcoated."USNationalLibraryofMedicine:DailyMed.AccessedDecember3,2014.http://dailymed.nlm.nih.gov/dailymed/drugInfo.cfm?setid=9c4bedb4-2d59-4fcd-aad7-fce988cd96d8.

26. Mylan Pharmaceuticals, Inc. 2014. "FLUPHENAZINE HYDROCHLORIDE- fluphenazine hydrochloride tablet, film coated." US National Library of Medicine: Daily Med. Accessed December 3, 2014. http://dailymed.nlm.nih.gov/dailymed/drugInfo.cfm?setid=a61e5bf9-b545-43e9-9f20-cdcb31abda91.

27. Mylan Pharmaceuticals, Inc. 2014. "HALOPERIDOL- haloperidol tablet." US National Library of Medicine: Daily Med. Accessed December 3, 2014. http://dailymed.nlm.nih.gov/dailymed/drugInfo.cfm?setid=c559b0b0-4087-d12a-e718-c18ccb6811e6.

28. Mylan Pharmaceuticals, Inc. 2014. "LOXAPINE- loxapine succinate capsule." US National Library of Medicine: Daily Med. Accessed December 3, 2014. http://dailymed.nlm.nih.gov/dailymed/drugInfo.cfm?setid=0c0a9ed3-20c8-48c2-bc18-8b0b4260e300.

29. Mylan Institutional Inc. 2012. "TRIFLUOPERAZINE HYDROCHLORIDE- trifluoperazine hydrochloride tablet, film coated." US National Library of Medicine: Daily Med. Accessed December 3, 2014. http://dailymed.nlm.nih.gov/dailymed/drugInfo.cfm?setid=f742a579-411a-4140-91c4-edc735d638fa.

30. National Alliance on Mental Illness (NAMI). 2015. "Psychosis." Accessed March 16, 2015. https://www.nami.org/Learn-More/Mental-Health-Conditions/Related-Conditions/Psychosis.

31. Nasrallah, H.A. 2007. "Atypical antipsychotic-induced metabolic side effects: insights from receptor-binding profiles." *Mol Psychiatry* 13(1):27–35.

32. Novartis Pharmaceuticals Corporation. 2015. "CLOZARIL- clozapine tablet." US National Library of Medicine: Daily Med. Accessed January 8, 2015. http://dailymed.nlm.nih.gov/dailymed/drugInfo.cfm?setid=5f0c6f5f-b906-4c8f-8580-3939a476a1c1.

33. Novartis Pharmaceuticals Corporation. 2014. "FANAPT- iloperidone tablet." US National Library of Medicine: Daily Med. Accessed December 11, 2014. http://dailymed.nlm.nih.gov/dailymed/drugInfo.cfm?setid=43452bf8-76e7-47a9-a5d8-41fe84d061f0.

34. Otsuka America Pharmaceutical, Inc. 2014. "ABILIFY- aripiprazole tablet." US National Library of Medicine: Daily Med. Accessed December 11, 2014. http://dailymed.nlm.nih.gov/dailymed/drugInfo.cfm?setid=c040bd1d-45b7-49f2-93ea-aed7220b30ac.

35. Perkins, Diana O., Hongbin Gu, Kalina Boteva, and Jeffrey A. Lieberman. 2005. "Relationship Between Duration of Untreated Psychosis and Outcome in First-Episode Schizophrenia: A Critical Review and Meta-Analysis." *American Journal of Psychiatry* 162(10):1785–1804. doi: doi:10.1176/appi.ajp.162.10.1785.

36. Pfizer, Inc. "GEODON- ziprasidone hydrochloride capsule." US National Library of Medicine: Daily Med. Accessed January 8, 2015. http://dailymed.nlm.nih.gov/dailymed/drugInfo.cfm?setid=8326928a-2cb6-4f7f-9712-03a425a14c37.

37. Pfizer, Inc. 2012. "NAVANE- thiothixene capsule." US National Library of Medicine: Daily Med. Accessed December 3, 2014. http://dailymed.nlm.nih.gov/dailymed/drugInfo.cfm?setid=3fe9b451-da9d-4790-947e-15a535b369a5.

38. Preston, John D., and James Johnson. 2011. *Clinical Psychopharmacology Made Ridiculously Simple.* 7th ed. 40–49. Miami: MedMaster Inc.

39. RxList. 2015. "Drugs A-Z List." Accessed March 25, 2015. http://www.rxlist.com/drugs/alpha_a.htm.

40. Saely, C. H., P. Rein, and H. Drexel. 2007. "The metabolic syndrome and risk of cardiovascular disease and diabetes: experiences with the new diagnostic criteria from the International Diabetes Federation." *Horm Metab Res* 39(9):642–650. doi: 10.1055/s-2007-985822.

41. Sandoz, Inc. 2011. "CHLORPROMAZINE HYDROCHLORIDE- chlorpromazine hydrochloride tablet, film coated." US National Library of Medicine: Daily Med. Accessed December 3, 2014. http://dailymed.nlm.nih.gov/dailymed/drugInfo.cfm?setid=f15e9f35-1e3e-4217-b8e2-1d6096dbee1b.

42. Sandoz, Inc. 2014. "PERPHENAZINE- perphenazine tablet, film coated." US National Library of Medicine: Daily Med. Accessed December 3, 2014. http://dailymed.nlm.nih.gov/dailymed/drugInfo.cfm?setid=6c76e98d-b8c3-441f-bac5-a9de6dc8f14f.

43. Schatzberg, A.F., and C.B. Nemeroff, eds. 2009. *The American Psychiatric Publishing Textbook of Psychopharmacology.* 4th ed. 531–668. Washington, DC: American Psychiatric Publishing.

44. Schatzberg, A.F., Jonathan O. Cole, and Charles DeBattista. 2010. *Manual of Clinical Psychopharmacology.* 7th ed. 169–259. Washington, DC: American Psychiatric Publishing.

45. Seeman, P. 2002. "Atypical antipsychotics: mechanism of action." *Can J Psychiatry* 47(1):27–38.

46. Stahl, S.M. 2008. *Essential Psychopharmacology: Neuroscientific Basis and Practical Applications.* 3rd ed. 79–236. New York: Cambridge Press.

47. Stahl, S.M. 2011. *Essential Psychopharmacology: the Prescriber's Guide.* 4th ed. 15–20, 47–52, 59–63, 97–101, 133–138, 349–353, 405–408, 427–433, 445–449, 463–467, 475–479, 481–485, 501–507, 519–525, 541–545, 559–563, 569–573, 575–578, 613–617, 645–650. Cambridge: Cambridge University Press.

48. Tandon, Rajiv, and Michael D. Jibson. 2002. "Extrapyramidal Side Effects of Antipsychotic Treatment: Scope of Problem and Impact on Outcome." *Annals of Clinical Psychiatry* 14(2):123–129. doi: 10.3109/10401230209149099.

49. Teva Select Brands. 2014. "ORAP- pimozide tablet." US National Library of Medicine: Daily Med. Accessed December 3, 2014. http://dailymed.nlm.nih.gov/dailymed/drugInfo.cfm?setid=fd9729c3-545f-4d34-9bc7-72b61e028fc4.

50. Truven Health Analytics. 2015. *Micromedex 2.0*. Accessed March 20, 2015. http://www.micromedexsolutions.com/home/dispatch.

51. UpToDate. 2015. Accessed March 12, 2015. http://www.uptodate.com/home.

52. US Food and Drug Administration. 2008. "Information for Healthcare Professionals: Conventional Antipsychotics." Accessed January 14, 2015. http://www.fda.gov/Drugs/DrugSafety/PostmarketDrugSafetyInformationforPatientsandProviders/ucm124830.htm.

53. US Food and Drug Administration. 2015. "Zyprexa Relprevv (Olanzapine Pamoate): Drug Safety Communication - FDA Investigating Two Deaths Following Injection." Accessed January 14, 2015. www.fda.gov/Safety/MedWatch/SafetyInformation/SafetyAlertsforHumanMedicalProducts/ucm357601.htm.

54. US National Library of Medicine. 2015. "Drugs and Lactation Database (LactMed)." Accessed February 3, 2015. http://toxnet.nlm.nih.gov/newtoxnet/lactmed.htm.

55. US National Library of Medicine. 2015. "Toxicology Data Network." Accessed March 17, 2015. http://toxnet.nlm.nih.gov.

56. Wegmann, J. 2008. *Psychopharmacology: Straight Talk on Mental Health Medications*. 9–28. Eau Claire: Pesi, LLC.

57. Zeier, K., R. Connell, W. Resch, and C. Thomas. 2013. "Recommendations for lab monitoring of atypical antipsychotics." *Current Psychiatry* 12(9):51–54.

Chapter 9
Side Effects of Psychiatric Medication

Psychiatric medications are associated with numerous side effects, which is one of the major causes of noncompliance.[13] To improve compliance, clinicians should educate the patient about potential side effects and suggest ways to combat them.

The most common side effects encountered in clinical practice caused or exacerbated by psychiatric medication include[28]:

- EPS
- Restless leg syndrome
- Tourette syndrome
- Sexual dysfunction
- Weight gain

Disorders/Side Effects Caused by Psychiatric Medication
Extrapyramidal Symptoms (EPS)[28,30]
Extrapyramidal symptoms (EPS) are abnormally-induced movement disorders caused by the antagonism of dopamine receptors by antipsychotic medications. EPS is more common with first-generation (typical) antipsychotics than second generation (atypical) antipsychotics.[30]

<u>Forms of EPS</u>
EPS include[28,30]:

- Akinesia
- Akathisia
- Dystonia
- Pseudoparkinsonism
- Tardive dyskinesia (TD)

Akinesia
Absence/impairment of voluntary movement[13]
Management:
- Modification of antipsychotic drug regimen
- Switch to a low-potency FGA or to SGA
Medications:
- Trihexyphenidyl, benztropine, diphenhydramine, etc.
Akathisia
A movement disorder characterized by feelings of inner restlessness and constant motion[30]
Symptoms: Feelings of anxiety, inability to relax, pacing, fidgeting, rocking movements, jitteriness
Management:
- Modification of antipsychotic drug regimen including reducing dose of culprit antipsychotic

- Switch to a low-potency FGA or to SGA with low potential of akathisia (e.g., quietapine)
- In severe cases, clozapine may be used[13]

Medications:

- Propranolol: non-selective β-adrenergic antagonist used as first-line anti-akathisia agent for decades—recommended dose 10–80 mg/day bid
- Mirtazapine: low-dose mirtazapine, 15 mg qd, has the most supportive evidence as initial treatment
- Mianserin: 15 mg qd
- Cyproheptadine: 8–16 mg/day
- Other options:
  - Anticholinergic agents (e.g., biperiden, trihexyphenidyl, benzatropine)
  - Benzos, alone or in combination

Important notes:

- Avoid co-administration of benzos with mirtazapine, mianserin, or cyproheptadine due to risk of CNS depression[27,30]

Dystonia

Sustained muscle contractions that cause twisting and repetitive movements[13,19]

Symptoms: Neck spasm, speech difficulties, uncontrolled blinking, uncontrolled tongue and jaw twisting

Treatment:

- Botulinum toxin for focal dystonias
- Trihexyphenidyl, benztropine, diphenhydramine, benzos

Pseudo-parkinsonism

Symptoms: Drug-induced Parkinson's-like symptoms such as masked face, tremors, shuffling gait, and cogwheel rigidity[13]

Treatment: Includes reducing dose or/and adding anticholinergic agents (e.g., biperiden, trihexyphenidyl, benztropine)

Tardive dyskinesia (TD)

Severe movement disorder developing months, years, or even decades after antipsychotic medication (especially with typical antipsychotics)

Symptoms: Facial grimacing, finger movement, jaw swinging, tremor, repetitive chewing, tongue thrusting

Treatment: Usually preventative[13,19,36]

Important notes: The risk of TD is greater in persons on antipsychotic drugs for long periods and who are over age 45

Medications for EPS

Amantadine[2,7,11,12,13,18,25,27,28,29,31,32,33,34,35]

Brand name: Symmetrel, Endantadine

FDA approved for: Parkinson's disease, influenza A treatment and prophylaxis, medication-induced EPS

Other potential uses (off-label): cocaine withdrawal, medication-induced sexual dysfunction, NMS, RLS

Medication forms: *Tab* (100 mg); *cap* (100mg); *oral sol* (50 mg/5 ml [480-ml bottle])

Dosage:

- Drug-induced EPS: 100 mg bid, can be increased based on tolerance/response to max 300 mg/day

MOA: May release dopamine and norepinephrine from storage sites and inhibit their reuptake

Pharmacokinetics: t_{max}=2–4 hrs, $t_{1/2}$=10–25 hrs

Warnings:

- May be fatal in overdose and increase the risk of suicide attempts
- May cause CHF, peripheral edema, orthostatic hypotension, and increase risk of seizures
- Can cause poor impulse control or impulsive behavior; use caution with prior history of psychotic or neurotic disorders
- Monitor for development of melanoma

Drug interactions:

- Use caution with CNS stimulant drugs
- Can increase risk of CNS effects if used with alcohol
- Use with potassium chloride can cause GI lesions
- Use with mefloquine can cause QT prolongation
- Reduce dose of anticholinergic drugs prior to initiation
- Increased plasma concentration with dyazide (triamterene/hydrochlorothiazide)
- Use with thioridazine may exacerbate tremor

Common side effects: Dizziness, hallucinations, headache, insomnia, lightheadedness, nausea, nervousness

Contraindications: Hypersensitivity, angle-closure glaucoma

Recommended lab tests: Serum creatinine, BUN

Overdose: Cardiac toxicity, hallucinations, psychosis, hypotension, acute lung injury, hypokalemia, lethargy, ataxia, and seizures; OD potentially fatal

Tapering/withdrawal: Increased risk of Parkinsonism and NMS with abrupt withdrawal; slow taper recommended

Special Populations:

Pregnancy: Risk Category C

Lactation: Contraindicated

Elderly: Lower dose recommended

Hepatic impairment: No dose adjustment necessary

Renal impairment: Lower dose based on renal function
Important notes:
* Useful for chorea associated with Huntington's Disease

Baclofen[2,7,11,12,13,18,23,25,27,28,31,33,34,35]
Brand name: Gablofen, Lioresal
FDA approved for: MS, muscle spasm, spasticity, spinal cord lesions
Other potential uses (off-label): Cerebral palsy, chronic hiccups, EPS
Medication forms: *Tab* (10, 20 mg); *oral sol* (5 mg/5 ml, 10 mg/5 ml, 10 mg/20 ml); *injectable* (0.05, 0.5, 2 mg/ml)
Dosage:
* Drug-induced EPS: 5 mg tid initially, max 40–80mg/day
MOA: Analogue of GABA; stimulates GABA-receptors and inhibits release of glutamate and aspartate
Pharmacokinetics: t_{max}=2 hrs, $t_{1/2}$=3–4 hrs
Warnings:
* May cause profound dizziness and drowsiness and impair mental/physical performance
* Ovarian cysts reported in MS patient
Drug interactions:
* Use with opiates, sodium oxybate, or other CNS depressants can cause severe CNS depression
Common side effects: Confusion, constipation, dizziness, drowsiness, fatigue, frequent urination, headache, hypotension, insomnia, nausea, sedation, weakness
Contraindications: Hypersensitivity
Recommended lab tests: EEG in patients with epilepsy
Overdose: Bradycardia, hypotension, coma, respiratory failure, seizures, mydriasis, flaccidity
Tapering/withdrawal: Slow tapering necessary; hallucinations and seizure can occur on abrupt withdrawal
Special populations
Pregnancy: Risk Category C
Lactation: Use caution
Elderly: Use caution
Hepatic impairment: No dose adjustment necessary
Renal impairment: Lower dose recommended

Benztropine[2,5,7,11,12,13,18,25,27,28,31,33,34,35]
Brand name: Cogentin
FDA approved for: Parkinsonism, tremor, EPS due to neuroleptic drugs

Other potential uses (off-label): Drooling
Medication forms: *Tab* (0.5, 1, 2 mg); *injectable sol* (1 mg/ml)
Dosage:

- Parkinsonism: 0.5–2 mg/day po/IV/IM hs or divided, max 6 mg/day
- Drug-induced EPS: 1–4 mg IV/IM/po qd or bid
- Acute dystonia: 1–2 mg IV, then 1–2 mg po bid

MOA: Antimuscarinic, antihistaminic, and local anesthetic effects; also blocks dopamine reuptake
Pharmacokinetics: t_{max}=1–2 hrs, $t_{1/2}$=12–24 hours
Warnings:

- Do not use for management of TD
- May aggravate myasthenia gravis
- Use caution in angle-closure glaucoma and BPH
- May impair mental/physical abilities
- Use caution during hot weather due to risk of anhidrosis

Drug interactions:

- Use with potassium chloride may result in risk of GI lesions
- May cause paralytic ileus, hyperthermia, and heat stroke with phenothiazines and/or TCAs

Common side effects: Blurred vision, constipation, drowsiness, dry mouth, hyperthermia, nausea, paralytic ileus, tachycardia, psychosis, urinary retention, vomiting
Contraindications: Hypersensitivity, children under 3 years
Recommended lab tests: None
Overdose: Agitated delirium, psychosis, hallucinations, seizures, hyperthermia, and coma **Tapering/withdrawal:** Gradual taper recommended
Special populations:
Pregnancy: Risk Category C
Lactation: Avoid
Elderly: Initiate at lower dose
Hepatic impairment: No dose adjustment necessary
Renal impairment: No dose adjustment necessary

Biperiden[2,7,11,12,13,18,25,27,28,31,33,34,35]
Brand name: Akineton
FDA approved for: Discontinued in US—Parkinsonism, drug-induced EPS
Other potential uses (off-label): Catatonia, drooling
Medication forms: *Tab* (2 mg); *injectable* (5 mg/ml)
Dosage:

- Drug-induced EPS: 2 mg bid–tid

MOA: Antagonism of acetylcholine at cholinergic receptors in the corpus striatum; also antisecretory, antispasmodic, mydriatic, and nicotinolytic activity

Pharmacokinetics: t_{max}=1.5 hrs, $t_{1/2}$=18–24 hrs

Warnings:

- Use caution in angle-closure glaucoma
- May worsen urinary obstruction in elderly patients

Drug Interactions:

- Use with potassium chloride may result in risk of GI lesions

Common side effects: Blurred vision, constipation, drowsiness, dry mouth, urinary retention

Contraindications: Hypersensitivity, bowel obstruction, megacolon

Recommended lab tests: None

Overdose: Delirium, psychosis, hallucinations, seizures, hyperthermia, and coma

Tapering/withdrawal: Gradual taper recommended

Special populations:

Pregnancy: Risk Category C

Lactation: Avoid

Elderly: Use caution

Hepatic/Renal impairment: Data unavailable; use caution

Important notes:

- May impair heat regulation

Diphenhydramine[11,18,27]

(Refer to *Chapter 10: Sleep Disorders and Hypnotics* for further details)

Other potential uses (off-label): Drug-induced EPS, morning sickness

Dosage:

- Parkinsonism
  - *Oral:* 25 mg tid initially, then 50 mg qid, can be increased based on tolerance/response to max 300 mg/day
  - *IM/IV:* 25–50 mg per dose, can be increased based on tolerance/response to max 400 mg/day

Trihexyphenidyl[2,7,11,12,13,18,21,25,27,28,31,33,34,35]

Brand name: Artane

FDA approved for: Parkinson's disease, drug-induced EPS

Other potential uses (off-label): Drooling

Medication forms: *Tab* (2, 5 mg); *elixir* (2 mg/5 ml)

Dosage:

- Parkinsonism: 1 mg/day initially, can be increased to 5–15 mg/day divided
- Drug-induced EPS: 5–15 mg/day divided tid–qid

MOA: Inhibits the parasympathetic nervous system; relaxes smooth muscles
Pharmacokinetics: t_{max}=1.3 hrs, $t_{1/2}$=33 hrs
Warnings:
- Use caution in myasthenia gravis, glaucoma, and GI obstruction disorders
- Use caution in BPH; can cause urinary retention, especially in elderly

Drug interactions:
- Intensified anticholinergic effects with MAOIs and TCA
- Involuntary movement is increased with levodopa
- Increased sedation with CNS depressants or alcohol
- Increased risk of TD with anticholinergics or neuroleptics

Common side effects: Blurred vision, constipation, dizziness, drowsiness, dry mouth, nausea, nervousness, urinary retention, vomiting
Contraindications: Hypersensitivity, angle-closure glaucoma
Recommended lab tests: LFTs, EKG, gonioscope evaluation prior to treatment initiation
Overdose: Agitated delirium, psychosis, hallucinations, seizures, hyperthermia, and coma **Tapering/withdrawal:** Gradual taper recommended; can cause NMS and exacerbate Parkinsonism upon abrupt withdrawal
Special populations:
Pregnancy: Risk Category B
Lactation: Avoid
Elderly: Lower dose recommended
Hepatic impairment: Lower dose recommended
Renal impairment: No dose adjustment necessary
Important notes:
- Use caution during hot weather due to risk of anhidrosis

Disorders Exacerbated by Psychiatric Medication

Restless Leg Syndrome[4,8,14,27]
Restless leg syndrome (RLS) is a neurologic, motor, and sensory impairment of the limbs primarily occurring in the evenings, often disturbing sleep.[14] Etiological factors include genetic predisposition, central dopaminergic pathway impairment, impaired iron metabolism/homeostasis, and use of psychiatric medications including neuroleptics and SSRIs.[4,8]
Symptoms: Irresistible urge to move legs, especially at night
Treatment:
- Stop medication(s) responsible for RLS
- Maintain proper sleep hygiene
- Avoid caffeine, alcohol, and nicotine

- Initiate iron supplementation if iron deficiency present
- Medications: ropinirole, pramipexole, bromocriptine [4]

Tourette Syndrome[19,26,27]

Tourette syndrome is an early-childhood-onset neuropsychiatric disorder involving motor and vocal tics which can create embarrassment for the individual and others.[19] The syndrome is more common in males than females.[27] Etiology includes genetic predisposition as well as the involvement of basal ganglia and dopamine.[26] Due to a lack of studies, infection cannot be ruled out as an etiological factor.

Symptoms: Tics (eye blinking, running), vocalizing repetitive words or phrases, vulgarity

Treatment:
- Family/patient education
- Medications (for severe cases)[26]:
  - Alpha-2 adrenergic agonists: clonidine, guanfacine
  - Dopamine-receptor blocking agents: neuroleptics
  - Clonazepam
  - Baclofen
  - Tetrabenazine

Sexual Dysfunction[1,13,15,22,27,29]

Psychiatric drugs are often associated with sexual dysfunction. Among antidepressants, those with strong serotonergic properties have the highest rate of sexual side effects.[15] SSRIs are notorious for causing sexual dysfunction due to reduced dopamine and norepinephine activity caused by serotonin inhibition.[1] Among antipsychotics, those with greater dopamine blockade can cause sexual dysfunction. Certain antidepressants (e.g., nefazodone, bupropion, mirtazapine, agomelatine, transdermal selegiline) and newer atypical antipsychotics are less likely to cause sexual side effects.[27] The frequency of sexual side effects from SSRI/SNRI antidepressants in males is extremely high at around 30–40%.[15,18]

Symptoms:
- *Males:* Decreased libido, erectile dysfunction, reduced spermatogenesis, gynecomastia, reduced ejaculation
- *Females:* Decreased libido, menstrual irregularities, galactorrhea

Treatment:
- Switch to a psychiatric drug that has low or no risk for sexual side effects
- Medication holidays on weekends or other times
- Medications: Amantadine, bethanechol, bromocriptine, bupropion, cyproheptadine, sildenafil citrate

Medications for Sexual Dysfunction
Amantadine[11,18,27]
(Refer to *Medications for EPS* in this chapter for further details)
Other potential uses (off-label): Medication-induced sexual dysfunction, cocaine withdrawal, NMS, RLS
Dosage:
- Medication-induced sexual dysfunction: 200 mg po daily

Bethanechol[2,7,11,12,13,16,18,25,27,28,31,33,34,35]
Brand name: Duvoid, Urecholine
FDA approved for: Bladder problems
Other potential uses (off-label): Sexual dysfunction
Medication forms: *Tab* (5, 10, 25, 50 mg)
Dosage:
- Sexual dysfunction:10–20 mg 2 hrs before sexual activity

MOA: Mixed central and peripheral cholinergic agonist; also has adrenergic effects
Pharmacokinetics: t_{max}=1–1.5 hrs, $t_{1/2}$=2 hrs
Warnings:
- May cause HSR and can cause UTIs from bladder contraction

Drug interaction:
- Use caution with ganglion-blocking compounds due to risk of hypotension
- Increased effect with ambenonium through synergism; may cause life-threatening side effects

Common side effects: Belching, bronchial constriction, colicky pain, diarrhea, flushing, headache, lacrimation, urinary frequency
Contraindications: Hyperthyroidism, peptic ulcer, asthma, bradycardia or hypotension, vasomotor instability, coronary-artery disease, AV-conduction defects, epilepsy, GI obstruction, Parkinsonism, hypersensitivity, bladder-neck obstruction
Recommended lab tests: LFTs, RFTs, hematological tests, biochemical tests
Overdose: Early signs include abdominal discomfort, salivation, flushing, sweating, nausea/vomiting
Tapering/withdrawal: Gradual taper recommended
Special populations:
Pregnancy: Risk Category C
Lactation: Avoid
Elderly: Effect unknown; use caution
Hepatic impairment: Data unavailable; use caution
Renal impairment: No dose adjustment necessary

Important notes:
- Administer carefully in cases of urinary retention, allergy, surgery, peritonitis, hyperthyroidism

Bromocriptine[2,7,11,12,13,18,20,25,27,28,31,33,34,35]

Brand name: Parlodel, Cycloset

FDA approved for: Parkinson's disease, acromegaly, hyperprolactinemia, type 2 diabetes

Other potential uses (off-label): Sexual dysfunction, alcohol dependence, cocaine withdrawal, NMS

Medication forms: *Snap-tab* (2.5 mg); *tab* (0.8 mg); *cap* (5 mg)

Dosage:
- Sexual dysfunction: 1.25–2.5 mg hs initially, can be increased based on tolerance/ response to max 30 mg

MOA: Agonist at monoamine receptors (D_1, D_2, 5-HT, α- and β-adrenergic receptors)

Pharmacokinetics: t_{max}=1–3 hrs, $t_{1/2}$=6–20 hrs

Warnings:
- May cause orthostasis; monitor BP regularly
- Evaluate pituitary gland before treatment of hyperprolactinemia
- Avoid driving or operating machinery due to somnolence and/or episodes of sudden sleep onset
- Monitor visual fields in macroprolactinoma treatment
- Use caution in patients with psychosis or cardiovascular disease

Drug interactions:
- Phenothiazines, haloperidol, metoclopramide may decrease efficacy
- Avoid with triptans or alcohol due to profound additive vasoconstriction and increased side effects
- Decreases efficacy of nitrates through antagonism
- Increased plasma levels with strong inhibitors of CYP3A4 (e.g., ketoconazole, HIV protease inhibitors)
- Use with macrolide antibiotics (e.g., erythromycin) and octreotide increase levels of bromocriptine

Common side effects: Abdominal cramps, constipation, dizziness, drowsiness, fatigue, headache, hypotension, lightheadedness, nasal congestion, nausea, vomiting

Contraindications: Uncontrolled hypertension, pregnancy, postpartum period in women with history of cardiac disease, hypersensitivity to ergot alkaloids

Recommended lab tests: Blood tests, LFTs, RFTs, serum prolactin levels, brain CT or MRI, fundus examination, pregnancy test

Overdose: Nausea, vomiting, constipation, diaphoresis, dizziness, pallor, severe hypotension, malaise, confusion, lethargy, drowsiness, delusions, hallucinations, repetitive yawning

Tapering/withdrawal: Gradual taper recommended

Special populations:

Pregnancy: Risk Category B

Lactation: Contraindicated

Elderly: Lower dose recommended

Hepatic impairment: Use caution

Renal impairment: No data available; use caution

Important notes:

- Excessive usage associated with uncontrollable sexual urges

Bupropion[11,18,27]

(Refer to *Chapter 4: Depressive Disorders and Antidepressants* for further details)

Other potential uses (off-label): ADHD, bipolar depression, sexual dysfunction

Dosage:

- Sexual dysfunction: 150–300 mg daily or 75–150 mg as needed

Cyproheptadine[1, 2,7,9,11,12,13,18,25,27,28,31,34,35]

Brand name: Periactin

FDA approved for: Seasonal allergies, conjunctivitis, dermatographism, angioedema

Other potential uses (off-label): Drug-induced sexual dysfunction, anorexia nervosa, loss of appetite

Medication forms: *Tab* (4 mg); *syrup* (2 mg/5 ml)

Dosage:

- Drug-induced sexual dysfunction: 4–12 mg 1–2 hrs before anticipated coitus or 2–16 mg/day

MOA: Antagonizes 5-HT_2 receptors; also has antihistaminic and anticholinergic properties

Pharmacokinetics: t_{max}=6–9 hrs, $t_{1/2}$=12 hrs

Warnings:

- Higher incidence of HSR
- May cause anticholinergic side effects, especially in elderly
- Use caution in history of bronchial asthma, increased IOP, hyperthyroidism, cardiovascular disease, or hypertension

Drug interactions:

- Do not prescribe within 2 weeks of using MAOIs
- Potentiates CNS-depressant actions of alcohol, barbiturates, sedatives, neuroleptics, and other CNS depressants

Common side effects: CNS depression, drowsiness, dry mouth, ECG changes, GI distress, heart block, hepatitis, impaired coordination, muscle weakness, nausea, psychosis, sedation, somnolence, weight gain

Contraindications: Hypersensitivity, newborn/premature infants, nursing mothers, elderly, angle-closure glaucoma, peptic ulcer, prostatic hypertrophy, bladder obstruction, concurrent MAOI use, pyloroduodenal obstruction

Recommended lab tests: Plasma cortisol level

Overdose: Hallucinations, depression, convulsion, respiratory or cardiac arrest, dry mouth, flushing, blurred vision, dizziness, hypotension

Tapering/withdrawal: Tapering recommended

Special populations:

Pregnancy: Risk Category B

Lactation: Contraindicated

Elderly: Contraindicated

Hepatic impairment: No dose adjustment necessary

Renal impairment: No dose adjustment necessary

Important notes:

- Drug of choice for sexual dysfunction caused by SSRIs

Sildenafil citrate[2,7,11,12,13,18,24,25,27,28,31,33,34,35]

Brand names: Revatio, Viagra

FDA approved for: Erectile dysfunction, pulmonary artery hypertension

Other potential uses (off-label): Drug-induced impotence, sexual dysfunction

Medication forms: *Tab* (20, 25, 50, 100 mg)*; injectable sol* (10 mg/12.5 ml)*; oral suspension* (10 mg/ml)

Dosage:

- Erectile dysfunction:
  - *Viagra:* 50 mg po 1 hr before sexual activity, can be increased based on tolerance/response to max 100 mg/day
  - *Revatio* 10 mg injection equals 20 mg oral Viagra

MOA: Inhibits PDE-5, causing increased levels of cGMP; relaxes smooth muscle and causes increased blood to corpus cavernosum

Pharmacokinetics: t_{max}=0.5–2 hrs, $t_{1/2}$=3–4 hrs, onset of action=60 min, duration of action=2–4 hrs, absorption slowed with high-fat meal

Warnings:

- Use caution with pre-existing cardiac disease (e.g., MI, CHF)
- May impair hearing and lead to tinnitus or incoordination
- May cause sudden visual loss due to ischemic optic neuropathy
- Advise patients to seek emergency treatment if erection lasts 4 hours or more
- Use caution with alpha-blockers or anti-hypertensive due to risk of hypotension

Drug interactions:
- Avoid with any other PDE-5 inhibitors and protease inhibitors
- Can potentiate hypotensive effects of nitrates, alpha-blockers, anti-hypertensives
- Increased exposure with CYP3A4 inhibitors (e.g., ritonavir, ketoconazole, itraconazole, erythromycin)

Common side effects: Abnormal vision, dyspepsia, flushing, headache, nasal congestion, nausea, rash

Contraindications: Hypersensitivity, concomitant nitrates

Recommended lab tests: Monitor BP and HR

Overdose: Similar to side effects of lower doses but rates and severities increased

Tapering/withdrawal: Gradual taper recommended

Special populations:

Pregnancy:
- Revatio: Risk Category B
- Viagra: Not for use in women

Lactation: Contraindicated

Elderly: Lower dose recommended

Hepatic impairment: Lower dose recommended

Renal impairment: Lower dose recommended

Important notes:
- Warn patients about the symptoms of priapism

Weight Gain[3,10,27]

Weight gain is the most common side effect of psychtropic medication use and should be considered worrisome, as it can cause many other systemic problems, including metabolic syndrome.[27] Psychiatric drugs interfere with CNS functions that regulate energy balance, appetite, and food cravings. Appetite and feeding are regulated via the hypothalamus by a complex group of neurochemicals.[10] Some psychotropics can cause weight gain despite reduced appetite by altering metabolic rates. Psychotropic-induced weight gain may be related to the their effects on peptide hormones (e.g., leptin, ghrelin, and adiponectin) and antagonism of H_1, $5-HT_{2C}$, and D_2 receptors.[3]

Treatment:
- Counsel all patients about healthy diet and regular exercise
- CBT may be a helpful intervention
- Dosage adjustments or cross-taper to more weight-neutral medication
- Sometimes patients may benefit from addition of a weight loss medication

Medications for Weight Gain

The drugs used to treat medication-induced weight gain are: amantadine, fluoxetine, and topiramate.

Amantadine[10,11,18,27,29]
(Refer to *Medications for EPS* in this chapter for further details)
Dosage:
- Drug-induced weight gain:100–300 mg daily

Fluoxetine (Prozac)[10,11,18,27]
(Refer to *Chapter 4: Depressive Disorders and Antidepressants* for further details)
Dosage:
- Drug-induced weight gain:20–60 mg daily

Important notes:
- Can lead to a mild degree of weight loss for 6 weeks in usual doses and up to 20 weeks in high doses but then a tolerance may develop

Topiramate (Topamax)[10,11,18,27]
(Refer to *Chapter 5: Bipolar Disorder and Mood Stabilizers* for further details)
Dosage:
- Drug-induced weight gain: 25–50 mg/day initially, increase to max 100–200 mg/day

Other weight-loss medications include[10,11,18,27]:
Benzphetamine (Didrex)[10]
Dosage: 25–50 mg po qd–tid

Diethylpropion (Tenuate)[10]
Dosage:
- *IR tab:* 25 mg tid for short-term use
- *XR tab:* 75 mg/day

Lorcaserin (Belviq)[10]
Dosage: 10 mg bid, max 20 mg/day

Metformin (Glucophage, Glumetza, Glucophage XR, Fortamet)[6]
Dosage: 500 mg bid or 850 mg/day

Naltrexone/bupropion ER (Contrave)[10]
Dosage: 1–2 (8 mg/90 mg) tab bid, max 32 mg/360 mg daily

Orlistat (Xenical, Alli)[10]
Dosage:
- Rx: 120 mg tid with each fat-containing meal
- OTC: 60 mg tid

Phendimetrazine (Bontril)[10]
Dosage:
- *IR tab:* 35 mg bid–tid 1 hr before meals
- *SR cap:* 105 mg/day before breakfast

Phentermine (Adipex-P, Suprenza)[10]
Dosage:
- *Tab*: 18.75–37.5 mg/daily
- *ODT cap*: 15–30 mg/daily (only for short-term use)

Phentermine/topiramate ER (Qsymia)[10]
Dosage: 3.75 mg/23 mg daily for 14 days, followed with 7.5 mg/46 mg daily for 12 weeks, max 15 mg/92 mg

References:

1. Aizenberg, D., Z. Zemishlany, and A. Weizman. 1995. "Cyproheptadine treatment of sexual dysfunction induced by serotonin reuptake inhibitors." *Clin Neuropharmacol* 18:320–324.

2. Albers, Lawrence J., Rhoda K. Hahn, and Christopher Reist. 2010. *Handbook of Psychiatric Drugs.* 2011 ed. 39–59. Current Clinical Strategies Publishing.

3. Allison, D. B., J. L. Mentore, M. Heo, L. P. Chandler, J. C. Cappelleri, M. C. Infante, and P. J. Weiden. 1999. "Antipsychotic-induced weight gain: a comprehensive research synthesis." *Am J Psychiatry* 156(11):1686–1696.

4. Aurora, R. Nisha, David A. Kristo, Sabin R. Bista, James A. Rowley, Rochelle S. Zak, Kenneth R. Casey, Carin I. Lamm, Sharon L. Tracy, and Richard S. Rosenberg. 2012. "Update to the AASM Clinical Practice Guideline: "The Treatment of Restless Legs Syndrome and Periodic Limb Movement Disorder in Adults—An Update for 2012: Practice Parameters with an Evidence-Based Systematic Review and Meta-Analyses" *Sleep* 35(8):1039–1062. doi: 10.5665/sleep.1986.

5. Bayshore Pharmaceuticals, LLC. 2014. "BENZTROPINE MESYLATE- benztropine mesylate tablet." US National Library of Medicine: Daily Med. Accessed December 18, 2014. http://dailymed.nlm.nih.gov/dailymed/drugInfo.cfm?setid=298f140d-b4e4-4cc6-a304-b32eaba3f0b0.

6. Bristol-Myers Squibb Company. 2014. "GLUCOPHAGE- metformin hydrochloride tablet, film coated." US National Library of Medicine: Daily Med. Accessed December 18, 2014. http://dailymed.nlm.nih.gov/dailymed/drugInfo.cfm?setid=4a0166c7-7097-4e4a-9036-6c9a60d08fc6.

7. Center Watch. 2015. "FDA Approved Drugs by Therapeutic Area." Accessed February 3, 2015. http://www.centerwatch.com/drug-information/fda-approved-drugs/therapeutic-area/17/psychiatry-psychology.

8. Chahine, L.M., and Z.N. Chemali. 2006. "Restless legs syndrome: a review." *CNS Spectr* 11(7):511–520. Accessed February 2, 2015. http://www.ncbi.nlm.nih.gov/pubmed/16816791.

9. C.O. Truxton, Inc. 2014. "CYPROHEPTADINE HYDROCHLORIDE - cyproheptadine hydrochloride tablet." US National Library of Medicine: Daily Med. Accessed December 18, 2014. http://dailymed.nlm.nih.gov/dailymed/drugInfo.cfm?setid=a071c63a-1162-4c1b-a73e-26068e0e9542.

10. Drugs.com. 2015. "Prescription Weight Loss Drugs." Accessed April 1, 2015. http://www.drugs.com/article/prescription-weight-loss-drugs.html.

11. Elsevier Gold Standard, Inc. 2015. "Clinical Pharmacology." Accessed March 12, 2015. https://www.clinicalpharmacology.com.

12. Epocrates. 2015. Accessed March 25, 2015. https://online.epocrates.com.

13. Gabbard, Glen O., ed. 2007. *Gabbard's Treatments of Psychiatric Disorders*. 4th ed. 641–655. Washington, DC: American Psychiatric Publishing.

14. Garcia-Borreguero, Diego, Ralf Kohnen, Michael H. Silber, John W. Winkelman, Christopher J. Earley, Birgit Högl, Mauro Manconi, Jacques Montplaisir, Yuichi Inoue, and Richard P. Allen. 2013. "The long-term treatment of restless legs syndrome/Willis–Ekbom disease: evidence-based guidelines and clinical consensus best practice guidance: a report from the International Restless Legs Syndrome Study Group." *Sleep Medicine* 14(7):675–684. doi: 10.1016/j.sleep.2013.05.016.

15. Gitlin, M. 2003. "Sexual dysfunction with psychotropic drugs." *Expert Opin Pharmacother* 4(12):2259–2269. doi: 10.1517/14656566.4.12.2259.

16. Lannett Company, Inc. 2014. "BETHANECHOL CHLORIDE- bethanechol chloride tablet." US National Library of Medicine: Daily Med. Accessed December 18, 2014. http://dailymed.nlm.nih.gov/dailymed/drugInfo.cfm?setid=cb6a43e9-5663-47e1-8f77-ed4cb806436d.

17. Medscape: Drugs & Diseases. 2015. "Dystonia Tardive" Accessed January 14, 2015. http://emedicine.medscape.com/article/287230-overview.

18. Medscape: Drugs & Diseases. 2015. "Psychiatrics." Accessed February 3, 2015. http://reference.medscape.com/drugs/psychiatrics.

19. Medscape: Drugs & Diseases. 2015. "Tourette Syndrome and Other Tic Disorders." Accessed February 10, 2015. http://emedicine.medscape.com/article/1182258-overview.

20. Mylan Pharmaceuticals, Inc. 2014. "BROMOCRIPTINE MESYLATE- bromocriptine mesylate tablet." US National Library of Medicine: Daily Med. Accessed December 18, 2014. http://dailymed.nlm.nih.gov/dailymed/drugInfo.cfm?setid=72d8eefe-c066-41b6-8922-9586f1cf47a1.

21. Natco Pharma Ltd. 2013. "TRIHEXYPHENIDYL HYDROCHLORIDE - trihexyphenidyl hydrochloride tablet." US National Library of Medicine: Daily Med. Accessed December 18, 2014. http://dailymed.nlm.nih.gov/dailymed/drugInfo.cfm?setid=b7e4200c-feff-4537-aad1-cf9989fd8c14.

22. Norden, M.J. 1994. "Buspirone treatment of sexual dysfunction associated with selective serotonin re-uptake inhibitors." *Depression* 2(2):109–112.

23. Novartis Pharmaceuticals Corporation. 2014. "LIORESAL- baclofen tablet." US National Library of Medicine: Daily Med. Accessed December 18, 2014. http://dailymed.nlm.nih.gov/dailymed/drugInfo.cfm?setid=c59b086d-8e2a-47fa-ae4f-135e65c37337.

24. Pfizer, Inc. 2014. "VIAGRA- sildenafil citrate tablet, film coated." US National Library of Medicine: Daily Med. Accessed December 18, 2014. http://dailymed.nlm.nih.gov/dailymed/drugInfo.cfm?setid=0b0be196-0c62-461c-94f4-9a35339b4501.

25. RxList. 2015. "Drugs A-Z List." Accessed March 25, 2015. http://www.rxlist.com/drugs/alpha_a.htm.

26. Scahill, Lawrence, Gerald Erenberg, Cheston M. Berlin, Cathy Budman, Barbara J. Coffey, Joseph Jankovic, Louise Kiessling, Robert A. King, Roger Kurlan, Anthony Lang, Jonathan Mink, Tanya Murphy, Samual Zinner, and John Walkup. 2006. "Contemporary assessment and pharmacotherapy of Tourette syndrome." *NeuroRx* 3(2):192–206. doi: 10.1016/j.nurx.2006.01.009.

27. Schatzberg, A.F., and C.B. Nemeroff, eds. 2009. *The American Psychiatric Publishing Textbook of Psychopharmacology*. 4th ed. 695–808. Washington, DC: American Psychiatric Publishing.

28. Schatzberg, A.F., Jonathan O. Cole, and Charles DeBattista. 2010. *Manual of Clinical Psychopharmacology*. 7th ed. 17–19, 281–357. Washington, DC: American Psychiatric Publishing.

29. Shrivastava, R.K., S. Shrivastava, N. Overweg, M. Schmitt. 1995. "Amantadine in the treatment of sexual dysfunction associated with selective serotonin reuptake inhibitors" [letter]. *J Clin Psychopharmacol* 15:83–84.

30. Stanilla, J.K., and G.M. Simpson. 2009. "Drugs to treat extrapyramidal side effects." In *The American Psychiatric Publishing Textbook of Psychopharmacology*. 4th ed. Edited by A.F. Schatzberg and C.B. Nemeroff. 69–92. Washington, DC: American Psychiatric Publishing.

31. Truven Health Analytics. 2015. *Micromedex 2.0*. Accessed March 20, 2015. http://www.micromedexsolutions.com/home/dispatch.

32. Upsher-Smith Laboratories, Inc. 2014. "AMANTADINE HYDROCHLORIDE- amantadine hydrochloride tablet." US National Library of Medicine: Daily Med. Accessed December 18, 2014. http://dailymed.nlm.nih.gov/dailymed/drugInfo.cfm?setid=63d9d4aa-5f92-45b0-98d0-d6ec38b727cb.

33. UpToDate. 2015. Accessed March 12, 2015. http://www.uptodate.com/home.

34. US National Library of Medicine. 2015. "Drugs and Lactation Database (LactMed)." Accessed February 3, 2015. http://toxnet.nlm.nih.gov/newtoxnet/lactmed.htm.

35. US National Library of Medicine. 2015. "Toxicology Data Network." Accessed March 17, 2015. http://toxnet.nlm.nih.gov.

36. Waln, Olga, and Joseph Jankovic. 2013. "An Update on Tardive Dyskinesia: From Phenomenology to Treatment." *Tremor Other Hyperkinet Mov* 3: doi: tre-03-161-4138-1.

Chapter 10
Sleep Disorders And Hypnotics

Sleep plays a vital role in restoring body systems, processing memory, and maintaining normal motor and cognitive function.[4] Sleep disorders are one of the most common problems in clinical practice.[10] Between 20–40% of US adults report difficulty sleeping, and approximately 20% experience chronic insomnia.[22,38] Between 50–70 million people in the US suffer from a chronic sleep disorder which affects their daily functioning, impairing their health and longevity.[10] Primary insomnia is more prevalent in women, with a female to male ratio of 3:2.[18]

Symptoms of insomnia include[4,10]:

- Difficulty initiating or maintaining sleep
- Excessive daytime sleepiness
- Early morning awakening
- Difficulty concentrating
- Irritability
- Fatigue
- Tiredness
- Snoring

Numerous psychiatric, medical, and environmental factors can cause sleep problems.[22] Such psychiatric conditions include depression, anxiety, mania, PTSD, substance abuse, and others.[18,38] Chronic medical conditions such as CHF, COPD, pain conditions, etc., are linked to sleep problems as well. Environmental issues such as stress, shift work, and poor sleep hygiene can also lead to poor sleep.[10]

Diagnosis of a sleep disorder is made after a clinical evaluation of sleep history and a detailed assessment of medical, substance abuse, and psychiatric history.[19] Management includes psychotherapy, pharmacotherapy, and helpful environmental changes.[22,38] Other modalities of treatment include biofeedback, sleep diaries, dietary modifications, exercise, and education about good sleep hygiene.[31] Sleep medication should be started at a low dose and maintained at the minimum effective dose for the shortest period of time.[19,33]

Hypnotics

Benzodiazepine Hypnotics
Benzodiazepines (benzos) are the most widely prescribed hypnotics in the US.[32] Drugs in this class exert their effects by enhancing GABA at $GABA_A$ receptors, which reduces neuronal activity, creating sedation and calming effects.

Class Profile[13,14,18,19,21,26,31,32,34,44]
MOA: Binds to benzodiazepine receptors at $GABA_A$, which is a major inhibitory neurotransmitter, resulting in decreased excitability of neurons and causing relaxation.

Warnings:

- Long-term use can cause dependence, tolerance, and withdrawal, even at therapeutic doses; gradual tapering is required due to risk of severe withdrawal symptoms, including seizure
- May cause CNS depression, impaired motor/cognitive performance, and memory loss
- Use with caution in patients with compromised pulmonary function, psychotic disorder, history of alcohol/substance abuse
- May cause emergence or worsening of depression; use with caution in patients with MDD or history of suicide ideations/attempts
- Can precipitate mania/hypomania and cause paradoxical reactions (aggression, hyperactivity)
- May increase seizure severity and/or frequency
- Use with alcohol can be deadly because they are cross-tolerant
- Evaluate for co-morbid diagnosis if insomnia persists after 7–10 days of use
- May cause severe anaphylactic/anaphylactoid reactions
- May prompt sleep-driving and eating while not fully awake
- Can reduce stage 4 (slow wave) sleep

Drug interactions:

- Increased CNS depression when taken with TCAs, MAOIs, anticonvulsants, antihistamines, alcohol, narcotics, methadone, barbiturates, opioid pain killers, buprenorphine, or other CNS depressants
- CYP3A inhibitors increase levels; inducers decrease levels
- Can cause seizures if used with flumazenil

Contraindications: Angle-closure glaucoma, untreated open-angle glaucoma, sleep apnea, myasthenia gravis, hypersensitivity, acute alcohol intoxication, concomitant use with sodium oxybate.

Recommended lab tests: Periodic LFTs, blood counts.

Overdose: Usually safe when used alone but potentially fatal with opiates and other CNS depressants. Symptoms include sedation, drowsiness, ataxia, slurred speech, and hypotonia.

Tapering/withdrawal: Slow taper needed if used for more than few weeks.

Special Populations:

Pregnancy: Risk Category D or X

Lactation: Avoid

Elderly: No dose adjustment necessary

Hepatic impairment: Use caution

Renal impairment: Use caution

Individual Drug Profiles

Estazolam [3,8,11,12,13,20,22,28,31,32,35,39,40,43]

Brand name: ProSom

FDA approved for: Short-term management of insomnia

Other potential uses (off-label): GAD

Medication forms: *Tab* (1, 2 mg)

Dosage:

- Sleep disorders:1–2 mg/day hs

MOA: Similar to *Benzo Class Profile*

Pharmacokinetics: t_{max}=2 hrs, $t_{1/2}$=10–24 hrs, metabolized primarily by liver

Warnings:

- Similar to *Benzo Class Profile*
- Can prompt amnesia

Drug interactions: Similar to *Benzo Class Profile*

Common side effects: Ataxia, dizziness, drowsiness, dry mouth, headache, hypokinesia, muscle weakness, somnolence

Contraindications: Pregnancy, concurrent use with ketoconazole or itraconazole

Important notes:

- Pregnancy risk Category X
- Long half-life; may accumulate in nightly administration causing cognitive/motor impairments
- Only administer if sleeping for 7–8 hours to avoid drowsiness and impaired performance

Flunitrazepam [11,20,35]

Brand name: Rohypnol

FDA approved for: None

Other potential uses (off-label): Drug withdrawal syndrome, insomnia, sleep disorder

Dosage:

- Insomnia: 1–2 mg hs

Important notes:

- Notoriously misused as a date rape drug due to potent hypnotic/amnestic effects

Flurazepam [3,8,11,12,13,20,22,28,31,32,35,39,40]

Brand name: Dalmane

FDA approved for: Insomnia characterized by difficulty falling asleep, frequent nocturnal awakening, and/or early morning awakening

Other potential uses (off-label): Anxiety
Medication forms: *Cap* (15, 30 mg)
Dosage:
- Sleep disorders: 15–30 mg/day hs

MOA: Similar to *Benzo Class Profile*
Pharmacokinetics: t_{max}=0.5–1 hr, $t_{1/2}$=2.3 hours, metabolized primarily by liver
Warnings: Similar to *Benzo Class Profile*
Drug interactions: Similar to *Benzo Class Profile*
Common side effects: Ataxia, confusion, depression, dizziness, drowsiness, fatigue, hangover, hyper-excitability, hypersalivation, hypotension, hypoventilation, lethargy, light-headedness, memory loss, sedation, somnolence
Contraindications:
- Similar to *Benzo Class Profile*
- Pregnancy

Lorazepam[11,20,35]
(Refer to *Chapter 6: Anxiety Disorders and Anxiolytics* for further details)
FDA approved for: Anxiety disorder, short-term relief of anxiety symptoms, anxiety associated with depressive symptoms, insomnia
Medication form: *Tab* (0.5, 1, 2 mg); *oral conc* (2 mg/ml); *injectable* (2, 4 mg/ml)
Dosage:
- Insomnia: 2–4 mg po qhs

Midazolam[3,5,8,11,12,13,20,22,28,31,32,35,39,40]
Brand name: Versed
FDA approved for: Sedation/anxiolysis/amnesia prior to or during diagnostic, therapeutic, or endoscopic procedures; preoperative amnesia; sedation amnesia
Other potential uses (off-label): Agitation, anxiety, insomnia, status epilepticus
Medication forms: Tab (7.5, 15 mg); *Injectable* (1, 5 mg/ml); *preservative-free injection* (2 mg/2ml); *syrup* (1, 2, 5 mg/ml)
Dosage:
- Insomnia: 7.5 mg to maximum of 15mg hs

MOA: Similar to *Benzo Class Profile*
Pharmacokinetics: t_{max} =approx 0.5 hr, $t_{1/2}$=2–6 hrs
Warnings:
- Similar to *Benzo Class Profile*
- **Black box warning:**
  - Associated with respiratory depression, airway obstruction, desaturation, hypoxia, and apnea when used concomitantly with other CNS depressants (e.g.,

opioids); should be used only in hospital or ambulatory care settings, including physicians' and dentists' offices, that can provide for continuous monitoring of respiratory and cardiac function

- Do not administer by rapid injection in neonates due to severe hypotension and seizure

Drug interactions: Similar to *Benzo Class Profile*

Common side effects: Apnea, ataxia, confusion, depression, dizziness, drowsiness, dry mouth, fatigue, hangover, headache, memory impairment, muscle weakness, nausea, nervousness, pain at injection site, psychomotor retardation, respiratory depression, slurred speech, somnolence

Contraindications: Similar to *Benzo Class Profile*

Important notes:
- Pregnancy risk Category D
- Very short acting drug; use only for patients with severe difficulty falling asleep
- Not effective for patients who have trouble staying asleep at night
- Indicated for acute management of psychosis or aggressive behavior alongside an antipsychotic

Quazepam[3,8,11,12,13,14,17,20,22,28,31,32,35,39,40]

Brand name: Doral, Dormalin

FDA approved for: Insomnia

Other potential uses (off-label): Anxiety disorders

Medication forms: *Tab* (7.5, 15 mg)

Dosage:
- Insomnia: 7.5–15 mg hs, may reduce dose after 1–2 nights

MOA: Similar to *Benzo Class Profile*

Pharmacokinetics: t_{max}=2 hrs, $t_{1/2}$=39 hrs

Warnings: Similar to *Benzo Class Profile*

Drug interactions: Similar to *Benzo Class Profile*

Common side effects: Dizziness, drowsiness, dry mouth, fatigue, headache, indigestion

Contraindications: Similar to *Benzo Class Profile*

Important notes:
- Unique mechanism of action compared to other benzos
- Next-day drowsiness can occur due to very long half-life[32]
- Fewer side effects than other benzos; less potential for dependence and rebound effects

Temazepam[2,3,8,11,12,13,20,22,28,31,32,35,39,40]

Brand name: Restoril

FDA approved for: Insomnia

Other potential uses (off-label): None
Medication forms: *Cap* (7.5, 15, 22.5, 30 mg)
Dosage:
- Insomnia: 15–30 mg qhs (use 7.5 mg qhs in debilitated patients)

MOA: Similar to *Benzo Class Profile*
Pharmacokinetics: t_{max}=1.5 hrs, $t_{1/2}$=8.8 hrs
Warnings: Similar to *Benzo Class Profile*
Drug interactions: Similar to *Benzo Class Profile*
Common side effects: Anxiety, dizziness, drowsiness, hangover, lethargy
Contraindications: Similar to *Benzo Class Profile*
Important notes[32]:
- Avoid in patients with hepatic dysfunction
- Preferred benzo, along with lorazepam, due to short half-life
- Should be taken approximately 1 hour before bedtime

Triazolam[3,8,11,12,13,20,22,27,28,31,32,35,39,40]
Brand name: Halcion
FDA approved for: Insomnia
Other potential uses (off-label): None
Medication forms: *Tab* (0.125, 0.25 mg)
Dosage:
- Insomnia: 0.125–0.25 mg qhs for 7–10 days

MOA: Similar to *Benzo Class Profile*
Pharmacokinetics: t_{max}=2 hrs, $t_{1/2}$=1.5–5.5 hrs
Warnings: Similar to *Benzo Class Profile*
Drug interactions:
- Similar to *Benzo Class Profile*
- Increased plasma concentration with isoniazid, OCP, ranitidine, grapefruit juice

Common side effects: Ataxia, dizziness, drowsiness, nausea, nervousness, vomiting
Contraindications:
- Similar to *Benzo Class Profile*
- Concurrent use with protease inhibitors

Important notes:
- Due to short half-life, not effective in patients with frequent nighttime awakening
- Significant abuse potential
- Prescribed to passengers for short/medium flight durations and jet lag
- The 0.5 mg tablet has been withdrawn by the FDA due to risk of anterograde amnesia

Non-Benzodiazepine Hypnotics

Non-benzodiazepine hypnotic drugs include[6,32,34]:

- Z drugs
- Melatonergic agents
- $GABA_B$ partial agonists
- Antihistamines
- Barbiturates
- Some antidepressants and other psychotropic agents
- OTC sleep medications

Z Drugs

Z drugs cause lower rebound insomnia and fewer airway problems than benzos.[29] Unlike benzos, however, these drugs are not potent muscle-relaxants or anticonvulsant agents.[32]

Eszopiclone[3,8,11,12,13,20,22,28,31,32,35,36,39,40,41]

Brand name: Lunesta

FDA approved for: Insomnia

Other potential uses (off-label): Insomnia in GAD, MDD, and menopause

Medication forms: *Tab* (1, 2, 3 mg)

Dosage:

- Insomnia: 1–3 mg hs

MOA: Binds to or interacts allosterically at the GABA-receptor complex domain

Pharmacokinetics: t_{max}=1 hr, $t_{1/2}$=6–9 hrs

Warnings:

- Use caution with prior MDD; may cause worsening of depression and suicidal tendencies
- May have CNS-depressant effects; impairs alertness and motor coordination, especially elderly and debilitated patients
- Must be taken just before going to bed; do not take immediately after meal
- Do not take during the night; sleep duration of 7–8 hours strongly recommended after intake
- Can lead to abnormal thinking and behavior
- Evaluate for comorbid conditions if insomnia persists after 7–10 days of use
- May cause severe anaphylactic/anaphylactoid reactions
- Associated with withdrawal effects
- Use caution in impaired hepatic function, metabolism, respiratory function, or hemodynamic responses

Drug interaction:

- Use with CNS depressants can cause additive CNS-depressant effects
- CYP3A4 inducers (e.g., rifampicin) can decrease exposure and effects; CYP3A4 inhibitors (e.g., ketoconazole) can increase exposure and effects

Common side effects: Dizziness, dry mouth, hallucination, headache, nervousness, rash, respiratory infection, somnolence, unpleasant metallic taste

Contraindications: Hypersensitivity, use with sodium oxybate

Lab tests needed: None

Overdose: Hypoxia, pulmonary edema, respiratory failure; OD rare

Tapering/withdrawal: Gradual taper recommended

Special populations:

Pregnancy: Risk Category C

Lactation: Avoid

Elderly: Lower dose recommended (1–2 mg/day)

Hepatic impairment: No dose adjustment necessary in mild to moderate, 1 mg/day recommended in severe

Renal impairment: No dose adjustment necessary

Important notes:

- First Z drug indicated for treatment of chronic insomnia
- Considered a better option in patients with drug-abuse history

Zaleplon[3,8,11,12,13,20,22,25,28,31,32,35,39,40,41]

Brand name: Sonata

FDA approved for: Insomnia

Other potential uses (off-label): None

Medication forms: *Cap* (5, 10 mg)

Dosage: 5–10 mg qhs, can be increased based on tolerance/response to max 20 mg/day

MOA: Binds to $GABA_{BZ}$ receptor complex responsible sedative, anxiolytic, muscle-relaxant, and anticonvulsant effects; also binds selectively to the $GABA_A$ omega-1 receptor

Pharmacokinetics: t_{max}=1 hr, $t_{1/2}$=1 hr, onset of action=0.5 hr, duration of action=7 hrs

Warnings:

- Use caution with prior MDD; may cause worsening of depression and suicidal tendencies
- May have CNS-depressant effects; impairs alertness and motor coordination, especially elderly and debilitated patients
- Loss of short-term and possibly long-term memory
- Can cause abnormal thinking and behavioral changes
- Associated with severe anaphylactic/anaphylactoid reactions
- Evaluate for comorbid conditions if insomnia persists after 7–10 day of treatment
- May worsen insomnia and impair motor/cognitive performance
- Use caution with impaired respiratory function, metabolism, or hemodynamic responses
- May prompt sleep-driving or eating while not fully awake

Drug interactions:
- Can potentiate effects of centrally acting drugs (e.g., neuroleptics, barbiturates, analgesics, antihistamines, alcohol)
- Use of CYP3A4 inducers may decrease plasma levels (up to 80% with rifampin); use of inhibitors may increase plasma levels
- Prescribe 5 mg when used with cimetidine due to decreased clearance

Common side effects: Abdominal pain, asthenia, dizziness, dysmenorrhea, headache, myalgia, nausea, somnolence

Contraindications: Hypersensitivity, use with sodium oxybate

Recommended lab tests: LFTs

Overdose: Hypotension, coma, respiratory depression; OD rare

Tapering/withdrawal: Gradual taper recommended

Special populations:

Pregnancy: Risk Category C

Lactation: Safe/preferred option

Elderly: Lower dose recommended (5 mg)

Hepatic impairment: 5 mg recommended in mild to moderate, avoid in severe

Renal impairment: No dose adjustment necessary in mild to moderate, lower dose recommended in severe

Important notes[32,35]:
- Preferred over benzos due to rapid onset, short duration of action, and good safety profile
- Popular choice for short-term sleep problems like jetlag
- Only hypnotic which can be taken during night that does not cause morning grogginess
- Lower risk dependency and minimal withdrawal effects

Zolpidem[3,8,11,12,13,20,22,28,30,31,32,35,39,40,41]

Brand name: Ambien, Ambien CR, Edluar, Intermezzo, Zolpimist

FDA approved for: Short-term treatment of insomnia characterized by difficulties with sleep initiation and difficulty returning to sleep in middle of night

Other potential uses (off-label): Long-term treatment of insomnia, medication-induced insomnia

Medication forms: *IR tab* (5, 10 mg); *CR tab* (6.25, 12.5 mg); *SL tab* (1.75, 3.5, 5, 10 mg); *oral spray* (5 mg/0.1 ml)

Dosage:
- Sleep initiation:
  - *IR tab, SL tab, oral spray:* 5 mg qhs for women, consider 5–10 mg qhs for men
  - *Ambien CR:* 6.25 mg po qhs for women; 6.25–12.5 mg po qhs for men

- Insomnia/night awakening (Intermezzo): 1.75 mg SL prn for women, 3.5 mg SL prn for men

MOA: Agonist at $GABA_A$ receptor complex, responsible for sedative, anticonvulsant, anxiolytic, and muscle-relaxant properties

Pharmacokinetics: t_{max}=0.5–1.5 hrs, $t_{1/2}$=2.5–3 hrs

Warnings:

- Use caution with prior MDD; may cause worsening of depression and suicidal tendencies
- Can induce abnormal thinking and behavior if used regularly
- Use caution with hemodynamic instability
- May have CNS-depressant effects; impairs alertness and motor coordination, especially elderly and debilitated patients
- Evaluate for co-morbid diagnosis if insomnia persists after 7–10 days of use
- May cause severe anaphylactic/anaphylactoid reactions
- May prompt sleep-driving or eating while not fully awake
- Risk of respiratory depression, withdrawal, and drowsiness leading to falls and severe injuries
- Effects slowed if taken with or immediately after meal

Drug interaction:

- Can potentiate effects of centrally acting drugs (e.g., neuroleptics, barbiturates, analgesics, antihistamine, alcohol)
- Increased plasma level with ketoconazole and decreased plasma level with rifampicin
- Effects reversed with flumazenil
- Decreased alertness with imipramine; impaired psychomotor performance with chlorpromazine

Common side effects: Amnesia, ataxia, diarrhea, confusion, dizziness, drowsiness, indigestion, nausea, sedation

Contraindications: Hypersensitivity

Recommended lab tests: LFTs

Overdose: Hypotension, coma, respiratory depression; OD rare

Tapering/withdrawal: Slow taper recommended

Special populations:

Pregnancy: Risk Category B

Lactation: Safe/preferred option

Elderly: Lower dose recommended (5 mg)

Hepatic impairment: 50% dose reduction recommended

Renal impairment: 50% dose reduction recommended

Important notes:

- Associated with temporary memory loss next day

- Take on empty stomach, as food can interfere with absorption
- In females, may linger in blood and impair alertness upon awakening
- SL administered during night to allow sleep resumption, whereas all other hypnotic agents must be administered prior to sleep
- The CR formulation has been approved by the FDA for insomnia for up to 6 months

Zopiclone[3,8,11,12,13,20,22,28,31,32,35,39,40,41]
Brand name: Imovane
FDA approved for: None
Other potential uses (off-label): Insomnia
Medication forms: *Tab* (3.5, 5, 7.5 mg)
Dosage:
- Insomnia: 5–7.5 mg hs

MOA: Similar to zaleplon
Pharmacokinetics: t_{max}=2 hrs, $t_{1/2}$=5 hrs
Warnings:
- Use cautiously in severe liver disease and history of substance abuse

Drug interactions: Similar to zaleplon
Common side effects: Ataxia, confusion, depression, dizziness, fatigue, forgetfulness, hyper-excitability, nervousness, sedation, slurred speech, weakness
Contraindications: Hypersensitivity
Recommended lab tests: None
Overdose: CNS depression, coma; OD potential fatal
Tapering/withdrawal: Gradual taper recommended
Special populations:
Pregnancy: No data; avoid
Lactation: Avoid
Elderly: Lower dose recommended (3.75 mg/day)
Hepatic impairment: Lower dose recommended (3.75 mg/day) in mild to moderate, avoid in severe
Renal impairment: Lower dose recommended (3.75 mg/day) in mild to moderate, avoid in severe
Important notes:
- Risk of tolerance increased with more frequent use, higher doses, and longer duration of use

Melatonergic Agents
Melatonin is a hormone produced in the pineal gland of the human brain, which helps to maintain circadian rhythms. It is available over the counter in pharmacies. The FDA

considers synthetic melatonin and melatonin-receptor agonists as food supplements.[13] These agents include and agomelatine, melatonin, and ramelteon.

Agomelatine[11,20,35]
(Refer to *Chapter 4: Depressive Disorders and Antidepressants* for further details)
FDA approved for: None (approved for MDD in Europe)
Other potential uses (off-label): Insomnia, MDD
Dosage:
- 25 mg/day hs initially, can be increased based on tolerance/response to max 50 mg/day

Melatonin[11,20,35]
(Refer to *Chapter 21: Dietary, Herbal, and OTC Medications in Psychiatry* for further details)
Dosage: 0.3–5 mg hs (usual dosage 3–5 mg hs)
Important notes:
- Used for insomnia and jet lag in children and adults
- Can treat delayed sleep-phase disorder and shift work disorder; not effective in short-term treatment of primary sleep disorders

Ramelteon[3,8,11,12,13,20,22,28,31,32,35,37,39,40,41]
Brand name: Rozerem
FDA approved for: Insomnia characterized by difficulty with sleep onset
Other potential uses (off-label): None
Medication forms: *Tab* (8 mg)
Dosage: 8 mg hs
MOA: Agonist MT_1 and MT_2 receptors but not MT_3
Pharmacokinetics: t_{max}=0.75 hr, $t_{1/2}$=1.2–6hrs
Warnings:
- Can cause cognitive and behavioral changes
- May cause severe anaphylactic/anaphylactoid reactions
- Evaluate for co-morbid conditions if insomnia persists after 7–10 days of treatment
- Can cause hallucinations or complex behaviors while not awake (including sleep-driving or eating)
- May worsen depression or suicidal thinking
- May impair mental alertness in hazardous activities (e.g., operating machinery, driving)
Drug interactions:
- Use caution with other CYP1A2, CYP3A4, and CYP2C9 enzyme inhibitor drugs, as they can increase levels

- Rifampin (strong CYP3A4 inducer) decreases exposure and effects
- Donepezil and doxepin increase systemic exposure
- Alcohol causes additive psychomotor impairment

Common side effects: Dizziness, dysgeusia, fatigue, headache, insomnia, nausea, somnolence

Contraindications: Angioedema, use with fluvoxamine, sleep apnea

Overdose: Drowsiness, CNS depression, hallucination; OD very rare

Tapering/withdrawal: Taper not necessary

Special populations:

Pregnancy: Risk Category C

Lactation: Avoid

Elderly: No dose adjustment necessary

Hepatic impairment: No dose adjustment necessary in mild to moderate, avoid in severe

Renal impairment: No dose adjustment necessary

Important notes[32]:

- Not classified as a controlled substance
- Should be taken 30 minutes before sleep
- Use caution with respiratory impairments, mental illness, sleep apnea, or liver disease
- Does not cause confusion and memory problems
- Not associated with high abuse potential, rebound insomnia, or tolerance
- May elevate prolactin levels in females and decrease testosterone levels in males

GABA-B Partial Agonists

Chloral hydrate[11,20,35]

Brand name: Noctec

Dosage: 500 mg to 1 g hs

Important notes:

- Discontinued due to very narrow therapeutic index

Sodium oxybate[3,8,11,12,13,15,20,22,28,31,32,35,39,40,41]

Brand name: Xyrem

FDA approved for: Cataplexy in narcolepsy, excessive daytime sleepiness associated with narcolepsy

Other potential uses (off-label): Insomnia, fibromyalgia

Medication forms: *Oral sol* (500 mg/ml)

Dosage:

- Insomnia: 4.5–9 g/night divided bid at 2.5–4 hrs apart

MOA: Selective partial agonist of $GABA_B$ receptor
Pharmacokinetics: t_{max}=25 min–1.25 hrs, $t_{1/2}$=20–60 min
Warnings:

- **Black box warning**: Because of the risks of CNS depression, abuse, and misuse, Xyrem is available only through a restricted distribution program called the Xyrem Success Program®, using a centralized pharmacy
- Risk of dangerous CNS adverse effects including respiratory depression, seizure, reduced consciousness, coma, and death, alone or in combination with another CNS depressant
- Observe closely for signs of misuse and abuse (Schedule III substance)
- Caution patients against hazardous activities requiring mental alertness or fine motor coordination within first 6 hours of dosing or after initiating treatment
- May cause or exacerbate depression and suicidality
- Can cause confusion, paranoia, parasomnias, hallucinations, agitation, and anxiety
- Monitor patients with hypertension, CHF, or impaired renal function due to high drug sodium level

Drug interactions:

- Avoid with other sedative hypnotics, alcohol, or other CNS depressants
- Use with divalproex sodium can increase effects; 20% does reduction recommended

Common side effects: Dizziness, enuresis, headache, nausea, somnolence, tremor, vomiting
Contraindications: Use of sedative hypnotic or alcohol, succinic semialdehyde deficiency
Overdose: Bradycardia, myoclonic movements, unconsciousness, delirium, coma; OD potentially fatal
Tapering/withdrawal: Taper not necessary
Special populations:
Pregnancy: Risk Category B
Lactation: Avoid
Elderly: Use lower dose
Hepatic impairment: Lower dose recommended (2.25 g/night divided)
Renal impairment: Use caution
Important notes:

- Also called GHB and is used as recreational drug, especially for club raves and date rape
- Potential of abuse by athletes due to increased growth-hormone release

Antihistamines

Antihistamines that are used as hypnotics include: diphenhydramine, doxylamine, hydroxyzine, and promethazine. These drugs are less dangerous than other hyponotics but may have prominent anticholinergic side effects. They may be useful in patients who are inclined to abuse sleep medications.[32]

Diphenhydramine[1, 3,8,11,12,20,22,28,31,32,35,39,40,41]
Brand name: Benadryl products and others
FDA approved for: Insomnia, allergic rhinitis, anaphylaxis, common cold, motion sickness, Parkinsonism, pruritus of skin
Other potential uses (off-label): Agitation in children, drug-induced EPS, morning sickness
Medication forms: *Tab* (25, 50 mg); *chew tab* (12.5 mg); *ODT* (25 mg); *cap* (25, 50 mg); *liq* (12.5/5ml); *strip* (25 mg); *injectable* (50 mg/ml)
Dosage:
• Insomnia: 25–50 mg po qhs
MOA: Competitively antagonizes histamine receptors, acts as central anti-muscarinic agent
Pharmacokinetics: t_{max}=2–4 hrs; $t_{1/2}$=9–12 hrs
Warnings:
• May cause anaphylactic reaction; use caution
• Use caution with lower-respiratory disease
• Can cause next day hangover in some patients
Drug Interactions:
• Increased effects with alcohol or other CNS depressants
Common side effects: Blurred vision, difficult urination, drowsiness, dry mouth, sedation, tachycardia
Contraindications: Children <1 year old, premature infants and neonates, hypersensitivity
Recommended lab tests: None
Overdose: Fixed/dilated pupils, flushing, GI symptoms, hallucinations, seizures
Tapering/withdrawal: Gradual taper recommended; sudden discontinuation causes anxiety, insomnia, and depression
Special populations:
Pregnancy: Risk Category B
Lactation: Injectable contraindicated, use oral with caution and at a lower dose
Elderly: Lower dose recommended
Hepatic impairment: Lower dose recommended
Renal impairment: No dose adjustment necessary
Important notes:
• Common OTC medication for insomnia
• Can be used for sedation and agitation in children
• Paradoxical excitation effects in young children

- Tolerance builds very quickly
- Avoid use among drivers/pilots due to sedative properties

Other antihistamines:
Doxylamine (Aldex AN, Unisom)[11,20,35]
Dosage: 25 mg po hs

Hydroxyzine (Atarax, Vistaril) [11,20,35]
(Refer to *Chapter 6: Anxiety Disorders and Anxiolytics* for further details)
Dosage: 50–100 mg po/IM hs

Promethazine (Phenergan) [11,20,35]
Dosage: 25–50 mg po/rectal/IM/IV hs
Important notes:
- Highly favored/misused by patients on methadone maintenance.

Barbiturates
These drugs are rarely used now due to their potential for dependence and their serious CNS depressant effects.[29,32] The barbiturate drugs that are approved for sedative/hypnotic use include:

Amobarbital[11,20,35]
Brand name: Amytal
Dosage: 65–200 mg qhs IV

Butabarbital[11,20,35]
Brand name: Butisol
Dosage: 50–100 mg qhs

Phenobarbital[11,20,35]
Brand Name: Luminal
Dosage: 100–200 mg (po/IM/IV) hs for max 2 weeks

Secobarbital [11,20,35]
Brand Name: Seconal
Dosage: 100 mg po qhs for max 2 weeks

Antidepressants and Other Psychotropics
Several psychotropic agents, especially TCAs, have antihistaminergic effects and are excellent hypnotics. [32]The majority of these drugs can potentially be used off-label for insomnia.[35]

Amitriptyline (Elavil)[11,20,35]
(Refer to *Chapter 4: Depressive Disorders and Antidepressants* for further details)
Dosage: 50-150 mg qhs

Doxepin (Sinequan, Silenor)[11,20,35]
(Refer to *Chapter 4: Depressive Disorders and Antidepressants* for further details)
Dosage: 10 mg qhs (Silenor: 3–6 mg qhs)

Mirtazapine (Remeron)[11,20,35]
(Refer to *Chapter 4: Depressive Disorders and Antidepressants* for further details)
Dosage: 7.5–45 mg po qhs

Trimipramine (Surmontil)[11,20,35]
(Refer to *Chapter 4: Depressive Disorders and Antidepressants* for further details)
Dosage: 50–150 mg po hs

Trazodone (Desyrel, Oleptro)[11,20,35]
(Refer to *Chapter 4: Depressive Disorders and Antidepressants* for further details)
Dosage: 50–100 mg po qhs

Gabapentin (Neurontin)[11,20,35]
(Refer to *Chapter 5: Bipolar Disorder and Mood Stabilizers* for further details)
Dosage: Up to 1800 mg po evenings for max 9 weeks

Pregabalin (Lyrica)[11,20,35]
(Refer to *Chapter 6: Anxiety Disorders and Anxiolytics* for further details)
Dosage: 150–300 mg hs

Clonidine (Catapres)[11,20,35]
(Refer to *Chapter 7: ADHD and Its Treatment* for further details)
Dosage: 0.1–0.3 mg hs

Over-the-Counter (OTC) Sleeping Medications
L-Tryptophan[11,20,35]
Dosage: 1–4 g hs
Important notes:
- Potentially free of dependence or abuse liability[32]
- Withdrawn due to eosinophilia-myalgia syndrome; only available for research

Melatonin
(Refer to *Melatonergic Agents* in this chapter for further details)

Valerian Extract[11,20,35]
(Refer to *Chapter 21: Dietary, Herbal and OTC Medications in Psychiatry* for further details)
Dosage: 400–600 mg/day hs

References:

1. AAA Pharmaceutical, Inc. 2013. "DIPHENHYDRAMINE- diphenhydramine hydrochloride capsule." US National Library of Medicine: Daily Med. Accessed December 16, 2014. http://dailymed.nlm.nih.gov/dailymed/drugInfo.cfm?setid=cda1a143-9063-49a6-a6ee-6a47fec25b10.

2. Actavis, LLC. 2013. "TEMAZEPAM; temazepam capsule." US National Library of Medicine: Daily Med. Accessed December 16, 2014. http://dailymed.nlm.nih.gov/dailymed/drugInfo.cfm?setid=a4370eb4-b00d-4247-af8d-980e59fbbec6.

3. Albers, Lawrence J., Rhoda K. Hahn, and Christopher Reist. 2010. *Handbook of Psychiatric Drugs.* 2011 ed. 39–59. Current Clinical Strategies Publishing.

4. American Psychiatric Association. 2013. *Diagnostic and Statistical Manual of Mental Disorders.* 5th ed. (DSM-5). Washington, DC: American Psychiatric Association.

5. Akorn, Inc. 2012. "MIDAZOLAM- midazolam hydrochloride injection." US National Library of Medicine: Daily Med. Accessed January 8, 2015. http://dailymed.nlm.nih.gov/dailymed/drugInfo.cfm?setid=737361a0-8db1-4d3c-ba5e-44df3f49fa22.

6. Avidan, Alon Y., and Phyllis C. Zee. 2011. *Handbook of Sleep Medicine.* 36–60. New York: Lippincott Williams & Wilkins.

7. BluePoint Laboratories. 2014. "PROMETHAZINE HYDROCHLORIDE- promethazine hydrochloride tablet." US National Library of Medicine: Daily Med. Accessed December 16, 2014. http://dailymed.nlm.nih.gov/dailymed/drugInfo.cfm?setid=44cd6d46-fbb9-4836-9426-d8ce2cb6d66d.

8. Center Watch. 2015. "FDA Approved Drugs by Therapeutic Area." Accessed February 3, 2015. http://www.centerwatch.com/drug-information/fda-approved-drugs/therapeutic-area/17/psychiatry-psychology.

9. Chattem, Inc. 2015. "UNISOM SLEEPTABS- doxylamine succinate tablet." US National Library of Medicine: Daily Med. Accessed January 8, 2015. http://dailymed.nlm.nih.gov/dailymed/drugInfo.cfm?setid=d5e3015c-49ae-4288-a78f-17a141f26817.

10. Colten, Harvey R., and Bruce M Altevogt, eds. 2006. *Sleep Disorders and Sleep Deprivation: An Unmet Public Health Problem,* U.S. Institute of Medicine Committee on Sleep Medicine and Research. Washington, DC: National Academies Press.

11. Elsevier Gold Standard, Inc. 2015. "Clinical Pharmacology." Accessed March 12, 2015. https://www.clinicalpharmacology.com.

12. Epocrates. 2015. Accessed March 25, 2015. https://online.epocrates.com.

13. Gabbard, Glen O., ed. 2007. *Gabbard's Treatments of Psychiatric Disorders*. 4th ed. 855–874. Washington, DC: American Psychiatric Publishing.

14. Hales, Robert. E., S. Yudofsky, and L. Roberts, eds. 2014. *The American Psychiatric Publishing Textbook of Psychiatry*. 6th ed. 607–650, 929–1004. Washington, DC: American Psychiatric Publishing.

15. Jazz Pharmaceuticals, Inc. 2014. "XYREM- sodium oxybate solution." US National Library of Medicine: Daily Med. Accessed December 16, 2014. http://dailymed.nlm.nih.gov/dailymed/drugInfo.cfm?setid=926eb076-a4a8-45e4-91ef-411f0aa4f3ca.

16. Kales, A. 1982. "Benzodiazepines in the treatment of insomnia." In *Pharmacology of Benzodiazepines*, edited by E. Usdin, P. Skolnick, J.F. Jr Tallman, T. Greenblatt and S.M. Paul, 199–217. New York: McMillan.

17. KLE 2, Inc. 2013. "Quazepam - quazepam tablet." U.S. National Library of Medicine: Daily Med. Accessed December 16, 2014. http://dailymed.nlm.nih.gov/dailymed/drugInfo.cfm?setid=6a8e1aff-a1ac-4f47-af33-d2fd23c631d6.

18. Lubit, R.H. 2015. "Sleep Disorders." Accessed February 3 2015. http://emedicine.medscape.com/article/287104-overview.

19. McVearry Kelso, C. 2014. "Primary Insomnia." Accessed March 12, 2015. http://emedicine.medscape.com/article/291573-overview.

20. Medscape: Drugs & Diseases. 2015. "Psychiatrics." Accessed February 3, 2015. http://reference.medscape.com/drugs/psychiatrics.

21. Medscape. 2015. "Psychiatry and Mental Health." Accessed March 12, 2015. http://www.medscape.com/psychiatry.

22. Medscape: Drugs & Diseases. 2015. "Sleep Disorders." Accessed January 14, 2015. http://reference.medscape.com/drugs/psychiatrics.

23. Mendelson, W.B., ed. 1992. "Current strategies in the treatment of insomnia." *J Clin Psychiatry* 53(12 suppl):1-45.

24. Nidhino, S.E., E. Mignot, and W.C. Dement. 1998. "Sedative-hypnotics." In *Textbook of Psychopharmacology*. 2nd ed., edited by A. F. Schatzberg and C. B. Nemeroff. 487–502. Washington, DC: American Psychiatric Publishing.

25. Pfizer, Inc. 2014. "SONATA- zaleplon capsule." US National Library of Medicine: Daily Med. Accessed December 16, 2014. http://dailymed.nlm.nih.gov/dailymed/drugInfo.cfm?setid=c8a6c478-1d05-47b2-c98d-99177395b762.

26. Preston, John D., and James Johnson. 2011. *Clinical Psychopharmacology Made Ridiculously Simple*. 7th ed. 1–79. Miami: MedMaster Inc.

27. Roxane Laboratories, Inc. 2015. "TRIAZOLAM- triazolam tablet." US National Library of Medicine: Daily Med. Accessed December 16, 2014. http://dailymed.nlm.nih.gov/dailymed/drugInfo.cfm?setid=db564864-17fc-4ba5-a438-a467ef57a0ca.

28. RxList. 2015. "Drugs A-Z List." Accessed March 25, 2015. http://www.rxlist.com/drugs/alpha_a.htm.

29. Sanger, D. J. 2004. "The pharmacology and mechanisms of action of new generation, non-benzodiazepine hypnotic agents." *CNS Drugs* 18(1 suppl):9-15; (1 discussion):41, 43–45.

30. Sanofi-Aventis, LLC. 2014. "AMBIEN- zolpidem tartrate tablet, film coated." US National Library of Medicine: Daily Med. Accessed December 16, 2014. http://dailymed.nlm.nih.gov/dailymed/drugInfo.cfm?setid=c36cadf4-65a4-4466-b409-c82020b42452.

31. Schatzberg, A.F., and C.B. Nemeroff, eds. 2009. *The American Psychiatric Publishing Textbook of Psychopharmacology*. 4th ed. 821–842, 1241–1266. Washington, DC: American Psychiatric Publishing.

32. Schatzberg, A.F., Jonathan O. Cole, and Charles DeBattista. 2010. *Manual of Clinical Psychopharmacology*. 7th ed. 431–461. Washington, DC: American Psychiatric Publishing.

33. Schutte-Rodin, S., L. Broch, D. Buysse, C. Dorsey, and M. Sateia. 2008. "Clinical guideline for the evaluation and management of chronic insomnia in adults." *J Clin Sleep Med* 4(5):487–504.

34. Stahl, S.M. 2008. *Essential Psychopharmacology: Neuroscientific Basis and Practical Applications*. 3rd ed. 444–470. New York: Cambridge Press.

35. Stahl, S.M. 2011. *Essential Psychopharmacology: the Prescriber's Guide*. 4th ed. 9–13, 91–95, 117–121, 129–132, 159–163, 377–379, 435–438, 497–500, 509–512, 555–558, 565–568, 609–612, 641–644, 651–654, 659–661. Cambridge: Cambridge University Press.

36. Sunovion. 2014. "LUNESTA- eszopiclone tablet, coated." US National Library of Medicine: Daily Med. Accessed December 16, 2014. http://dailymed.nlm.nih.gov/dailymed/drugInfo.cfm?setid=fd047b2b-05a6-4d99-95cb-955f14bf329f.

37. Takeda Pharmaceuticals U.S.A, Inc. 2010. "ROZEREM- ramelteon tablet, film coated." US National Library of Medicine: Daily Med. Accessed December 16, 2014. http://dailymed.nlm.nih.gov/dailymed/drugInfo.cfm?setid=9de82310-70e8-47b9-b1fc-6c6848b99455.

38. Taylor, Renée R. 2006. "Sleep Dysfunction: Diagnostic Categories, Prevalence, and Associated Conditions." In *Cognitive Behavioral Therapy for Chronic Illness and Disability*, 279–297. New York: Springer.

39. Truven Health Analytics. 2015. *Micromedex 2.0*. Accessed March 20, 2015. http://www.micromedexsolutions.com/home/dispatch.

40. UpToDate. 2015. Accessed March 12, 2015. http://www.uptodate.com/home.

41. US National Library of Medicine. 2015. "Drugs and Lactation Database (LactMed)." Accessed February 3, 2015. http://toxnet.nlm.nih.gov/newtoxnet/lactmed.htm.

42. US National Library of Medicine. 2015. "Toxicology Data Network." Accessed March 17, 2015. http://toxnet.nlm.nih.gov.

43. Watson Laboratories, Inc. 2010. "ESTAZOLAM- estazolam tablet." US National Library of Medicine: Daily Med. Accessed December 16, 2014. http://dailymed.nlm.nih.gov/dailymed/drugInfo.cfm?setid=a1e3b4bf-22e9-430a-a768-4d86ae886c9e.

44. Wegmann, J. 2008. *Psychopharmacology: Straight Talk on Mental Health Medications.* 93–108. Eau Claire: Pesi, LLC.

45. Zhang, B., and Y. K. Wing. 2006. "Sex differences in insomnia: a meta-analysis." *Sleep* 29(1):85–93

Chapter 11-1
Substance Use Disorders And Their Treatment

Substance use disorders involve the recurrent use of alcohol and/or drugs in a way that causes clinically and functionally-significant impairment.[35] These disorders have emerged as a major public health problem in the US, with a total cost of over $600 billion annually.[29] This figure does not account for these disorders vicious impact on public health and society.[23] Drugs and alcohol are implicated in 40% of all hospital admissions as well as in 25% of all emergency room visits and deaths.[23] Alcohol intoxication is associated with approximately 50% of all motor vehicle accidents, domestic violence cases, and murders.[23] Additionally, there are 23.9 million illicit drug users in the US.[24] Substance abuse is responsible for numerous problems, including dangerous medical and psychiatric conditions, academic and occupational difficulties, poor peer and family relationships, crime involvement, accidents, injuries, and traffic fatalities.[29] The multifactorial etiology of substance abuse includes genetics, psychiatric disorders, and psychosocial risk factors.

DSM-5 Changes
Substance abuse and substance dependence have been combined into individual disorders specific to each substance of abuse within a new "addictions and related disorders" category, which is divided into mild, moderate, and severe subtypes.[3] Whereas DSM-IV diagnostic criteria required only one symptom, a DSM-5 diagnosis now requires at least two, even for mild substance use disorder.[3]

Types of Disorders[3,35]:
- Alcohol-Related Disorders
- Caffeine-Related Disorders
- Cannabis Use Disorder
- Hallucinogen-Related Disorders
- Inhalant-Related Disorders
- Opioid-Related Disorders
- Sedative-, Hypnotic-, or Anxiolytic-Related Disorders
- Stimulant-Related Disorders
- Tobacco-Related Disorders
- Other (or Unknown) Substance-Related Disorders

Management of Substance Abuse Disorders
Management of these disorders includes pharmacological, psychological and psychosocial treatment. Pharmacological treatments involve medications that treat intoxication and withdrawal states, prevent relapse, treat co-occurring psychiatric conditions, and provide maintenance support.[29] Substance abuse disorders require continuous monitoring and long-term treatments similar to the management of other chronic illnesses.[29,31]

Healthcare providers must ensure the proper identification, counseling, education, and treatment of patients with substance abuse disorders.

Psychosocial Treatments[2,11]:

- Cognitive behavioral therapies (CBT)
- Motivational enhancement therapy (MET)
- Behavioral therapies
- 12-step facilitation (TSF)
- Psychodynamic/interpersonal therapy (IPT)

Drugs of Abuse:

- *Detoxable drugs of abuse:* Alcohol, benzodiazepines/sedative hypnotics, opiates
- *Non-detoxable drugs of abuse:* Angel's trumpet, PCP, cocaine, marijuana, ecstasy, amphetamines, ketamine, LSD, mushrooms, steroids, Triple C's (Coricidin Cough & Cold), inhalants, bath salts, K2/spice

Management of Intoxication and Withdrawal

Alcohol[2,4,9,10,11,15,16,18,19,21,23,32,36,37]

Intoxication: Ataxia, confusion, difficulty walking, dilated pupils, disinhibition, disorientation, drowsiness, euphoria, memory loss, poor judgment, slurred speech, vomiting

Withdrawal sx: Anxiety, confusion, depression, fatigue, insomnia, irritability, nightmares, sweating, tachycardia, tremors

Alcohol withdrawal treatment:[4] Acute withdrawal can be life-threatening. The best validated tool is the Clinical Institute Withdrawal Assessment for Alcohol-Revised (CIWA-Ar).

- *Outpatient treatment* [4]: (CIWA-Ar) symptom scale scores <12 can often be managed as outpatients
  - Vitamin B1: 100mg/day along with multivitamin supplement and folic acid 1 mg po qd
  - Benzos:
    - Chlordiazepoxide: 50–100 mg q6hr for 4 doses, then 25–50 mg q6hr for 8 doses
    - or
    - Diazepam:10–20 mg q6hr for 4 doses, then 5–10 mg q6hr for 8 doses
    - or
    - Lorazepam: 2–4 mg q6hr for 4 doses, then 1–2 mg q6hr for 8 doses
- *Inpatient Treatment*[32]: (CIWA-Ar) symptom scale scores of >15 may require inpatient treatment

Maintenance treatment of alcohol dependence[32]:

- CBT, family therapy groups, meetings, sponsorship, 12-step program such as Alcoholics Anonymous (AA)

- Medications like disulfiram, naltrexone, acamprosate, etc.

Benzodiazepines[2,11,21,24,32,35]
(Refer to *Chapter 6: Anxiety Disorders and Anxiolytics* for further details)
Intoxication: Agitation, amnesia, blurred vision, difficulty concentrating, disinhibition, drowsiness, hostility, irritability, poor judgment, sleepiness, slurred speech, unsteadiness
Withdrawal sx: Anxiety, difficulty concentrating, dry retching, hand tremors, headache irritability, nausea, palpitations, panic attacks, sleep disturbance, sweating
Medication for withdrawal: Long-acting benzos
Benzo withdrawal treatment:
- Prolonged taper with currently prescribed benzo; can be reduced rapidly by 50% of initial dose, then 10% reduction/month
- Conversion to long-acting benzo (clonazepam, chlordiazepoxide)
- Conversion to non-benzo (e.g., carbamazepine, phenobarbital)

Hallucinogens[2,11,17,24,32,35]
Forms:
- Natural: peyote, psilocybin, DMT (dimethyltryptamine)
- Synthetic: LSD (lysergic acid diethylamide), DOM, MDA, MDMA (ecstasy), PCP, ketamine
Intoxication: Arrhythmia, diaphoresis, hallucination, heightened perception, hyperreflexia, hypertension, hyperthermia, pupil dilation, tachycardia, seizure, visual illusion
Withdrawal: Rare

Inhalants[2,21,24,32,35]
Forms: Glues, aerosols, vapors
Intoxication: Apprehension, ataxia, disinhibition, dizziness/lightheadedness, drowsiness, euphoria, headaches, impaired vision, irritability, memory/thought impairment, nausea, slurred speech,
Withdrawal: Anxiety, depression, dizziness, headache, insomnia, irritability, tremors
Medication: None

Marijuana[2,11,21,24,32,35]
Intoxication: Delayed reflex, erythemic eyes, excessive sleepiness, inappropriate laughter, lack of motivation, weight gain/loss
Withdrawal: Aggression, decreased appetite, insomnia, irritability, restlessness
Medication:
- No FDA approved medications

- Candidates: dronabinol, nabilone, rimonabant, lofexidine, N-acetylcysteine (NAC) can aid detoxification for cannabis use disorder

Opiates[2,6,11,13,17,19,21,27,28,32,35,36]

Forms: Buprenorphine, codeine, meperidine, fentanyl, heroin, hydrocodone, methadone, morphine, oxycodone, oxycontin

Intoxication: Coma, contracted pupils, coughing/snorting, diaphoresis, hypersomnolence, loss of appetite, miosis, twitching, unresponsive pupils, vomiting

Withdrawal: Abdominal cramping, agitation, anxiety, diarrhea, goose bumps, hot/cold sweats, insomnia, muscle aches and pains, nausea, runny nose, teary eyes, vomiting, yawning[32]

Acute withdrawal treatment:

- Withdrawal is not life-threatening
- Methadone (a long-acting opiate): 10 mg po in liquid/crushed tablet form, evaluate q4hr and administer additional 10 mg methadone if >2 of 4 objective withdrawal criteria met; stabilization dose reduced by 5 mg/day until complete withdrawal
- Clonidine attenuates noradrenergic hyperactivity; initiate at 0.1–0.2 mg qid and taper over 5–7 days, watch for bradycardia
- Buprenorphine: dose varies; loading dose 8–32 mg, then taper by 2 mg every other day

Maintenance therapy for opioid dependence[32]:

- Methadone maintenance is the most commonly used although it is being replaced by buprenorphine
- LAAM is longer-acting than methadone and can be used 3x/week
- Buprenorphine: recommended dose 8–32 mg/day
- Naltrexone maintenance: 50 mg/day, can be given 3x/week

Stimulants[2,11,17,21,32,34,35]

Forms: Cocaine, methamphetamine, methylphenidate, amphetamine, ephedrine, khat

Intoxication: Anger, anxiety, arrhythmia, chest pain, confusion, decreased appetite, enhanced vigor, euphoria, hyperactivity, hypertension, impaired judgment, restlessness, paranoia, seizure

Withdrawal: Abdominal cramps, depression, diarrhea, drowsiness, headache, increased appetite

Medication:

- None FDA-approved for cocaine dependence
- Medications such as topiramate, disulfiram, modafinil, can help those who fail to respond to psychosocial therapy alone
- Imipramine, desipramine, venlafaxine may aid depressed cocaine-dependent patients

Management of intoxication/withdrawal[2]:
- Self-limiting; usually requires only supportive care
- Acutely agitated patients may benefit from benzo sedation

Psychotherapy:
- CBT
- Behavioral therapy
- 12-step-oriented individual drug counseling
- Self-help group

Medications

Acamprosate[1,5,7,8,10,11,16,20,30,31,32,34,38,39,40]

Brand name: Campral

FDA approved for: Alcohol dependence, maintenance of alcohol abstinence

Other potential uses (off-label): None

Medication forms: *Tab* (333 mg)

Dosage:
- Alcohol abuse: 666 mg po tid

MOA: Interaction with glutamate and GABA neurotransmitter systems centrally, which lowers neuronal excitability

Pharmacokinetics: t_{max}=3–8 hrs, $t_{1/2}$=20–33 hrs

Warnings:
- Can create emergence of alcohol withdrawal
- Does not stop withdrawal symptoms
- May cause increased suicidal tendencies

Drug interactions:
- No significant interactions

Common side effects: Anxiety, asthenia, depression, diarrhea, dizziness, flatulence, insomnia, nausea, pruritus

Contraindications: Hypersensitivity, renal impairment

Lab tests recommended: BUN/Creatinine

Overdose: Diarrhea; OD rare

Tapering/withdrawal: None

Special populations:

Pregnancy: Risk Category C

Lactation: Avoid

Elderly: No dose adjustment necessary

Hepatic impairment: No dose adjustment necessary

Renal impairment: 333 mg tid recommended in mild to moderate, contraindicated in severe

Important notes:
- Can reduce craving for alcohol in motivated patients
- Since it is not metabolized through liver, it can be taken by patients with liver disease

Buprenorphine and Suboxone[1,5,7,8,11,20,27,30,31,32,34,38,39,40]

Brand name: Subutex, Suboxone, Zubsolv, Bunavail

FDA approved for: Opioid dependence (induction and maintenance)

Other potential uses (off-label): Pain control

Medication forms:
- Buprenorphine monotherapy: *SL tab* (2, 8 mg)
- Buprenorphine/naloxone: *Tab* (2/0.5, 8 mg/2 mg); *SL tab* (1.4/0.36, 5.7/1.4, 8.6/2.1, 11.4mg/2.9mg); *SL film* (2/0.5, 4/1, 8/2, 12 mg/3 mg); *buccal film* (2.1/0.3, 4.2/0.7, 6.3 mg/1 mg)

Dosage:
- Induction (Subutex):
  - *Day 1:* 4 mg SL initially, may repeat if needed, max 8 mg SL
  - *Day 2:* 4–16 mg SL, switch to buprenorphine/naloxone for unsupervised maintenance
- Induction (Suboxone):
  - *Day 1:* 2 mg/0.5 mg or 4 mg/1 mg SL, increase by 2–4 mg increments of buprenorphine at 2 hr intervals to max 8 mg/2 mg (buprenorphine/naloxone)
  - *Day 2:* Up to 16 mg/4 mg SL as a single daily dose
  - *Day 3*: Adjust dose to level that suppresses withdrawal
- Maintenance (Suboxone): 16–32mg/4mg day
- Maintenance (Zubsolv): 2.8/0.72 mg to 17.1/4.2 mg (target 11.4/2.8 mg/day)
- Maintenance (Bunavail): 2.1/0.3 mg to 12.6/2.1 mg (target 8.4/1.4 mg/day)

MOA:
- Buprenorphine: Partial agonist at mu-opioid receptor and antagonist at K-opioid receptor
- Naloxone: Antagonist at mu-opioid receptors

Pharmacokinetics:
- Buprenorphine: t_{max}=1.53–1.72 hrs, $t_{1/2}$=16–42 hrs
- Naloxone: t_{max}=0.77–0.81 hrs, $t_{1/2}$=1.9–12 hrs

Warnings:
- Buprenorphine is a schedule III controlled substance with the potential for addiction, abuse, and misuse, which can lead to overdose and death
- Can lead to respiratory depression; use caution with alcohol intoxication, withdrawal, DT, and respiratory- and CNS-depressing agents

- Use caution in hypothyroidism, myxedema, adrenocortical insufficiency, severe renal impairment, urethral stricture, comatose patients, severe hepatic impairment, head injury, intracranial lesions, and intracranial hypertension
- Severe, possibly fatal, respiratory depression in children
- Risk of opioid withdrawal syndrome with parenteral misuse of Suboxone SL film
- Risk of neonatal withdrawal if used during pregnancy
- Not for use as an analgesic; reported deaths of opioid-naive individuals with 2 mg SL
- Caution patients about risks of driving or operating hazardous machinery

Drug interactions:
- With CYP3A4 inhibitors or inducers, potential for over or under dosing, respectively
- Use caution in patients receiving benzos as it can be fatal; reduce dose with CNS depressants
- Avoid with alvimopan due to increased plasma levels of buprenorphine

Common side effects: Abdominal pain, constipation, headache, hyperhidrosis, insomnia, nausea, pain, rhinitis, vomiting, withdrawal

Contraindications: Hypersensitivity

Recommended lab tests: LFTs

Overdose: CNS depression, coma, respiratory depression, and hypotension

Tapering/withdrawal: Slow taper recommended

Special populations:

Pregnancy: Risk Category C

Lactation: Use caution

Elderly: Use caution

Hepatic impairment: Use caution in mild to moderate, avoid in severe

Renal impairment: No dose adjustment necessary

Important notes:
- Buprenorphine in combination with naloxone reduces the possibility of parenteral misuse by producing withdrawal symptoms when injected
- Only use for dependence on short-acting opioids (heroin); generally not for dependence on long-acting opioids (methadone)
- Monotherapy recommended for long-acting opioid induction
- May transfer patients on methadone maintenance once methadone dose is 30 mg/day
- Can be used as maintenance for patients with chronic pain and undergoing detoxification

Chlordiazepoxide[7,18,20,34]
(Refer to *Chapter 6: Anxiety Disorders and Anxiolytics* for further details)
FDA approved for: Anxiety disorder, alcohol withdrawal, pre-operative apprehension
Medication forms: *Cap* (5, 10, 25 mg)
Dosage:
- Acute alcohol withdrawal: 50–100 mg IV/IM/po, can be increased based on tolerance/response to max 300 mg/day

Disulfiram[1,5,7,8,11,20,30,31,32,34,37,38,39,40]
Brand name: Antabuse
FDA approved for: Alcoholism
Other potential uses (off-label): Cocaine dependence
Medication forms: *Tab* (250, 500 mg)
Dosage:
- 250 mg po qd initially for 1–2 weeks, range 125–500 mg, maintenance 250 mg po qd, max 500 mg/day

MOA: Irreversibly inhibits enzyme responsible for ethanol oxidation, leading to acetaldehyde accumulation
Pharmacokinetics: t_{max}=4 hrs, $t_{1/2}$=20–33 hrs
Warnings:
- **Black box warning:** Should never be administered to a patient in a state of alcohol intoxication or without his/her full knowledge
- Avoid in patients with recent history of MI or coronary artery inclusion
- May lead to liver toxicity and has potential for new abuse
- Risk of disulfiram-alcohol reaction: flushing, throbbing headache, respiratory difficulty, nausea, copious vomiting, sweating, thirst, chest pain, dyspnea, tachycardia, hypotension, syncope, blurred vision, confusion
- Use caution in DM, hypothyroidism, epilepsy, cerebral damage, chronic/acute nephritis, hepatic insufficiency
- Evaluate for rubber-contact dermatitis (HSR to thiuram derivatives)
- Avoid exposure to ethylene dibromide

Drug interactions:
- Should be used with caution in patients receiving phenytoin
- Can lead to gait and mental-status abnormalities if used with isoniazid
- Anticoagulants doses need to be adjusted on beginning or stopping disulfiram
- Avoid use of alcohol-based preparations and solutions

Common side effects: Drowsiness, headache, hepatitis, impotence, lethargy, metallic taste, optic neuritis, peripheral neuropathy, skin eruptions
Contraindications:

- Patients receiving paraldehyde/metronidazole, ETOH, or ETOH-containing preparations
- Psychoses, myocardial disease, hypersensitivity

Recommended lab tests: Periodic LFTs and CBC

Overdose: CNS depression, coma, respiratory depression, and hypotension; OD can be fatal

Tapering/withdrawal: None recommended

Special populations:

Pregnancy: Risk Category C, although methadone preferred

Lactation: Avoid

Elderly: Lower dose recommended

Hepatic impairment: Use caution

Renal impairment: No dose adjustment necessary

Important notes:

- Do not start treatment unless patient has been alcohol-free for at least 24 hours
- Should be used for only highly motivated patients in addition to other modalities

Flumazenil[1,5,7,8,11,20,22,30,31,32,34,38,39,40]

Brand name: Romazicon

FDA approved for: Drug overdose, reversal of benzo activity, overdose of GABA medications

Other potential uses (off-label): Addiction disorders, antihistamine-induced coma,

Medication forms: *Injectable sol* (0.1 mg/ml)

Dosage:

- Benzo overdose: 0.2 mg over 15–30 s initially; if no change in 30 s, give 0.3 mg over 30 sec 1 min later
  - Repeat doses: 0.5 mg over 30 sec at 20-min intervals to max 3 mg/hr

MOA: Competitively inhibits benzo site on GABA/benzodiazepine receptor complex

Pharmacokinetics: Rapid onset of 1–2 min, $t_{1/2}$=53 min

Warnings:

- **Black box warning:** Has been associated with the occurrence of seizures, most frequently in patients who have been on benzodiazepines for long-term sedation or in overdose cases where patients are showing signs of serious cyclic antidepressant overdose; individualize dose and be prepared to manage seizures
- Do not use for reversal of respiratory depression due to benzos; treat serious respiratory depression due to benzos with appropriate ventilator support
- Risk of seizures if used in patients with concurrent major sedative-hypnotic withdrawal, recent therapy with repeated benzo doses, myoclonic jerking or seizure activity, and concurrent cyclic-antidepressant poisoning

- Can cause hypoventilation and return of sedation; use caution in ICU
- Used as adjunct; not a substitute for proper airway management, assisted breathing, circulatory access and support, or internal decontamination by lavage and charcoal
- Use caution in head injury, alcoholism and other drug dependence
- May cause pain with injection

Drug interactions:
- Avoid with TCAs; increases availability of these agents and causes toxicity
- Avoid until effects of neuromuscular blockers have been fully reversed
- Use caution in cases of mixed-drug overdose, as toxic effects (e.g., convulsion and cardiac dysrhythmia) of other drugs can cause reversal of effect by flumazenil
- Blocks effects of non-benzo agonists at benzo receptors (e.g., zopiclone)
- Avoid in epileptic patients receiving benzos

Common side effects: Agitation, blurred vision, dizziness, headache, injection-site pain, nausea, seizure, sweating, visual disturbance, vomiting

Contraindications: Hypersensitivity to flumazenil and benzos, in patients given benzos to treat life-threatening conditions (e.g., intracranial pressure, status epilepticus), TCA overdose

Recommended lab tests: ECG

Overdose: Precipitated withdrawal, seizures; OD rare

Tapering/withdrawal: Gradual taper recommended

Special populations:

Pregnancy: Risk Category C

Lactation: Use caution

Elderly: No dose adjustment necessary

Hepatic impairment: Lower dose recommended

Renal impairment: No dose adjustment necessary

Important notes:
- Only $GABA_A$-receptor antagonist available primarily by injection
- Good choice for minimizing severity of drinking

Levacetylmethadol[1,5,7,8,11,20,30,31,32,34,38,39,40]

Brand name: OrLAAM

FDA approved for: Opioid dependence

Other potential uses (off-label): Opioid withdrawal

Medication forms: *Conc* (10 mg/ml)

Dosage:
- Opioid dependence: 20–40 mg 3x/week initially, use 60–90 mg for maintenance

MOA: Acts as synthetic methadone and mu agonist

Pharmacokinetics: t_{max}=1.5–2 hrs, $t_{1/2}$=2.6–4 days

Warnings:

- QT prolongation and torsade de pointes have been reported
- Physiological dependence can develop
- Should not be used for any type of pain

Drug interactions: Concurrent use of CNS depressants

Common side effects: Abdominal cramps, arthralgia, asthenia, back pain, chills, edema, vomiting

Contraindications: Hypersensitivity, QTc prolongation,

Overdose: CNS depression, somnolence, coma, apnea; OD rare

Tapering/withdrawal: Gradual taper recommended

Special populations:

Pregnancy: Risk Category C

Lactation: Avoid

Elderly: Lower dose recommended

Hepatic impairment: Lower dose recommended

Renal impairment: No dose adjustment needed

Important notes:

- Synthetic opiate agonist with longer duration of action due to active metabolites
- Should be reserved for those patients who don't respond to other treatments

Methadone[1,5,6,7,8,11,20,28,30,31,32,34,38,39,40]

Brand name: Dolophine, Methadose, Diskets

FDA approved for: Opioid dependence, opioid detoxification, chronic pain (moderate to severe)

Other potential uses (off-label): Neuropathic pain

Medication forms: *Tab* (5, 10 mg); *ODT* (40 mg); *oral sol* (5, 10 mg/5 ml); *oral conc sol* (10 mg/ml); *injectable sol* (10 mg/ml)

Dosage:

- Opioid abuse: 20–30 mg po in demonstrated withdrawal, 80–120 mg/day maintenance
- Short-term detox: 15–40 mg po qd or minimum necessary to suppress withdrawal for 2–3 days, then decrease by max 20% daily as tolerated

MOA: Synthetic opioid analgesic; is an agonist at the mu receptor and also acts as an antagonist at the N-methyl-D-aspartate (NMDA) receptor

Pharmacokinetics: t_{max}=1–7hrs, $t_{1/2}$=8–59 hrs

Warnings:

- **Black box warning:**
  - Use of methadone hydrochloride increases the risk of opioid addiction, abuse, or misuse, which may cause overdose and death; only approved hospitals

and pharmacies can dispense oral methadone for the treatment of narcotic addiction

- Can cause life-threatening and fatal cases of respiratory depression, even when used as recommended
- Accidental ingestion of even one dose (especially by children) can result in fatal OD
- Not for acute or post-operative pain
- Can cause life-threatening QTc prolongation and serious arrhythmias
- Use during pregnancy can result in life-threatening neonatal withdrawal
- For detoxification and maintenance of opioid dependence, methadone should be administered in accordance with the treatment standards cited in 42 CFR Section 8, including limitations on unsupervised administration

- Life-threatening respiratory depression more likely in elderly, cachectic, or debilitated patients or those with chronic pulmonary disease
- Avoid abrupt discontinuation in physically dependent patients
- Has hypotensive effect; risk of orthostatic hypotension and syncope
- Monitor patients with head injury or increased ICP for sedation, respiratory depression
- May impair mental/physical abilities; use caution with potentially hazardous activities

Drug interactions:
- Avoid with rasagaline and selegiline, as both increase drug levels
- Affects hepatic enzyme CYP2D6, increasing plasma levels of medications metabolized by CYP2D6
- Increased plasma level and toxicity with agents that inhibit CYP3A4 (e.g., ketoconazole)
- CYP3A4 inducers decrease levels and drug effects
- Avoid with alvimopan due to increased drug activity
- Use with CNS depressants may cause profound sedation, respiratory depression, death
- Antiretroviral agents increase clearance and decrease drug plasma levels; alternatively, methadone increase risk of elevated plasma levels and toxicity of antiretroviral agents
- Use extreme caution when prescribing alongside any drug known to prolong QT interval
- Avoid with mixed agonist/antagonist and partial-agonist opioid analgesics due to reduced analgesic effects of drug or precipitation of withdrawal symptoms
- Use caution with anticholinergic drugs due to risk of urinary retention and reduced gastric motility

Common side effects: Constipation, dizziness, drowsiness, nausea, sedation, sweating, vomiting

Contraindications: Hypersensitivity, paralytic ileus, CNS depression, severe bronchial asthma

Recommended lab tests: EKG when using with antipsychotics

Overdose: Coma, respiratory depression, pulmonary edema, bradycardia, hypotension, QT prolongation, torsade de pointes, arrhythmias, syncope, rhabdomyolysis, seizure, cardiac arrest; OD potentially fatal

Tapering/withdrawal: Gradual taper over 3–6 months with 5–10 mg weekly reduction recommended

Special populations:

Pregnancy: Risk Category C

Lactation: Use caution and monitor closely

Elderly: Lower dose recommended

Hepatic impairment: No dose adjustment necessary in mild to moderate, lower dose recommended in severe

Renal impairment: No dose adjustment necessary in mild to moderate, lower dose recommended in severe

Important notes:

- Synthetic opiate analgesic primarily used for opioid dependence
- Alcohol, benzos, and cocaine frequently abused among patients on methadone maintenance
- Promethazine and clonidine misuse is also common among methadone pupulation
- Purpose of methadone maintenance and related programs is to stabilize patients to improve psychosocial functioning and to limit criminal activity and medical complications[32]

Naltrexone[1,5,7,8,11,19,20,30,31,32,34,36,38,39,40]

Brand name: ReVia (oral), Vivitrol (injection)

FDA approved for: Alcohol dependence, opiate dependence

Other potential uses (off-label): Opiate and nicotine withdrawal

Medication forms: *Tab* (50 mg); *suspension* (380 mg/vial)

Dosage:

- Opioid dependence:
  - Patient must be opioid-free for 7–10 days with negative naloxone challenge to avoid opioid withdrawal
  - *Oral:* 25 mg initially, then observation for 1 hr, then 50 mg qd starting on day 2
  - *IM:* 380 mg in gluteal muscle every 4 weeks
- Alcohol dependence:

- *Oral:* 50 mg qd for ≤12 weeks
- *IM:* 380 mg in gluteal muscle every 4 weeks

MOA: Pure opioid antagonist; blocks opioid effects through competitive binding at opioid receptors

Pharmacokinetics: t_{max}=1 hr (oral)/2 days (injectable), $t_{1/2}$=4 hrs (oral)/5–10 days (injectable)

Warnings:
- May increase depression and suicidal tendencies with long-term abuse of opioids or other substances
- Accidental ingestion can lead to severe withdrawal symptoms
- Risk of vulnerability to opioid overdose, precipitated opioid withdrawal, and hepatotoxicity
- Dangerous if reversal of ReVia blockade needed for pain management

Drug interactions:
- Avoid with other opioid analgesics due to antagonized effects
- Avoid with disulfiram due to possibility of hepatotoxicity
- Patients on ReVia do not benefit from opioid-containing medications
- May cause lethargy and somnolence with thioridazine

Common side effects: Abdominal cramps, allergic reaction, anxiety, decreased appetite, depression, dizziness, fatigue, headache, insomnia, joint pain, injection site reactions, myalgia, nausea, pruritus, rash, vomiting

Contraindications:
- Current dependence on opioids or acute opiate withdrawal; only administer when patient is free of opioid for >1 week
- Failure of naloxone challenge test or positive urine screen for opioids
- Hypersensitivity to naltrexone or any other diluent components

Recommended lab tests: Urine screen for opioids, naloxone challenge

Overdose: Tremor, hypotension, tachycardia, dizziness, insomnia, fatigue, and agitation

Tapering/withdrawal: Taper usually not required

Special populations

Pregnancy: Risk Category C

Lactation: Expressed in low amounts; use caution

Elderly: No data available; use caution

Hepatic impairment: No dose adjustment necessary in mild to moderate, avoid in severe

Renal impairment: No dose adjustment necessary in mild to moderate, avoid in severe

Important notes:
- Inform patients and/or caregivers about the serious risks associated with the use of naltrexone, including injection-site reactions

Nicotine Replacement Therapy (NRT)[1,5,7,8,11,12,20,30,31,32,34,38,39,40]

Brand name: Nicorette, Nicoderm, Nicotrol, Nicotrol NS

FDA approved for: Nicotine dependence

Other potential uses (off-label): Tourette syndrome, ulcerative colitis

Medication forms: *Transdermal patch* (5, 10, 15 mg worn over 16 hrs and 7, 14, 21 mg worn over 24 hours); *chewing gum* (2, 4 mg); *SL tab* (2 mg); *lozenge* (1, 2, 4 mg); *inhalation cartridge plus mouthpiece* (10 mg/cartridge [4 mg delivered]); *metered nasal spray* (0.5 mg dose/spray)

Dosage[11]:

- Gum:
  - *<25 cigarettes/day:* 2 mg every 1–2 hours for 6 weeks, then gradually taper for weeks 7–12
  - *≥25 cigarettes/day:* 4 mg every 1–2 hours for 6 weeks, then gradually taper for weeks 7–12
- Lozenge:
  - *First cigarette over 30 min after waking:* 2 mg every 1–2 hours for weeks 1–6, every 2–4 hours for weeks 7–9, and every 4–8 hours for weeks 10–12
  - *First cigarette within 30 min of waking:* 4 mg with same tapering schedule as above
- Patch:
  - *>10 cigarettes/day:*
    - 21/14/7-mg regimen: 21-mg patch/day for 6 weeks, then 14-mg patch/day for 2 weeks, then 7-mg patch/day for 2 weeks
    - 15/10/5-mg regimen: 15-mg patch/day for 6 weeks, then 10-mg patch/day for 2 weeks, then 5-mg patch/day for 2 weeks
  - *<45 kg or ≤10 cigarettes per day:*
    - 14/7-mg regimen: 14-mg patch/day for 6 weeks, then 7 mg patch/day for 2 weeks
    - 10/5-mg regimen: 10-mg patch/day for 6 weeks, then 5 mg patch/day for 2 weeks
- Inhaler: 6–16 cartridges/day for 3–6 weeks, then taper dose from weeks 6–12
- SL tab: One or two 2-mg tab/hour, max 80 mg/day (40 tab)
- Nasal spray: 1 spray (0.5 mg) per nostril as required, max 2x per hour and 64 sprays/day

MOA: Acts as an agonist at the nicotinic-cholinergic receptors in the autonomic ganglia, adrenal medulla, neuromuscular junctions, and brain

Pharmacokinetics: t_{max}=15 min (oral, inhalation)/4–15 min (intranasal)/6–12 hrs (transdermal), $t_{1/2}$=1–2 hrs (oral, inhalation, intranasal)/4 hrs (transdermal), nicotine spray delivers fastest nicotine

Warnings:
- Avoid in patients with menthol sensitivity or with active gum disease
- Use caution in patients with cardiac arrhythmia, PVD, HTN, and those requiring sodium-restricted diet
- Use utmost caution and consult healthcare provider in pregnant and breastfeeding women
- Use caution with prescription medication for asthma or depression

Drug interactions:
- Adjust dosage of following agents with NRT use: acetaminophen, caffeine, imipramine, lorazepam, pentazocine, theophylline, insulin, adrenergic antagonists, propranolol or other beta-blockers
- Reduce dosage of other antidepressant agents and anti-asthmatic drugs with NRT use

Common side effects: Anorexia, cough, diarrhea, dizziness, headache, heartburn, indigestion, nausea, rash

Contraindications: Hypersensitivity, cardiac problems

Recommended lab tests: HR, BP

Overdose: Seizures, confusion, weakness, bradycardia, hypotension

Tapering/withdrawal: Gradual taper recommended

Special populations

Pregnancy: Risk Category D

Lactation: Avoid any form of nicotine

Elderly: Use caution

Hepatic impairment: Use caution

Renal impairment: Use caution

Varenicline[1,5,7,8,11,20,25,30,31,32,34,38,39,40]

Brand name: Chantix

FDA approved for: Smoking cessation

Other potential uses (off-label): Nicotine withdrawal

Medication forms: *Tab* (0.5, 1 mg)

Dosage:
- Smoking cessation: 1-week titration in 12-week treatment
  - *Day 1–3:* 0.5 mg/day
  - *Day 4–7:* 0.5 mg bid
  - *Day 8–end of treatment:* 1 mg bid

MOA: Partial agonist at $\alpha_4\beta_2$-nicotine acetylcholine receptors; prevents nicotine from binding

Pharmacokinetics: t_{max}=2–4 hrs, $t_{1/2}$=24 hrs

Warnings:

- **Black box warning**: Monitor for serious neuropsychiatric symptoms including changes in behavior, hostility, agitation, depressed mood, and suicide-related events (e.g., ideation, behavior, and attempted suicide), which have occurred in patients taking or discontinuing varenicline; risks should be weighed against the benefits of its use
- Associated with accidental injury (e.g., traffic accidents)
- Risk of cardiovascular events (e.g., MI, stroke) and angioedema
- May cause HSR and serious skin reactions

Drug interactions:

- Renal clearance decreased by cimetidine
- Interaction with alcohol increases effects
- Smoking cessation with varenicline may alter pharmacokinetics/pharmacodynamics of certain drugs; adjust dose accordingly

Common side effects: Abdominal pain, abnormal dreams, constipation, flatulence, headache, insomnia, nausea, suicidal ideations, vomiting

Contraindications: Hypersensitivity

Recommended lab tests: None

Overdose: Agitation, confusion, tachycardia

Tapering/withdrawal: Gradual taper recommended

Special populations:

Pregnancy: Risk Category C

Lactation: Avoid

Elderly: No dose adjustment necessary

Hepatic impairment: No dose adjustment necessary

Renal impairment: No dose adjustment necessary in mild to moderate, max 0.5 mg bid in severe

Important notes:

- Commence treatment 1 week before smoking quit date; continue 12 weeks after quitting
- Can be used along with Zyban for smoking cessation

References:

1. Albers, Lawrence J., Rhoda K. Hahn, and Christopher Reist. 2010. *Handbook of Psychiatric Drugs*. 2011 ed. 39–59. Current Clinical Strategies Publishing.

2. American Psychiatric Association (APA). 2005. *Practice Guideline for the Treatment of Patients with Substance Use Disorders*. 2nd ed. Washington, DC: American Psychiatric Publishing.

3. American Psychiatric Association (APA). 2013. *Diagnostic and Statistical Manual of Mental Disorders.* 5th ed. (DSM-5®). Washington, DC: American Psychiatric Publishing.

4. Asplund C., Aaronson J., and Aaronson H. 2004. "3 regimens for alcohol withdrawal and detoxification." Accessed January 14, 2015. http://www.jfponline.com/home/article/3-regimens-for-alcohol-withdrawal-and-detoxification.

5. Center Watch. 2015. "FDA Approved Drugs by Therapeutic Area." Accessed February 3, 2015. http://www.centerwatch.com/drug-information/fda-approved-drugs/therapeutic-area/17/psychiatry-psychology.

6. Drugs.com. 2015. "Methanadone (Oral Route)." Accessed January 14, 2015. http://www.drugs.com/cons/methadone.html.

7. Elsevier Gold Standard, Inc. 2015. "Clinical Pharmacology." Accessed March 12, 2015. https://www.clinicalpharmacology.com.

8. Epocrates. 2015. Accessed March 25, 2015. https://online.epocrates.com.

9. Etherington, J. M. 1996. "Emergency management of acute alcohol problems. Part 1: Uncomplicated withdrawal." *Can Fam Physician* 42:2186–2190.

10. Forest Laboratories, Inc. 2012. "CAMPRAL - acamprosate calcium tablet, delayed release." US National Library of Medicine: Daily Med. Accessed December 5, 2014. http://dailymed.nlm.nih.gov/dailymed/drugInfo.cfm?setid=1c427b06-32d4-482f-bb83-71e386c1e203.

11. Gabbard, Glen O., ed. 2007. *Gabbard's Treatments of Psychiatric Disorders.* 4th ed. 193–294. Washington, DC: American Psychiatric Publishing.

12. GlaxoSmithKline Consumer Healthcare LP. 2014. "NICORETTE- nicotine lozenge." US National Library of Medicine: Daily Med. Accessed December 5, 2014. http://dailymed.nlm.nih.gov/dailymed/drugInfo.cfm?setid=991704ed-781a-489b-8b56-0b558e8fc385.

13. Gold, M.S., D.E. Redmond Jr., and H.D. Kleber. 1978. "Clonidine in opiate withdrawal." *Lancet* 1:929–930.

14. Hales, Robert. E., S. Yudofsky, and L. Roberts, eds. 2014. *The American Psychiatric Publishing Textbook of Psychiatry.* 6th ed. 735–814, 929–1004. Washington, DC: American Psychiatric Publishing.

15. Mann, K. 2004. "Pharmacotherapy of alcohol dependence: a review of the clinical data." *CNS Drugs* 18:485–504.

16. Mason, B.J. 2005. "Acamprosate in the treatment of alcohol dependence." *Expert Opinion on Pharmacotherapy* 6:2103–2115.

17. Medscape: Drugs & Diseases. 2013. "Alcohol and Substance Abuse Evaluation." Accessed January 14, 2015. http://emedicine.medscape.com/article/805084-overview.

18. Medscape: Drugs & Diseases. 2015. "Chlordiazepoxide (Rx) - Librium." Accessed January 14, 2015. http://reference.medscape.com/drug/librium-chlordiazepoxide-342899.

19. Medscape: Drugs & Diseases. 2015. "Naltrexone (Rx) - ReVia, Vivitrol, Depade." Accessed January 14, 2015. http://reference.medscape.com/drug/vivitrol-revia-naltrexone-343333.

20. Medscape: Drugs & Diseases. 2015. "Psychiatrics." Accessed February 3, 2015. http://reference.medscape.com/drugs/psychiatrics.

21. Medscape. 2015. "Psychiatry and Mental Health." Accessed March 12, 2015. http://www.medscape.com/psychiatry.

22. Mylan Institutional, LLC. 2014. "FLUMAZENIL- flumazenil injection, solution." US National Library of Medicine: Daily Med. Accessed December 5, 2014. http://dailymed.nlm.nih.gov/dailymed/drugInfo.cfm?setid=f5716b57-6e5c-4c89-9d4e-5be0bc86c5be.

23. National Institute on Alcohol Abuse and Alcoholism (NIAAA). 2015. Accessed February 3, 2015. http://www.niaaa.nih.gov.

24. National Institute on Drug Abuse (NIDA). 2015. Accessed February 3, 2015. www.drugabuse.gov.

25. Pfizer Inc. 2014. "CHANTIX- varenicline tartrate tablet, film coated." US National Library of Medicine: Daily Med. Accessed December 5, 2014. http://dailymed.nlm.nih.gov/dailymed/drugInfo.cfm?setid=f0ff4f27-5185-4881-a749-c6b7a0ca5696.

26. Preston, John D., and James Johnson. 2011. *Clinical Psychopharmacology Made Ridiculously Simple.* 7th ed. 1–79. Miami: MedMaster Inc.

27. Reckitt Benckiser Pharmaceuticals, Inc. 2014. "SUBOXONE- buprenorphine hydrochloride and naloxone hydrochloride film, soluble." US National Library of Medicine: Daily Med. Accessed December 5, 2014. http://dailymed.nlm.nih.gov/dailymed/drugInfo.cfm?setid=8a5edcf9-828c-4f97-b671-268ab13a8ecd.

28. Roxane Laboratories, Inc. 2014. "DOLOPHINE- methadone hydrochloride tablet." US National Library of Medicine: Daily Med. Accessed December 5, 2014. http://dailymed.nlm.nih.gov/dailymed/drugInfo.cfm?setid=7a4840d6-98e3-4523-81a0-ef0b3a47d0c2.

29. Ruiz, Pedro, Eric C. Strain, and John G. Langrod. 2007. *The Substance Abuse Handbook.* 203–224. New York: Lippincott Williams & Wilkins.

30. RxList. 2015. "Drugs A-Z List." Accessed March 25, 2015. http://www.rxlist.com/drugs/alpha_a.htm.

31. Schatzberg, A.F., and C.B. Nemeroff, eds. 2009. *The American Psychiatric Publishing Textbook of Psychopharmacology.* 4th ed. 1007–1026, 1213–1230. Washington, DC: American Psychiatric Publishing.

32. Schatzberg, A.F., Jonathan O. Cole, and Charles DeBattista. 2010. *Manual of Clinical Psychopharmacology.* 7th ed. 565–588. Washington, DC: American Psychiatric Publishing.

33. Stahl, S.M. 2008. *Essential Psychopharmacology: Neuroscientific Basis and Practical Applications.* 3rd ed. 537–575. New York: Cambridge Press.

34. Stahl, S.M. 2011. *Essential Psychopharmacology: the Prescriber's Guide.* 4th ed. 1–3, 9–13, 91–95, 117–121, 129–132, 159–163, 377–379, 409–412, 435–438, 497–500, 565–568, 609–612, 631–633. Cambridge: Cambridge University Press.

35. Substance Abuse and Mental Health Services Administration (SAMHSA). 2015. Accessed February 3, 2015. http://www.samhsa.gov/disorders/substance-use.

36. Teva Women's Health, Inc. 2013. "REVIA- naltrexone hydrochloride tablet, film coated." US National Library of Medicine: Daily Med. Accessed December 5, 2014. http://dailymed.nlm.nih.gov/dailymed/drugInfo.cfm?setid=0d929bf5-2eaa-4679-8334-1ac159b2b55c.

37. Teva Women's Health, Inc. 2014. "ANTABUSE- disulfiram tablet." US National Library of Medicine: Daily Med. Accessed December 5, 2014. http://dailymed.nlm.nih.gov/dailymed/drugInfo.cfm?setid=f0ca0e1f-9641-48d5-9367-e5d1069e8680.

38. Truven Health Analytics. 2015. *Micromedex 2.0.* Accessed March 20, 2015. http://www.micromedexsolutions.com/home/dispatch.

39. UpToDate. 2015. Accessed March 12, 2015. http://www.uptodate.com/home.

40. US National Library of Medicine. 2015. "Drugs and Lactation Database (LactMed)." Accessed February 3, 2015. http://toxnet.nlm.nih.gov/newtoxnet/lactmed.htm.

41. US National Library of Medicine. 2015. "Toxicology Data Network." Accessed March 17, 2015. http://toxnet.nlm.nih.gov.

42. Wegmann, J. 2008. *Psychopharmacology: Straight Talk on Mental Health Medications.* 93–108. Eau Claire: Pesi, LLC

Chapter 11-2
Benzodiazepine Use And Abuse

Generally producing immediate effects, benzos are prescribed for short-term, intermittent, and as-needed use.[9] They work as hypnotics at higher doses, anxiolytics in moderate doses, and sedatives in lower doses. Benzos have a high addictive potential and dependence and tolerance can develop with long-term use, even at therapeutic doses.[17] Special attention should be given to a patient's addiction history before prescribing these medications. Understanding the abuse pattern of benzos and being familiar with alternative anxiolytic/hypnotic agents will enable healthcare providers to maximize treatment results and reduce their medical-legal liability.[10]

MOA: These drugs act on the benzodiazepine receptor that modulates GABA.[5,14]

Types:

- *High-potency:* Alprazolam, lorazepam, triazolam
- *Low-potency:* Oxazepam, temazepam
- *Long half-life:* Chlordiazepoxide, clonazepam, clorazepate, diazepam, flurazepam

Clinical use:

- Helpful for various conditions, including[3,7,14]:
  - Insomnia
  - Detoxification
  - Acute mania and agitation associated with psychiatric conditions
  - Anxiety disorders: GAD, panic disorder, phobias, OCD
  - Akathisia associated with neuroleptic use
  - Catatonia or mutism, convulsive disorders, impulse control disorders
  - Spasticity and seizures

Abuse

Benzos are relatively inexpensive, widely prescribed, and can be legally obtained. Four of them (alprazolam, clonazepam, diazepam, and lorazepam) are among the top 100 most commonly prescribed medications.[9,10] Poly-drug abuse accounts for 80% of benzo abuse, as the drug is often paired with opioids.[3,9] The rapid onset of short-acting benzos makes them a favorite for addicts, and high-dose benzo abuse is especially prevalent in patients taking methadone.[8,9] Medical prescriptions constitute the primary source of supply for abusers.[9] Benzos may be a factor in road accidents, particularly when used with other sedative drugs or alcohol.[4] Although benzo overdose is not lethal generally, overdose may be fatal when benzos are paired with another sedative (including methadone).[4]

Symptoms: Amnesia, blurred vision, confusion, disturbing dreams, drowsiness, hostility, irritability, poor coordination, reduced inhibition and impaired judgment.[7,10,15]

Risk factors: Although genetic factors may contribute to developing addiction, environmental and psychosocial factors also play a significant role. Some of the risk factors include low socioeconomic status, unemployment, peer pressure, inappropriate dosages, negligent prescription practices, history of substance abuse, use of high-dose or short-acting potent benzos, long-term use, and dependent personality.[4,7,10]

Withdrawal

Approximately 50% of patients on benzos for more than four months have reported withdrawal symptoms.[13,14] Symptoms include: anxiety, panic attack, insomnia, restlessness, excitability and dysphoria, poor memory and concentration, tremor, palpitation, sweating, depersonalization and derealization, hallucinations, formication, sensory hypersensitivity, psychosis, confusion, delirium, and convulsions.[2,3,17]

Management of Withdrawal

Pharmacologic Treatment[1,10,14,17]

Tapering: Gradual prolonged decrease of current dose; rapid reduction of up to 50% of initial dose, then 10% reduction per week.

Conversion to long-acting benzo: A shift from short-acting benzos such as lorazepam or alprazolam to longer-acting ones such as clonazepam can be attempted if tapering the shorter-acting drug causes uncomfortable symptoms. The longer-acting benzo can be tapered gradually.[14]

Substituting phenobarbital/carbamazepine: The pentobarbital tolerance test followed by phenobarbital is now rarely used.[14] Carbamazepine has mixed results during withdrawal from alprazolam and other short-acting benzos but 200-800 mg/day prior to taper has shown longer abstinence post-taper than placebo.

Psychological Therapy

Counseling and support with cognitive, behavioral, and group therapy.[7,10]

Prescription Guidelines

Prescribing maintenance benzos for chronic anxiety disorders in patients with serious substance-abuse disorders can be a very risky protocol.[9] To make matters worse, some of these patients may be getting medications on the street as well. At the same time, some substance abuse patients likely have severe anxiety disorders and may not respond to usual medications, especially non-benzos, and may respond better to a prescribed, well-monitored low-dose benzo regimen.[14] Controlled-substance over-prescriptions are a leading cause of physician investigation, which creates an unfortunate paradox for physicians: the desire to relieve anxiety must be weighed against the fear of creating addictions.[10] These competing concerns can make physicians reluctant to prescribe benzos to patients with legitimate illnesses who are then left undertreated or feeling stigmatized.[10] Implementing a few basic safeguards can optimize risk-management. These safeguards include writing "tamper-resistant" prescriptions, treatment contracts, consulting with peers, and monitoring prescriptions via state prescription-drug monitoring programs (PDMP) that list all controlled medications prescribed to the patient.[17]

Signs of a dependent/drug seeking patient[4,10,17]

- May be doctor shopping; goes to multiple providers for same prescription
- Insists on receiving a particular medications on the first visit
- Insists that nothing else has worked and that they have tried everything
- Complains of having side effects to all non-benzo medications
- Claims to have high tolerance to medications and insists on higher dosage
- Loses prescriptions before the prescription is due for refill
- Arrives after hours and claims to be from out of town
- Very resistant to tapering or change of dosage
- Increases dosage on his/her own and gives rationale for it
- Routinely complains about having withdrawal and seizures without benzos
- Sells/forges prescriptions or may use the prescriptions of others

Important notes[7,9,14,17]

- Gradually taper with high doses and use adjuvant medications
- Explain risk of dependence associated with long-term use to patients
- Avoid in known substance abusers unless justified with clear documentation
- Use lowest dose with shortest duration necessary
- First treat anxiety with non-benzos and non-pharmacological means (e.g., CBT)
- Communicate with other healthcare-team members (e.g., methadone-prescribers, pain clinics)
- Use regular toxicology tests to screen for other substances
- Monitor for memory impairment, especially in elderly patients
- Fatal overdoses often involve alcohol, with or without opiates
- Oxazepam, clorazepate, and chlordiazepoxide may have lower reinforcing effects[9]

References:

1. American Psychiatric Association (APA). 2005. *Practice Guideline for the Treatment of Patients with Substance Use Disorders.* 2nd ed. Washington, DC: American Psychiatric Publishing.

2. American Psychiatric Association (APA). 2013. *Diagnostic and Statistical Manual of Mental Disorders.* 5th ed. (DSM-5®). Washington, DC: American Psychiatric Publishing.

3. Ashton, C. Heather. 2002. "Benzodiazepines: How They Work and How to Withdraw." Newcastle University. Accessed March 12, 2015. http://www.benzo.org.uk/manual.

4. Benzodiazepines Addiction Treatment. 2009. "Benzodiazepines Drug Addiction Rehab." Accessed February 3, 2015. http://www.benzosrehab.com.

5. Campo-Soria, Claudia, Yongchang Chang, and David S. Weiss. 2006. "Mechanism of action of benzodiazepines on GABA(A) receptors." *British Journal of Pharmacology* 148(7):984–990. doi: 10.1038/sj.bjp.0706796.

6. Etherington, J. M. 1996. "Emergency management of acute alcohol problems: Part 1: Uncomplicated withdrawal." *Can Fam Physician* 42:2186–2190.

7. Gabbard, Glen O., ed. 2007. *Gabbard's Treatments of Psychiatric Disorders*. 4th ed. 193–294. Washington, DC: American Psychiatric Publishing.

8. Iguchi, M. Y., R. R. Griffiths, W. K. Bickel, L. Handelsman, A. R. Childress, and A. T. McLellan. 1989. "Relative abuse liability of benzodiazepines in methadone maintained populations in three cities." *NIDA Res Monogr* 95:364–365.

9. Longo, Lance P., and Brian Johnson. 2000. "Addiction: Part I. Benzodiazepines – Side Effects, Abuse Risk and Alternatives." *Am Fam Physician* 61(7):2121–2128.

10. Longo, Lance P., Ted Parran, Jr., Brian Johnson, and W. Kinsey. 2000. "Addiction: Part II. Identification and Management of the Drug-Seeking Patient." *Am Fam Physician* 61(8):2401–2408.

11. National Drug Intelligence Center (NDIC). 2011. *The Economic Impact of Illicit Drug Use on American Society*. United States Department of Justice. Accessed March 31, 2015. http://www.justice.gov/archive/ndic/pubs44/44731/44731p.pdf.

12. Ries, R.K., P.P. Roy-Byrne, N.G. Ward, V. Neppe, and S. Cullison. 1989. "Carbamazepine treatment for benzodiazepine withdrawal." *Am J Psychiatry* 146:536–537.

13. Ruiz, P., Strain, E., and Langrod J. 2007. *Substance Abuse Handbook*. 1st ed. Philadelphia, PA: Lippincott Williams & Wilkins.

14. Schatzberg, A.F., Jonathan O. Cole, and Charles DeBattista. 2010. *Manual of Clinical Psychopharmacology*. 7th ed. 565–588. Washington, DC: American Psychiatric Publishing.

15. Scher, Lorin. 2014. "Sedative, Hypnotic, Anxiolytic Use Disorders Clinical Presentation." Accessed March 12, 2015. http://emedicine.medscape.com/article/290585-clinical.

16. US National Library of Medicine. 2015. "Toxicology Data Network." Accessed March 17, 2015. http://toxnet.nlm.nih.gov.

17. Uhlenhuth, E.H., ed. 1999. "Benzodiazepine Dependence and Withdrawal: Myths and Management." *J Clin Psychopharmacol* 19(2 suppl):1S–29S.

Chapter 12
Dementia-Related Disorders And Cognitive Enhancers

Cognition refers to brain processes involved in memory, attention, perception, executive function, language, and psychomotor function. Cognitive impairment involves reversible or irreversible mental deterioration and confusion which can interfere with social and occupational functioning.[2,3] Cognitive-enhancing drugs are used to treat cognitive deficits in patients suffering from the effects of Alzheimer's, stroke, ADHD, or aging.[14] Cognitive impairments are often prolonged and progressive and some patients may require constant assistance and supervision. This often places an enormous physical, emotional, and psychological strain on caregivers.

Alzheimer's disease (AD) is a common neurocognitive disorder with symptoms of marked cognitive and behavioral impairment.[2,3] It is among the top five leading causes of death in patients over 65.[14]

Changes in DSM-5
The DSM-5 diagnoses of dementia and amnestic disorder are included under the newly named Neurocognitive Disorder (NCD).[3] According to the APA, the term dementia can still be used to refer to this condition.[3] The major change in this category of disorders is the addition of "mild neurocognitive disorder," stressing the need for early detection and treatment before these conditions progress to a "major neurocognitive disease" or other serious, debilitating impairments.[4]

DSM-5 major and mild neurocognitive disorders[3,4]:
- Includes dementia and amnestic disorders
- Divided by etiologies:
    - Major or mild neurocognitive disorder due to Alzheimer's disease
    - Major or mild frontotemporal neurocognitive disorder
    - Major or mild neurocognitive disorder due to Lewy bodies
    - Vascular disease
    - Traumatic brain injury
    - Substance/medication use
    - HIV
    - Prion disease
    - Parkinson's
    - Huntington's
    - Another medical condition
    - Multiple etiologies

- Specifiers:
  - With or without behavioral disturbance
  - Current severity (for major neurocognitive disorders): mild, moderate, or severe
- Delirium: Criteria updated and clarified based on currently available evidence

Treatment

Cognitive impairment demands a thorough psychiatric, neurological, and general medical evaluation of the nature and cause of the cognitive deficits and any associated non-cognitive symptoms.[5] An individualized, multimodal treatment approach is crucial.[5] Management includes supportive therapy and pharmacologic management.[5,14] Medications such as neuroleptics, benzos, and cholinesterase inhibitors are commonly used.[5] Supportive therapy includes psychotherapy, nutrition, multivitamins reorientation, and memory cues using family photos, calendars, and caregiving.[14,21] It is important to note that anticholinergic agents can further impair cognition in patients with dementia.[19]

Medications

Cholinesterase inhibitors and NMDA-receptor antagonists are used to treat cognitive impairment.[26] Functional symptoms of impairment involving personality and behavior may also improve with the help of cognitive enhancers, but there is no evidence that they prevent or slow neurodegeneration or alter the course of the underlying disease.[16,27]

Cholinesterase Inhibitors

Cholinesterase inhibitors increase acetylcholine availability and enhance cholinergic neurotransmission by decreasing the cholinesterase-mediated degradation of acetylcholine in the synaptic cleft.[6,14] At least six months of use is needed before there are observable effects of these medications on cognitive function.[6] The cholinesterase inhibitors used for cognitive enhancement are: donepezil (Aricept), galantamine (Razadyne), and rivastigmine (Exelon).

Donepezil[1,8,10,11,12,14,20,24,25,26,29,30,31,32,33]
Brand names: Aricept, Aricept ODT
FDA approved for: Treatment of mild, moderate, or severe dementia (Alzheimer's type)
Other potential uses (off-label): Multi-infarct and Lewy body dementia
Medication forms: *Tab* (5, 10, 23 mg); *ODT* (5, 10 mg)
Dosage:
- Alzheimer's disease:
  - *Mild-to-moderate:* 5 mg qhs initially, can be increased based on tolerance/response to 10 mg/day after 4–6 weeks
  - *Severe:* 10–23 mg/day

MOA: Reversible acetylcholinesterase (AChE) inhibitor; increases the concentration of acetylcholine through the reversible inhibition of its hydrolysis by acetylcholinesterase

Pharmacokinetics: t_{max}=3–4 hrs, $t_{1/2}$=70 hrs

Warnings:

- Use caution in patients with a history of asthma or obstructive pulmonary disease
- Risk of exaggerated muscle relaxation during anesthesia
- Can have vagotonic effects on the SA and AV nodes causing bradycardia, heart block
- May cause increased GI secretion; avoid in active or occult GI bleeding
- Dose of 23 mg/day associated with weight loss and increased side effects
- May cause bladder outflow obstructions and generalized convulsions

Drug interactions:

- Can potentiate the action of fluoxetine
- Can lower seizure threshold when combined with bupropion
- Metabolism decreased with inhibitors of CYP2D6 and CYP3A4
- Can interfere with anticholinergic medications
- Synergistic effects with succinylcholine, similar neuromuscular blocking agents, or cholinergic agonists

Common side effects: Cramps, diarrhea, fatigue, headache, insomnia, nausea, vomiting

Contraindications: Hypersensitivity

Recommended lab tests: Weight

Overdose: Miosis, flushing, bradycardia, bronchospasm, sweating, lacrimation, hypotension, and/or seizure

Tapering/withdrawal: Slow taper recommended

Special populations:

Pregnancy: Risk Category C

Lactation: Avoid

Elderly: Lower dose recommended especially in women of low body weight

Hepatic impairment: Lower dose recommended

Renal impairment: No dose adjustment necessary

Important notes:

- Start at low dose and slowly titrate to avoid side effects

Galantamine[1,8,11,12,14,18,20,24,25,26,29,30,31,32,33]

Brand names: Razadyne, Razadyne ER

FDA approved for: Mild-to-moderate dementia (Alzheimer's disease)

Other potential uses (off-label): Multi-infarct and Parkinson's dementia

Medication forms: *Tab* (4, 8, 12 mg); *ER cap* (8, 16, 24 mg); *liq* (4mg/ml [100 ml bottle])

Dosage:

- Alzheimer's disease:
  - *IR:* 4 mg bid initially, can be increased based on tolerance/response to maintenance 8–12 mg bid
  - *ER:* 8 mg qam initially, maintenance 16–24 mg qam

MOA: Increases acetylcholine levels by reversibly inhibiting the neurotransmitter's hydrolysis by acetylcholinesterase; activity at nicotinic receptors enhances release of acetylcholine and other neurotransmitters, boosting attention and improving behavior

Pharmacokinetics: t_{max}=1 hr, $t_{1/2}$=7 hrs

Warnings:

- Risk of serious skin reactions (including SJS)
- Caution in patients with a history of asthma or obstructive pulmonary disease
- Risk of exaggerated muscle relaxation during anesthesia
- Can have vagotonic effects on the SA and AV nodes causing bradycardia, heart block
- May cause increased GI secretion; avoid in active or occult GI bleeding
- May cause bladder outflow obstructions and generalized convulsions

Drug interactions:

- Metabolism decreased with inhibitors of CYP2D6 and CYP3A4
- Can interfere with anticholinergic medications
- Synergistic effects with succinylcholine, similar neuromuscular blocking agents, or cholinergic agonists
- Cimetidine can increase levels when combined

Common side effects: Decreased appetite, diarrhea, dizziness, headache, nausea, vomiting, weight loss

Contraindications: Hypersensitivity

Recommended lab tests: Weight

Overdose: Sweating, vomiting, bradycardia, syncope

Tapering/withdrawal: Gradual taper recommended

Special populations:

Pregnancy: Risk Category C

Lactation: Avoid

Elderly: Lower doses in patients with low body weight

Hepatic impairment: Lower dose recommended in mild to moderate, avoid in severe

Renal impairment: Lower dose recommended in mild to moderate, avoid in severe

Cardiac impairment: Use caution

Important notes:
- Treats cognitive, behavioral, and psychological symptoms of Alzheimer's dementia
- Advise patients to take with food to minimize GI side effects

Rivastigmine[1,8,11,12,14,22,24,25,26,29,30,31,32,33]

Brand names: Exelon, Exelon Patch

FDA approved for: Mild-to-moderate dementia of Alzheimer's type and dementia associated with Parkinson's disease

Other potential uses (off-label): Cognitive impairment due to other dementias

Medication forms: *Cap* (1.5, 3, 4.5, 6 mg); *liq* (2mg/ml [120 ml bottle]); *transdermal patch* (9 mg/5 cm² [4.6 mg/24 hr], 18 mg/10 cm² [9.5 mg/24 hr], 27 mg/15 cm² [13.3mg/24 hr])

Dosage:
- Alzheimer's dementia:
  - *Oral (mild-to-moderate dementia):* 1.5 mg bid initially, can be increased based on tolerance/response to maintenance 3–6 mg bid
  - *Transdermal:* Apply 4.6 mg/24 hr initially, use 9.5-13.3 mg/24 hr for mild to moderate or 13.3 mg/24 hr in severe

MOA: Inhibits the hydrolytic action of cholinesterase, resulting in increased acetylcholine concentrations

Pharmacokinetics: t_{max}=8–16 hrs, $t_{1/2}$=3 hrs

Warnings:
- May cause acute dermatitis; discontinue if disseminated hypersensitivity skin reaction occurs and only reinstate oral dose after negative allergy testing
- Can cause or exacerbate EPS
- Caution in patients with a history of asthma or obstructive pulmonary disease
- Risk of exaggerated muscle relaxation during anesthesia
- Can have vagotonic effects on the SA and AV nodes causing bradycardia, heart block
- May cause bladder outflow obstructions and generalized convulsions
- GI adverse reactions include significant nausea, vomiting, diarrhea, anorexia/decreased appetite, ulcers, and weight loss; may result in serious dehydration
- May cause increase GI secretion; avoid in active or occult GI bleeding

Drug interactions:
- Can increase risk of QT prolongation with other QT-prolonging drugs (e.g., amifamridine, piperquine)
- Increased risk of EPS when used with metoclopramide; avoid
- Avoid with cholinomimetic and anticholinergic drugs unless clinically necessary
- Avoid concurrent use with beta-blockers due to additive effects

Common side effects: Asthenia, confusion, diarrhea, dizziness, headache, indigestion, malaise, nausea, vomiting

Contraindications: Hypersensitivity, history of application-site reaction with transdermal patch (allergic contact dermatitis) without negative allergy testing

Recommended lab tests: LFTs, weight

Overdose: HTN, drowsiness, colic, diaphoresis

Tapering/withdrawal: Gradual taper recommended

Special populations:

Pregnancy: Risk Category B

Lactation: Avoid

Elderly: Lower dose recommended in patients with low body weight

Hepatic/Renal impairment: No dose adjustment necessary

Important notes:

- Increased incidence of nausea during titration; usually improves during maintenance
- Advise patients to take with food
- Transdermal patch should be applied to dry skin at same time every day in different body locations
- Trace aluminum in some transdermal patches; ask patient to disclose that information if he or she needs an MRI

N-Methyl-D-Aspartate (NDMA) Receptor Antagonists

Chronic activation of NMDA receptors in the CNS leading to neuronal excitotoxicity may be partially responsible for the neurodegeneration and symptoms of AD. Memantine is proposed to reduce chronic activation by acting as an NMDA-receptor antagonist.[16,27] Because of their different mechanisms of action, the use of cholinesterase inhibitors with memantine has been suggested for patients with moderate-to-severe AD.[8]

Memantine[1,8,11,12,13,14,20,24,25,26,29,30,31,32,33]

Brand names: Namenda, Namenda XR

FDA approved for: Moderate-to-severe dementia (Alzheimer's type)

Other potential uses (off-label): Vascular dementias

Medication forms: *Tab* (5, 10 mg); *ER cap* (7, 14, 21, 28 mg); *oral sol* (2 mg/ml)

Dosage:

- Alzheimer's dementia
  - *IR:* 5 mg qd initially, increase based on tolerance/response (>5 weeks) to target dosage of 20 mg/day divided bid for maintenance
  - *ER:* 7 mg qd initially, use target dosage of 28 mg qd for maintenance

MOA: Noncompetitive NMDA receptor antagonist; also blocks the 5-hydroxytryptamine-3 receptor and nicotinic acetylcholine receptors and prevents excitatory amino acid neurotoxicity

Pharmacokinetics: t_{max} =3–7 hrs, $t_{1/2}$=60–80 hrs

Warnings: Toxicity due to UTI and renal tubular acidosis

Drug interactions:

- Reduced elimination with drugs that raise urine pH
- Increased serum concentration with bupropion

Common side effects: Confusion, constipation, cough, dizziness, hallucination, headache

Contraindications: Hypersensitivity

Lab tests recommend: Serum creatinine

Overdose: GI symptoms, confusion, muscle weakness, hypertension

Tapering/withdrawal: Slow taper recommended

Special populations:

Pregnancy: Risk Category B

Lactation: Avoid

Elderly: No dose adjustment needed

Hepatic impairment: No dose adjustment necessary in mild to moderate, use caution in severe

Renal impairment: No dosage adjustment necessary in mild to moderate, max 5 mg bid in severe

Important notes:

- Combining memantine and donepezil may be mildly more useful than either alone

Stimulants

Most stimulant drugs can be utilized as cognitive enhancers. Please see *Chapter 7: ADHD and Its Treatment* for full details on these medications.

Amphetamine-based stimulants include:

- Adderall
- Adderall XR
- Dexedrine

- Dexedrine Spansule
- Dextrostat

- Vyvanse

Methylphenidate-based stimulants include:

- Focalin
- Focalin XR
- Methylin
- Methylin ER

- Metadate ER
- Metadate CD
- Ritalin
- Ritalin SR

- Ritalin LA
- Concerta
- Quillivant XR
- Daytrana

Other Medications

Caprylidene[1,8,11,12,14,20,24,25,26,29,30,31,32,33]

Brand names: Axona

FDA approved for: Dietary management of the metabolic processes associated with mild-to-moderate Alzheimer's disease

Medication forms: *Oral powder* (40 g/packet)

Dosage: 40 g/day

MOA: Provides medium-chain triglycerides to the body that can be metabolized into ketone bodies which may be utilized by the brain as an alternative source of fuel

Pharmacokinetics: Processed by lipase in gut and absorbed into the portal vein

Warnings: Use caution with GERD, stomach problems, IBS; can cause nausea, diarrhea, gas, heartburn

Drug interactions: None

Common side effects: Diarrhea, dyspepsia, flatulence, headache, nausea

Contraindications: Proven allergy to milk or soy

Recommended lab tests: None

Overdose: Severe GI symptoms

Tapering/withdrawal: Tapering not needed

Special populations:

Pregnancy: Risk Category C

Lactation: Avoid

Elderly: Lower dose recommended

Hepatic impairment: No data available

Renal impairment: No data available

L-methylfolate[1,8,11,12,14,20,24,25,26,29,30,31,32,33,34]

Brand names: Deplin

FDA approved for: Megabalastic anemia, adjunctive treatment in depression and schizophrenia

Other potential uses (off-label): As a cognitive enhancer, depression

Medication forms: *Tab* (7.5, 15 mg)

Dosage: 7.5–15 mg/day

MOA: May increase monoamine synthesis and augment antidepressant therapy in patients with depression; normalizes high homocysteine levels

Pharmacokinetics: t_{max}=1–3 hrs, $t_{1/2}$=3 hrs

Warnings: Caution in patients with history of anemia or bipolar illness or low levels of vitamin B12

Drug interactions:

- Use with anticonvulsants increases the metabolism of circulating folate
- Use with L-dopa, isotretinoin, triamterene, metformin, methylprednisolone, colchicine, OCP, and trimethoprim may decrease plasma folate levels
- High levels of folic acid may decrease serum levels of pyrimethamine
- Smoking and alcohol reduce serum folate levels

Common side effects: Abdominal distention, anorexia, confusion, difficulty concentrating, excitement, flatulence, irritability, nausea

Contraindications: Hypersensitivity
Recommended lab tests: CBC
Overdose: Effects not known
Tapering/withdrawal: Tapering not needed
Special populations:
Pregnancy: Risk Category A
Lactation: Generally safe
Elderly: No dose adjustment necessary
Hepatic/Renal impairment: Max 40 mg/day

Modafinil[1,8,9,11,12,14,20,24,25,26,29,30,31,32,33]
Brand names: Provigil
FDA approved for: Narcolepsy, excessive somnolence due to OSA or shift work sleep disorder
Other potential uses (off-label): ADHD, cocaine abuse, depression, fatigue due to HIV, improving brain function, weight loss
Medication forms: *Tab* (100, 200 mg)
Dosage:
- Depression:100 mg qam initially, can be increased based on tolerance/response to max 400 mg/day
- Narcolepsy/improving brain function: 200 mg qam initially, can be increased based on tolerance/response to max 400 mg/day
- Shift work sleep disorder: 200 mg 1 hour prior to patient's work shift

MOA: Antagonist at α_1-adrenergic receptors; has some actions similar to sympathomimetic agents
Pharmacokinetics: t_{max}=2–4 hrs, $t_{1/2}$=15 hrs, food slows absorption
Warnings:
- Can cause depression, mania, psychosis, and cardiac problems
- May cause angioedema/anaphylactoid reactions (HSR); rare risk of serious rash(including SJS)
- May not result in normalized wakefulness; assess for and advise patients of risk of persistent sleepiness
- May alter judgment, thinking, or motor skills; use caution when operating an automobile or machinery
- Periodically assess CPAP compliance in sleep apnea

Drug interactions:
- May reduce efficacy of aripiprazole
- Increased plasma levels and toxicity with inhibitors of CYP3A4
- Decreases effectiveness of OCP

- Avoid with MAOIs due to increased toxicity through synergism

Common side effects: Anxiety, backache, diarrhea, dizziness, headache, indigestion, insomnia, nausea, nervousness, rhinitis

Contraindications: Hypersensitivity

Recommended lab tests: CBC, LFTs, BP

Overdose: Severe hypertension and tachycardia, agitated delirium and hallucinations; OD rare

Tapering/withdrawal: Tapering not needed

Special populations:

Pregnancy: Risk Category C

Lactation: Avoid

Elderly: Lower dose recommended

Hepatic impairment: Lower dose recommended

Renal impairment: No dose adjustment necessary

Important notes:

- For sleepiness, higher doses may be more effective than lower doses

References:

1. Albers, Lawrence J., Rhoda K. Hahn, and Christopher Reist. 2010. *Handbook of Psychiatric Drugs.* 2011 ed. 107–110. Current Clinical Strategies Publishing.

2. Anderson, H. 2014. "Alzheimer Disease." Accessed March 12, 2015. http://emedicine.medscape.com/article/1134817-overview.

3. American Psychiatric Association (APA). 2013a. *Diagnostic and Statistical Manual of Mental Disorders.* 5th ed. (DSM-5®). Washington, DC: American Psychiatric Publishing.

4. American Psychiatric Association (APA). 2013b. "Updates to Neurocognitive Disorders in DSM-5 and DSM-5 Desk Reference." Accessed January 14, 2015. http://www.dsm5.org/Documents/IMPORTANT-NeurocogCodingNoteUpdates-10-18-13.pdf.

5. American Psychiatric Association (APA). 2015. "American Psychiatric Association Practice Guidelines." Accessed February 3, 2015. http://psychiatryonline.org/guidelines.

6. Birks, J. 2006. "Cholinesterase inhibitors for Alzheimer's disease." *Cochrane Database Syst Rev* (1):CD005593. Accessed February 2, 2015. http://www.ncbi.nlm.nih.gov/pubmed/16437532.

7. Buccafusco, J.J. 2009. "Emerging cognitive enhancing drugs." *Expert Opin Emerg Drugs* 14(4):577–589. Accessed February 2, 2015. http://ncbi.nlm.nih.gov/pubmed/19772371.

8. Center Watch. 2015. "FDA Approved Drugs by Therapeutic Area." Accessed February 3, 2015. http://www.centerwatch.com/drug-information/fda-approved-drugs/therapeutic-area/17/psychiatry-psychology.

9. Cephalon, Inc. 2013. "PROVIGIL- modafinil tablet." US National Library of Medicine: Daily Med. Accessed November 21, 2014. http://dailymed.nlm.nih.gov/dailymed/drugInfo.cfm?setid=e16c26ad-7bc2-d155-3a5d-da83ad6492c8.

10. Eisai, Inc. 2014. "ARICEPT- donepezil hydrochloride tablet, film coated." US National Library of Medicine: Daily Med. Accessed November 21, 2014. http://dailymed.nlm.nih.gov/dailymed/drugInfo.cfm?setid=98e451e1-e4d7-4439-a675-c5457ba20975.

11. Elsevier Gold Standard, Inc. 2015. "Clinical Pharmacology." Accessed March 12, 2015. https://www.clinicalpharmacology.com.

12. Epocrates. 2015. Accessed March 25, 2015. https://online.epocrates.com.

13. Forest Laboratories, Inc. 2013. "NAMENDA - memantine hydrochloride tablet." US National Library of Medicine: Daily Med. Accessed November 21, 2014. http://dailymed.nlm.nih.gov/dailymed/drugInfo.cfm?setid=b9f27baf-aa2a-443a-9ef5-e002d23407ba.

14. Gabbard, Glen O., ed. 2007. *Gabbard's Treatments of Psychiatric Disorders.* 4th ed. 139–192. Washington, DC: American Psychiatric Publishing.

15. GlaxoSmithKline, PLC. 2014. "LOVAZA- omega-3-acid ethyl esters capsule, liquid filled." US National Library of Medicine: Daily Med. Accessed December 2, 2014. http://dailymed.nlm.nih.gov/dailymed/drugInfo.cfm?setid=5ada82f0-a5fd-46c9-aecc-f106f614c9f0.

16. Hales, Robert. E., S. Yudofsky, and L. Roberts, eds. 2014. *The American Psychiatric Publishing Textbook of Psychiatry.* 6th ed. 815–850, 1233–1251. Washington, DC: American Psychiatric Publishing.

17. Herrmann, N., S.A. Chau, I. Kircanski, and K.L. Lanctot. 2011. "Current and emerging drug treatment options for Alzheimer's disease." *Drugs* 71(15):2031–2065. Accessed February 2, 2015. http://www.ncbi.nlm.nih.gov/pubmed/21985169.

18. Janssen Pharmaceuticals, Inc. 2014. "RAZADYNE- galantamine hydrobromide tablet, film coated." US National Library of Medicine: Daily Med. Accessed November 21, 2014. http://dailymed.nlm.nih.gov/dailymed/drugInfo.cfm?setid=ec9b5a9c-8caf-4f9b-8c1b-209b2de556dc.

19. Kannayiram, A. 2013. "Delirium." Accessed March 12, 2015. http://emedicine.medscape.com/article/288890-overview.

20. Medscape: Drugs & Diseases. 2015. "Psychiatrics." Accessed February 3, 2015. http://reference.medscape.com/drugs/psychiatrics.

21. Medscape. 2015. "Psychiatry and Mental Health." Accessed March 12, 2015. http://www.medscape.com/psychiatry.

22. Novartis Pharmaceuticals Co. 2014. "EXELON- rivastigmine tartrate capsule." US National Library of Medicine: Daily Med. Accessed November 21, 2014. http://dailymed.nlm.nih.gov/dailymed/drugInfo.cfm?setid=f1e28b44-3897-4788-9659-f5d6bce4d91e.

23. Preston, John D., and James Johnson. 2011. *Clinical Psychopharmacology Made Ridiculously Simple.* 7th ed. 1–79. Miami: MedMaster Inc.

24. RxList. 2015. "Drugs A-Z List." Accessed March 25, 2015. http://www.rxlist.com/drugs/alpha_a.htm.

25. Schatzberg, A.F., and C.B. Nemeroff, eds. 2009. *The American Psychiatric Publishing Textbook of Psychopharmacology.* 4th ed. 843–860, 987–1001. Washington, DC: American Psychiatric Publishing.

26. Schatzberg, A.F., Jonathan O. Cole, and Charles DeBattista. 2010. *Manual of Clinical Psychopharmacology.* 7th ed. 625–630. Washington, DC: American Psychiatric Publishing.

27. Sink, K.M., K.F. Holden, and K. Yaffe. 2005. "Pharmacological treatment of neuropsychiatric symptoms of dementia." *JAMA* 293(5):596–608. Accessed February 2, 2015. http://jama.jamanetwork.com/article.aspx?articleid=200265.

28. Stahl, S.M. 2008. *Essential Psychopharmacology: Neuroscientific Basis and Practical Applications*. 3rd ed. 503–536. New York: Cambridge Press.

29. Stahl, S.M. 2011. *Essential Psychopharmacology: the Prescriber's Guide*. 4th ed. 81–83, 165–169, 349–351, 355–358, 399–403, 527–531. Cambridge: Cambridge University Press.

30. Truven Health Analytics. 2015. *Micromedex 2.0*. Accessed March 20, 2015. http://www.micromedexsolutions.com/home/dispatch.

31. UpToDate. 2015. Accessed March 12, 2015. http://www.uptodate.com/home.

32. US National Library of Medicine. 2015. "Drugs and Lactation Database (LactMed)." Accessed February 3, 2015. http://toxnet.nlm.nih.gov/newtoxnet/lactmed.htm.

33. US National Library of Medicine. 2015. "Toxicology Data Network." Accessed March 17, 2015. http://toxnet.nlm.nih.gov.

34. Virtus Pharmaceuticals. 2012. "L-METHYLFOLATE CALCIUM- levomefolate calcium tablet, coated." US National Library of Medicine: Daily Med. Accessed November 21, 2014. http://dailymed.nlm.nih.gov/dailymed/drugInfo.cfm?setid=2ebbba9c-9451-4b87-87b0-31546c37cef6.

Chapter 13
Psychiatric Medication Use In Pregnancy And Lactation

Pregnant or lactating women with existing psychiatric disorders can present a unique challenge for physicians. Since at least two simultaneous medical conditions are involved, the administration of psychiatric medications in these cases becomes a complex clinical, ethical, and legal situation.[16] These scenarios warrant a careful analysis of the risk to benefit ratio to ensure both fetal and maternal safety.[2]

The interplay between psychiatric disorders and pregnancy is quite significant, as noted by the following[5,9,10,16,17,21]:

- 14–20% of expectant mothers suffer from MDD during pregnancy[16,21]
- Postpartum depression may affect up to 10–22% of adult and 26% of adolescent mothers[16,21]
- Pregnant bipolar patients are likely to relapse without continued pharmacotherapy, as indicated by an 84–100% recurrence rate[10,16]
- 19% of patients with panic disorder experience increased panic attacks during pregnancy, 30% experience reduced attacks, while 51% experience no change[5,10,16]
- The postpartum period dramatically increases a mother's odds of psychiatric hospitalization; 13% of all female hospitalizations occur during the first year after parturition[9,16]

FDA Pregnancy Ratings[2,8,16]

Due the absence of adequate data, the FDA has not approved any psychiatric medication for use during pregnancy.[8] Nevertheless, the risk of untreated psychiatric disorders during pregnancy may often outweigh the unknown risk of medication use. It is estimated that one third of all pregnant women are exposed to a psychiatric medication at some point during pregnancy.[2]

The categories established by the FDA to indicate the safety of medications during pregnancy are as follows[2,8,16]:

- **A** *Controlled studies show no risk*: Adequate, well-controlled studies have failed to demonstrate fetal risk
- **B** *No evidence of risk in humans:* Animal findings show risk, but human findings do not; or if no adequate human studies exist, animal findings are negative
- **C** *Risk cannot be ruled out:* Human studies are lacking, and animal studies are positive for fetal risk or are also lacking; however, potential benefits may justify potential risks
- **D** *Positive evidence of risk:* Investigational or post-marketing data show risk to the fetus; potential benefits may outweigh risks

- **X** *Contraindicated in pregnancy:* Studies in animals or humans, or investigational or post-marketing reports demonstrate fetal risk which clearly outweighs any benefit to the patient

Table 13.1: Psychiatric Drugs According to Pregnancy Risk Category[1,6,7,8,9,11,13,15,16,17,18,19,20]

Category	Medications
A	**Cognitive Enhancers:** L-methylfolate **Hypnotics:** Doxylamine
B	**Antidepressants:** Maprotiline **Antipsychotics:** Clozapine, Lurasidone **Anxiolytics:** Buspirone **Cognitive Enhancers:** Memantine, Rivastigmine **Hypnotics:** Diphenhydramine, Sodium oxybate, Zolpidem **Others:** Bromocriptine, Cyproheptadine, Sildenafil citrate, Trihexyphenidyl
C	**ADHD Medications:** Amphetamine-based stimulants, Atomoxetine, Methylphenidate-based stimulants **Antidepressants:** *SSRIs:* Citalopram, Escitalopram, Fluoxetine, Fluvoxamine, Sertraline *SNRIs:* Desvenlafaxine, Duloxetine, Levomilnacipran, Milnacipran, Venlafaxine *SARIs:* Nefazodone, Trazodone, Vilazodone *Others:* Bupropion, Mirtazapine, Vortioxetine *MAOIs:* Isocarboxazid, Moclobemide, Phenelzine, Tranylcypromine, Selegiline *TCAs:* Amitriptyline, Amoxapine, Clomipramine, Desipramine, Doxepin **Antipsychotics:** *Atypical:* Asenapine, Aripiprazole, Iloperidone, Olanzapine, Paliperidone, Quetiapine, Risperidone, Ziprasidone *Typical:* Chlorpromazine, Fluphenazine, Haloperidol, Loxapine, Molindone, Perphenazine, Pimozide, Thiothixene, Thioridazine, Trifluoperazine **Anxiolytics:** Prazosin, Propranolol, Hydroxyzine, Pregabalin, Tiagabine **Cognitive Enhancers:** Caprylidene, Donepezil, Galantamine, Modafinil **Hypnotics:** Eszopiclone, Ramelteon, Zaleplon **Mood stabilizers:** Gabapentin, Lamotrigine, Oxcarbazepine **Others:** Acamprosate, Amantadine, Baclofen, Benztropine, Biperiden, Bethanechol, Buprenorphine, Disulfiram, Flumazenil, Levacethylmethadol, Methadone, Naltrexone, Varenicline
D	**Antidepressants:** Paroxetine **Benzos:** Alprazolam, Chlordiazepoxide, Clonazepam, Clorazepate, Diazepam, Lorazepam, Midazolam, Oxazepam **Mood stabilizers:** Lithium, Carbamazepine, Topiramate, Valproate **Others:** Nicotine Replacement Therapy (NRT)
X	**Benzos:** Estazolam, Quazepam, Temazepam, Triazolam

Medication Use in Pregnancy and Lactation

Antidepressants[1,2,12,14,16,17, 21,22,23]

- These medications have been widely studied compared to other psychotropics.[17]
- These drugs carry some risk of congenital malformation, persistent pulmonary hypertension in newborns, loss of pregnancy, perinatal toxicity, and neurobehavioral sequelae.[22]
- The lowest possible dosage should be used during pregnancy.
- SSRIs have not been shown to significantly increase the risk of teratogenesis.
- All SSRIs are considered pregnancy risk Category C except for paroxetine which is Category D.
- Paroxetine has been associated with some risk of cardiac defects.
- Third-trimester SSRI exposure may cause neonatal abstinence syndrome (NAS) manifested by jitteriness, poor muscle tone, weak or absent cry, hypoglycemia, low Apgar scores, seizures, and possible cardiac abnormalities.[2]
- Most antidepressants can be used while nursing with few problems if the mother's needs outweigh the risk to the infant.

Antipsychotics[1,2, 9,12,16,17,22]

- There has been no significant teratogenesis reported with use of some of the typical antipsychotics, especially chlorpromazine, haloperidol, and perphenazine.[2]
- There is limited safety data on atypicals and although some reports indicate that olanzapine, risperidone, quetiapine, and clozapine may be associated with increased rates of low-birth weight, data does not demonstrate any increased risk of teratogenesis.[2]
- Of the atypicals, quetiapine appears to have the least placental transfer and olanzapine the most.
- Atypicals carry other risks in pregnancy, including gestational diabetes and large-for-gestation-age infants.
- No long-term studies of children exposed to atypicals have been conducted; routine use during pregnancy/lactation depends on risk to benefit analysis.

Mood Stabilizers[1,2,5,9,12,17,22]

- Lithium is generally contraindicated during pregnancy; exposure during the first trimester is associated with fetal cardiac problems.
- Lithium is highly concentrated in breast milk and thus is contraindicated during lactation.
- Most anticonvulsants are Category D, and exposure to these drugs (e.g., valproate, phenytoin, carbamazepine) during first trimester is strongly associated with neural-tube defects; should be avoided during pregnancy and lactation.

- Newer anticonvulsants such as Trileptal (oxcarbazepine) and Neurontin (gabapentin) do not seem to increase risk of major birth defects.
- There is some evidence that Lamictal may increases the risk of cleft palate and cleft lip.

Anxiolytics[1,2,9,12,16,17,22]

- Benzos must be avoided at all costs, especially in the first and second trimesters.
- Most of the benzos have Category X or D designation.
- First trimester use of benzos can cause of orofacial malformation in the fetus.
- Other significant consequences of benzo use during pregnancy include neonatal CNS depression and neonatal abstinence syndrome (NAS).

Pregnancy-Related Psychiatric Disorders

Postpartum Blues[9,10,16,17,21,23]

Also known as baby blues or maternal blues, this disorder is seen in 75–80% of mothers post-delivery. It is likely caused by hormonal fluctuations post-delivery due to placental separation.[23]
Symptoms: Usually mild and include anxiety, irritability, lethargy, and tearfulness. Symptoms usually subside in the following weeks, and pharmacotherapy is rarely required. If not resolved within two to three weeks, patients should be evaluated for depression.
Treatment: Reassurance.

Postpartum Depression[9,10,16,17,21,23]

According to the Centers for Disease Control and Prevention (CDC), 8–19% of women experience post-partum depressive symptoms.[3,16] Treatment should be considered after weighing the risk to benefit ratio in accordance with the patient's severity of symptoms.
Symptoms: Appetite changes, depressed mood, fatigue, insomnia, loss of pleasure, thoughts of death or suicide; feelings of worthlessness, hopelessness, and helplessness.
Treatment:

- Non-pharmacologic treatment strategies such as individual/group psychotherapy may be effective in mild/moderate depressive symptoms
- If non-pharmacological treatments are not effective, pharmacological therapy should be added
- Medication:
  - *SSRIs:* First-line agents (fluoxetine, sertraline, paroxetine)
  - *SNRIs:* Venlafaxine, duloxetine
  - *TCAs:* Nortriptyline
  - *Others:* Mirtazapine
- Other non-pharmacologic modalities: ECT, CBT, interpersonal therapy

Postpartum Psychosis[9,10,16,17]

Postpartum psychosis can occur suddenly following childbirth and usually begins within 1–3 months of delivery. Its incidence is less than 1 in 1000 deliveries and is more common in primi-para mothers.

Symptoms: Auditory hallucinations, delusions, disorganized speech, euphoric mood, extreme fear, homicidal ideations towards the child, irritability, mutism, negligence towards the child, thought disorder, violence.

Treatment:

- Antipsychotics including Haldol (haloperidol), Zyprexa (olanzapine), Seroquel (quetiapine), and Abilify (aripiprazole)
- Severe over-activity and delusions may require rapid tranquilization with neuro-leptic drugs
- Mood stabilizing drugs (lithium, Depakote) may be useful in postpartum period, although they have potential teratogenic effects if used early in pregnancy
- ECT is highly effective and safe

Principles of Management[1,2,9,10,12,16,17,23]

- Risk-benefit ratio assessment: Consider maternal psychiatric history, potential harm of untreated illness, and potential adverse effects of fetal exposure to different classes of drugs.
- Mild/moderate psychiatric illness: Employ non-pharmacological treatment modalities such as psychotherapy, stress-reduction strategies, psychosocial support.
- Severe/disabling psychiatric illness: Use medication only if risks to the mother and infant are less severe than those of untreated illness.
- Prescribe the lowest effective dose.
- Avoid any drug which has potential for birth defects, especially lithium, anticonvulsants, and benzos.[17]
- Choose medication based on greatest safety, lowest FDA risk category, and fewest side effects.
- The goal of treatment during pregnancy is symptom remission; inadequate treatment only puts the mother and infant at risk of both drug exposure and continued illness.
- Obtain documented informed consent from patients and/or their family before starting any medications.[17]

References:

1. American College of Obstetricians and Gynecologists (ACOG). 2008. "Use of psychiatric medications during pregnancy and lactation." Washington, DC: American College of Obstetricians and Gynecologists (ACOG). Practice bulletin(92):1–20.

2. Armstrong, Carrie. 2008. "ACOG Guidelines on Psychiatric Medication Use During Pregnancy and Lactation." *Am Fam Physician.* 78(6):772–778. Accessed April 29, 2013. http://www.aafp.org/afp/2008/0915/p772.html.

3. Centers for Disease Control and Prevention (CDC). 2013. "Depression Among Women of Reproductive Age." Division of Reproductive Health, National Center for Chronic Disease Prevention and Health Promotion. Accessed March 23, 2015. http://www.cdc.gov/reproductivehealth/depression.

4. Developmental and Reproductive Toxicology/Environmental Teratology Information Center (DART*/ETIC). 2015. "Drugs and Lactation Database (LactMed)." Accessed February 4, 2013. http://toxnet.nlm.nih.gov/newtoxnet/lactmed.htm.

5. Dodd, S., and M. Berk. 2006. "The safety of medications for the treatment of bipolar disorder during pregnancy and the puerperium." *Curr Drug Saf* 1(1):25–33.

6. Elsevier Gold Standard, Inc. 2015. "Clinical Pharmacology." Accessed March 12, 2015. https://www.clinicalpharmacology.com.

7. Epocrates. 2015. Accessed March 25, 2015. https://online.epocrates.com.

8. Focus Information Technology, Inc (FIT). 2010. "FDA Use-in-Pregnancy Ratings." Perinatology. Accessed March 17, 2015. http://www.perinatology.com/exposures/Drugs/FDACategories.htm.

9. Hales, Robert. E., S. Yudofsky, and L. Roberts, eds. 2014. *The American Psychiatric Publishing Textbook of Psychiatry.* 6th ed. 1319–1352. Washington, DC: American Psychiatric Publishing.

10. Levey, L., K. Ragan, A. Hower-Hartley, D.J. Newport, and Z.N. Stowe. 2004. "Psychiatric disorders in pregnancy." *Neurol Clin* 22(4):863–893.

11. Medscape. 2015. "Psychiatry and Mental Health." Accessed March 12, 2015. http://www.medscape.com/psychiatry.

12. Menon, S.J. 2008. "Psychotropic medication during pregnancy and lactation." *Arch Gynecol Obstet* 277(1):1–13.

13. Motherisk. 2013. Accessed February 3, 2015. http://www.motherisk.org.

14. Ray, Shona, and Zachary N. Stowe. 2013. "The use of antidepressant medication in pregnancy." *Clinical Obstetrics & Gynaecology: Best Practice & Research.* Accessed February 3, 2015. http://dx.doi.org/10.1016/j.bpobgyn.2013.09.005.

15. RxList. 2015. "Drugs A-Z List." Accessed March 25, 2015. http://www.rxlist.com/drugs/alpha_a.htm.

16. Schatzberg, A.F., and C.B. Nemeroff, eds. 2009. *The American Psychiatric Publishing Textbook of Psychopharmacology.* 4th ed. 1373–1412. Washington, DC: American Psychiatric Publishing.

17. Schatzberg, A.F., Jonathan O. Cole, and Charles DeBattista. 2010. *Manual of Clinical Psychopharmacology.* 7th ed. 595–602. Washington, DC: American Psychiatric Publishing.

18. Truven Health Analytics. 2015. *Micromedex 2.0.* Accessed March 20, 2015. http://www.micromedexsolutions.com/home/dispatch.

19. UpToDate. 2015. Accessed March 12, 2015. http://www.uptodate.com/home.

20. US National Library of Medicine. 2015. "Drugs and Lactation Database (LactMed)." Accessed February 3, 2015. http://toxnet.nlm.nih.gov/newtoxnet/lactmed.htm.

21. Varkukla, M., A.C. Viguera, and L. Gonsalves. 2009. "Depression and pregnancy." *Compr Ther* 35:44–49.

22. Wegmann, J. 2008. *Psychopharmacology: Straight Talk on Mental Health Medications.* 109–112. Eau Claire: Pesi, LLC.

23. Yonkers, K.A., K.L. Wisner, D.E. Stewart, T.F. Oberlander, D.L. Dell, N. Stotland, S. Ramin, L. Chaudron, and C. Lockwood. 2009. "The management of depression during pregnancy: a report from the American Psychiatric Association and the American College of Obstetricians and Gynecologists." *Gen Hosp Psychiatry* 31:403–413.

Chapter 14
Psychiatric Medication Use In Children And The Elderly

Generalist clinicians frequently encounter youth and elderly patients with psychiatric disorders. These patients often require treatment deviations from those for adults because they have different physiological processes which may render these age-groups more vulnerable to the adverse effects of medications.[9] Consequently, choosing psychiatric medications in these populations requires appropriate and up-to-date psychopharmacological understanding and significant caution.[23]

Children and Adolescents

Black Box Warning Regarding Antidepressant Use in Children[15,30]
The warning applies to any and all use of antidepressant drugs in children and adolescents. The black box warning includes the following statement:

> *Antidepressants increased the risk of suicidal thinking and behavior in children, adolescents, and young adults in short-term studies with major depressive disorder (MDD) and other psychiatric disorders. This risk must be balanced with the clinical need. Monitor patients closely for clinical worsening, suicidality, or unusual changes in behavior. Families and caregivers should be advised of the need for close observation and communication with the prescriber.*[22,30]

Medications[9,19,23]
Diagnosing mental illness in children and adolescents can be difficult, as these groups may have different methods of coping and handling stress and may not communicate their feelings effectively. There is also a lack of reliable data available for psychopharmacology in children and adolescents.[22,32] Clinicians must demonstrate clinical insight during the diagnosis and treatment of psychiatric disorders in pediatric patients, being mindful of the physiological and psychological differences in children compared to adults. Since there is not much data on the long-term effects of psychiatric medications in children, medications should only be used if their benefits clearly outweigh any risks.[23] Medications should usually be initiated at a lower dosage, but children may need a higher dosage at times, as they are rapid metabolizers.[23]

Stimulants
These are the major medication class prescribed for children and youth.[23] Please refer to *Chapter 7: ADHD and Its Treatment* for further details.
Amphetamine-based stimulants include[23]:

- Adderall
- Adderall XR
- Dexedrine
- Dexedrine Spansule
- Dextrostat
- Vyvanse

Methylphenidate-based stimulants include[23]:

- Focalin
- Focalin XR
- Methylin
- Methylin ER
- Metadate ER
- Metadate CD

- Ritalin
- Ritalin SR
- Ritalin LA
- Concerta
- Quillivant XR
- Daytrana

Antidepressants

- SSRIs are considered the medication of choice for depression in children and adolescents.[23]
- Prescribers, especially primary-care physicians, are reluctant and frankly fearful at times to prescribe antidepressants due to potential risk of liability associated with the black box warning.[23]
- As suicidal ideation may emerge during the early phases of treatment, close supervision and frequent visits throughout early treatment are required.[32]

Table 14.1: FDA-Approved Antidepressants in Children/Adolescents[2,19,22]

Disorder	Ages ≥6 yrs	≥7	≥8	≥10	≥12
Depression					Amitriptyline Imipramine
MDD			Fluoxetine		Escitalopram
OCD	Sertraline	Fluoxetine	Fluvoxamine	Clomipramine	
Enuresis	Imipramine				

Antipsychotics

- It is imperative to obtain documented informed consent from the patient's parents/ legal guardians, as the safety and efficacy of antipsychotics in children has been long debated.
- All pediatric patients on antipsychotics should be routinely monitored carefully, particularly for metabolic syndrome.[23]
- Sedative first generation antipsychotics (typicals) may interfere with learning and have a higher risk of EPS.[9,23]
- Although weight gain and metabolic syndrome are the major concerns with atypicals, they can be useful in the treatment of developmental disorders like autism.[9,23]

- The use of antipsychotics to control the behavior of angry, impulsive children and adolescents without psychosis is not well-validated, but its utility is supported by most clinicians.[23]

Table 14.2: FDA-Approved Second Generation (Atypical) Antipsychotics in Children/ Adolescents[3,8]

Medications	Autism Irritability/ Aggression	Bipolar Mania/Mixed	Schizophrenia
Aripiprazole	Ages 6–17 yrs	10–17	13–17
Olanzapine		13–17	13–17
Paliperidone			12–17
Quetiapine		10–17	13–17
Risperidone	5–16	10–17	13–17

Table 14.3: FDA-Approved First Generation (Typical) Antipsychotics in Children/ Adolescents[3]

Medications	Schizophrenia	Severe behavioral/ hyperactivity problems
Chlorpromazine		ages ≥6 mo–12 yrs
Haloperidol	ages ≥3 yrs	ages ≥3 yrs
Pimozide		ages ≥12 yrs (Tourette Syndrome)

Mood Stabilizers[10,19,22,23]

- Studies suggest that lithium is well-tolerated and effective in treating a variety of mood disorders in children and adolescents including bipolar depression, mood liability, explosive violent behavior, and others.[23] It is the only medication approved for treating mania in adolescents[22]; however, it has been found to be associated with multiple side effects, and data on its long-term safety and efficacy is unclear.[23]
- Carbamazepine has been reported to be efficacious in treatment of conduct disorder and intermittent explosive disorder.
- Valproate has been found to be effective in bipolar disorder and aggressive behavior[23]; however, it has also been associated with serious adverse events such as hepatic failure and pancreatitis.[23,32]

- Use of lamotrigine in pediatric bipolar disorder is still debated, but some open-label studies suggest its benefits for the treatment of bipolar depression. Children are at a higher risk of developing a rash while taking lamotrigine than adults.[23]
- Oxcarbazepine is often used as mood stabilizer due to its more favorable side effect profile.

Mood stabilizers used in children/adolescents include[10,19,22,23]:

- Lithium
- Valproate
- Carbamazepine
- Risperidone
- Quetiapine
- Olanzapine
- Lamotrigine
- Oxcarbazepine

Anxiolytics

- SSRIs—especially citalopram, escitalopram, fluoxetine, and sertraline—are the first-choice psychotropic medications for the treatment for anxiety.[19,22]
- Outside of their occasional use in the treatment of severe anxiety in adolescents, benzos are best avoided in this population.[32]
- The efficacy of buspirone in the treatment of childhood anxiety disorder has some supportive evidence.[23]
- Sedating antihistamines such as diphenhydramine and hydroxyzine have been postulated to have some anxiolytic effects; however, they have been associated with anticholinergic adverse effects and cognitive impairment.[23]
- Most antianxiety medications prescribed for youth are off-label—that is, they have not received an FDA treatment indication for use in pediatric patients.

Antianxiety medications often prescribed for youth include[19,22,23]:

- Escitalopram
- Fluoxetine
- Sertraline
- Alprazolam
- Citalopram
- Clonazepam
- Lorazepam
- Hydroxyzine
- Diphenhydramine
- Buspirone
- Clomipramine

Elderly Patients

Black Box Warning Regarding Antipsychotic Use in the Elderly[29]

This warning applies to all antipsychotics and includes the following statement:

> *Elderly patients with dementia-related psychosis treated with atypical antipsychotic drugs are at an increased risk of death compared with placebo. Although the causes of death in clinical trials were varied, most of the deaths appeared to be either cardiovascular (e.g. heart failure, sudden death) or infectious (e.g. pneumonia) in nature. Observational studies suggest that antipsychotic drugs may increase mortality. It is unclear from the observational studies to what extent these mortality findings may be attributed to the antipsychotic drug as opposed to patient characteristics.*[2]

Medications

The elderly are more sensitive to the effects of medication, and appropriate dosing in this population requires vigilance due to the physiological changes associated with aging. Slower metabolism, decreased cardiovascular competence, and inefficient hepatic conjugation and renal clearance can potentially increase the concentration of certain medications in the elderly.[22,23] In most cases, the usual dosage in the elderly should be half of the usual adult dose.[16,17] The elderly also tend to self-medicate with OTCs and herbal supplements, increasing their risk of drug interactions, and this should be addressed carefully by the prescriber.[18,32] It is also important for clinicians to know that suicide disproportionately impacts older adults, accounting for 14% of all suicides.[21] Clinicians must consider important comorbid factors in this population such as altered mental states, memory loss, confusion, noncompliance, and misuse of prescription drugs. As a rule, a medication regimen should be kept simple and should be initiated at lower doses and increased gradually as tolerated.[32]

Antidepressants[1,9,17,18,22,23]

- SSRIs—particularly citalopram, sertraline, and escitalopram—are first-line medications for treating geriatric depression.[23] Citalopram and escitalopram have the fewest drug interactions.

- Bupropion, venlafaxine, and mirtazapine are also considered safe treatment options.

- Mirtazapine is better tolerated in elderly patients and has sedating, anti-anxiety, and weight-gaining effects.[1,23]

- Trazodone is a moderately effective antidepressant in elderly depressed patients and acts as an excellent hypnotic.[23]

- TCAs should be avoided in geriatric patients; if used, the clinician should also consider prescribing nortriptyline or desipramine and initiating at lower doses.[9,18]

- ECT is a viable option for treatment-resistant depression in this population.

Hypnotics and Anxiolytics[4,11,17,21,22,23]

- The use of these drugs (by age group) is greatest among seniors and continues to increase.

- For sleep disorders, behavioral interventions must be used and other systemic and psychiatric causes must be ruled out before resorting to medication.[17]

- Anxiety should be treated with SSRIs, SNRIs, mirtazapine, or Buspar (buspirone).

- Although Zolpidem is widely used by physicians, Zaleplon is a more prudent choice as it is better tolerated by patients due to its shorter half-life.[4,23]

- Trazodone remains an important hypnotic; however, it increases the risk of orthostatic hypotension when used in higher doses.
- Mirtazapine is comparable to trazodone in its efficacy, without the increased risk of orthostatic hypotension, and thus, may be a more prudent choice in certain cases as it can increase appetite.[22,23]
- Ramelteon is preferred to others hypnotics, as it does not contribute to confusion, amnesia, or orthostatic hypotension. However, due to lower efficacy, it is not preferred by all clinicians.[23]
- Benzos must be used only if absolutely necessary at the lowest effective dose and only until the primary medication starts working. When using benzos, consider short-acting ones such as temazepam and lorazepam at lower doses for 2–4 weeks only.[22,23] Benzo use in older adults increases the risk of cognitive impairment, sedation, falls, paradoxical behavioral, and disinhibition.[11]

Mood Stabilizers[17,21,22,23]

- Lithium excretion occurs at slower rate in the elderly[22]; treatment should be initiated at a lower dose of 150–300 mg/day.[23]
- Elderly patients are at a higher risk for lithium toxicity due to concomitant use of drugs such as NSAIDS, thiazide diuretics, and ACE inhibitors.[23]
- Valproate at lower doses seems to be better tolerated in this population than lithium; however, its adverse effect of hepatotoxicity is of concern.
- Carbamazepine should be avoided due to its severe adverse effect profile and interaction potential.[23]
- Gabapentin is well-tolerated in geriatric patients but is a weak mood stabilizer; may be more useful for geriatric agitation, anxiety, and pain conditions.[23]
- Lamotrigine should be used at low doses with gradual titration.
- Atypical antipsychotics can be used as mood stabilizers; they are well-tolerated and efficacious.[23]

Antipsychotics[16,17,23,24,25,29]

- These medications carry a black box warning for elderly patients with dementia regarding the increased risk of death due to cardiovascular problems and infections.[24,25,29] Because of the black box warning, monitor ECG continuously in elderly patients who are receiving antipsychotics (both FGA and SGA) for QTc prolongation.[16] Regular monitoring of potassium and magnesium is also recommended.
- Elderly patients are at higher risk of serious adverse effects associated with antipsychotics, including orthostatic hypotension, EPS, and TD.[23,25]
- Low doses of Risperdal (0.25–2 mg), quetiapine (12.5–150 mg), aripiprazole (2–10 mg), and haloperidol(0.25–2 mg) are preferred choices for this population.[16,17,23]

Cognitive enhancers
(Refer to *Chapter 12: Dementia-Related Disorders and Cognitive Enhancers* for further details)

Commonly used drugs for dementia-related disorders include donepezil, rivastigmine, galantamine, and memantine.[9,17,22]

Treatment of Agitation in the Elderly
(Refer to *Chapter 16: Psychiatric Emergencies and Their Management* for further details)

Treating the underlining cause of agitation is essential.[22] If restraints are needed, use mittens, elbow restraints, a Posey vest, or other measures.

Medications include[9,13]:

- Haloperidol: 1–2 mg po/sq q4–6 hrs
- Olanzapine: 2.5–5 mg daily
- Risperdal: 0.5 mg bid
- Quetiapine: 12.5–25 mg bid

References:

1. Alam, Abdulkader, Zoya Voronovich, and Joseph A. Carley. 2013. "A Review of Therapeutic Uses of Mirtazapine in Psychiatric and Medical Conditions." *The Primary Care Companion for CNS Disorders* 15(5):PCC.13r01525. doi: 10.4088/PCC.13r01525.

2. Centers for Medicare and Medicaid Services (CMS). 2013a. "Antidepressant Medications: Use in Pediatric Patients." Accessed April 2, 2015. http://www.cms.gov/medicare-medicaid-coordination/fraud-prevention/medicaid-integrity-education/pharmacy-education-materials/downloads/ad-pediatric-factsheet.pdf.

3. Centers for Medicare and Medicaid Services (CMS). 2013b. "Atypical Antipsychotic Medications: Use in Pediatric Patients." Accessed April 2, 2015. http://www.cms.gov/medicare-medicaid-coordination/fraud-prevention/medicaid-integrity-education/pharmacy-education-materials/downloads/atyp-antipsych-pediatric-factsheet.pdf.

4. Danjou, P., I. Paty, R. Fruncillo, P. Worthington, M. Unruh, W. Cevallos, and P. Martin. 1999. "A comparison of the residual effects of zaleplon and zolpidem following administration 5 to 2 h before awakening." *British Journal of Clinical Pharmacology* 48(3):367–374. doi: 10.1046/j.1365-2125.1999.00024.x.

5. Dworkin, Robert H., Alec B. O'Connor, Joseph Audette, Ralf Baron, Geoffrey K. Gourlay, Maija L. Haanpää, Joel L. Kent, Elliot J. Krane, Alyssa A. LeBel, Robert M. Levy, Sean C. Mackey, John Mayer, Christine Miaskowski, Srinivasa N. Raja, Andrew S. C. Rice, Kenneth E. Schmader, Brett Stacey, Steven Stanos, Rolf-Detlef Treede, Dennis C. Turk, Gary A. Walco, and Christopher D. Wells. 2010. "Recommendations for the Pharmacological Management of Neuropathic Pain: An

Overview and Literature Update." *Mayo Clinic Proceedings* 85(3 Suppl):S3–S14. doi: 10.4065/mcp.2009.0649.

6. Elsevier Gold Standard, Inc. 2015. "Clinical Pharmacology." Accessed March 12, 2015. https://www.clinicalpharmacology.com.

7. Epocrates. 2015. Accessed March 25, 2015. https://online.epocrates.com.

8. Fraguas, D., C. U. Correll, J. Merchan-Naranjo, M. Rapado-Castro, M. Parellada, C. Moreno, and C. Arango. 2011. "Efficacy and safety of second-generation antipsychotics in children and adolescents with psychotic and bipolar spectrum disorders: comprehensive review of prospective head-to-head and placebo-controlled comparisons." *Eur Neuropsychopharmacol* 21(8):621–645. doi: 10.1016/j.euroneuro.2010.07.002.

9. Hales, Robert. E., S. Yudofsky, and L. Roberts, eds. 2014. *The American Psychiatric Publishing Textbook of Psychiatry*. 6th ed. 1189–1352. Washington, DC: American Psychiatric Publishing.

10. Kafantaris, V. 1995. "Treatment of bipolar disorder in children and adolescents." *J Am Acad Child Adolesc Psychiatry* 34:732–741.

11. Madhusoodanan, S. and O.J. Bogunovic. 2004. "Safety of benzodiazepines in the geriatric population." *Expert Opin Drug Saf* 3:485–493.

12. McLaren, K.D., and Marangell, L.B. 2004. "Special considerations in the treatment of patients with bipolar disorder and medical co-morbidities." *Annals of General Hospital Psychiatry* 3:7. Accessed February 3, 2015. http://www.general-hospital-psychiatry.com/content/3/1/7.

13. Medscape: Drugs & Diseases. 2015. "Psychiatrics." Accessed February 3, 2015. http://reference.medscape.com/drugs/psychiatrics.

14. Medscape. 2015. "Psychiatry and Mental Health." Accessed March 12, 2015. http://www.medscape.com/psychiatry.

15. National Institute of Mental Health (NIMH). 2015. "Antidepressant Medications for Children and Adolescents: Information for Parents and Caregivers." Accessed February 5, 2015. http://www.nimh.nih.gov/health/topics/child-and-adolescent-mental-health/antidepressant-medications-for-children-and-adolescents-information-for-parents-and-caregivers.shtml.

16. Neil, W., S. Curran, and J. Wattis. 2003. "Antipsychotic prescribing in older people." *Age & Aging.* 32(5):475-483.

17. Peterson, J. F., G. J. Kuperman, C. Shek, M. Patel, J. Avorn, and D. W. Bates. 2005. "Guided prescription of psychotropic medications for geriatric inpatients." *Archives of Internal Medicine* 165(7):802–807. doi: 10.1001/archinte.165.7.802.

18. Rasimas, J.J. 2011. "Medical toxicology." In *The American Psychiatric Publishing Textbook of Psychosomatic Medicine: Psychiatric Care of the Medically Ill*. 2nd ed. Edited by J.L. Levenson, 929–953. Washington, DC: American Psychiatric Publishing.

19. Rosenberg, D.R., J. Holttum, and S. Gershon. 1994. *Textbook of Pharmacotherapy for Child and Adolescent Psychiatric Disorders*. 3–509. New York: Brunner/Mazel.

20. RxList. 2015. "Drugs A-Z List." Accessed March 25, 2015. http://www.rxlist.com/drugs/alpha_a.htm.

21. Salzman, C.A. 1990. "Practical considerations in the pharmacologic treatment of depression and anxiety in the elderly." *J Clin Psychiatry* 51(1 suppl):21–26.

22. Schatzberg, A.F., and C.B. Nemeroff, eds. 2009. *The American Psychiatric Publishing Textbook of Psychopharmacology*. 4th ed. 1309–1440. Washington, DC: American Psychiatric Publishing.

23. Schatzberg, A.F., Jonathan O. Cole, and Charles DeBattista. 2010. *Manual of Clinical Psychopharmacology*. 7th ed. 603–624. Washington, DC: American Psychiatric Publishing.

24. Schneider, L.S., K.S. Dagerman, and P. Insel. 2005. "Risk of death with atypical antipsychotic drug treatment for dementia." *JAMA* 294:1935–1943.

25. Steinberg, Martin, and Constantine G. Lyketsos. 2012. "Atypical Antipsychotic Use in Patients with Dementia: Managing Safety Concerns." *The American Journal of Psychiatry* 169(9):900–906. doi: 10.1176/appi.ajp.2012.12030342.

26. Truven Health Analytics. 2015. *Micromedex 2.0*. Accessed March 20, 2015. http://www.micromedexsolutions.com/home/dispatch.

27. UpToDate. 2015. Accessed March 12, 2015. http://www.uptodate.com/home.

28. University of Washington: Psychiatry Clerkship. 2007. "Lectures." Accessed February 3, 2015. http://depts.washington.edu/psyclerk/lectures.html.

29. US Food and Drug Administration (FDA). 2008. "Information for Healthcare Professionals: Conventional Antipsychotics." Accessed April 18, 2015. http://www.fda.gov/Drugs/DrugSafety/PostmarketDrugSafetyInformationforPatientsandProviders/ucm124830.htm.

30. US Food and Drug Administration (FDA). 2009. "Labeling Change Request Letter for Antidepressant Medications." Center for Drug Evaluation and Research. Accessed March 24, 2015. http://www.fda.gov/Drugs/DrugSafety/InformationbyDrugClass/ucm096352.htm.

31. US National Library of Medicine. 2015. "Toxicology Data Network." Accessed March 17, 2015. http://toxnet.nlm.nih.gov.

32. Wegmann, J. 2008. *Psychopharmacology: Straight Talk on Mental Health Medications*. 112–123. Eau Claire: Pesi, LLC.

Chapter 15
Psychiatric Medication Use In Comorbid Medical Conditions-Hepatic, Renal, HIV

Progressive diseases involving the liver, kidneys, or immune system can alter the metabolism of psychiatric medications by affecting their absorption, distribution, and elimination.[7] Selection and dosing of psychiatric medications should be performed carefully to minimize adverse effects in medically ill patients.

Hepatic Disorder
Severe liver dysfunction alters the metabolism and protein-binding capacity of drugs. In patients with hepatic impairment, initiate at low doses and titrate gradually for any drug that is primarily metabolized by the liver.[7,14]

Table 15.1: Psychiatric Medication Recommendations
in Hepatic Disorders[2,3,4,6,7,9,10,12,13,14,16,17,18]

	No Dose Adjustment	Lower Dose Recommended	Use Caution	Avoid
Antidepressants	• Levomilnacipran • Milnacipran* • Vilazodone* • Vortioxetine*	• Bupropion *(reduce by 50%)* • Citalopram *(20 mg/day max)* • Desvenlafaxine *(50 mg/day)* • Doxepin • Escitalopram *(10 mg/day max)* • Fluoxetine • Fluvoxamine • Imipramine • Milnacipran *(if LFTs 5x normal)* • Paroxetine *(10 mg/day initially, max 40 mg/day)* • Reboxetine • Venlafaxine *(reduce by 50%*)* • Vilazodone**	• Amitriptyline • Amoxapine • Clomipramine • Desipramine • Milnacipran** • Mirtazapine • Sertraline • Trazodone • Venlafaxine**	• Agomela-tine** • Duloxetine • MAOIs • Nefazodone • Vortioxetine**
Mood Stabilizers	• Gabapentin • Lamotrigine* • Lithium • Oxcarbazepine* • Topiramate*	• Lamotrigine (reduce by 25-50%**) • Topiramate**	• Carbamazepine*	• Carbamaze-pine** • Oxcarbaze-pine** • Valproate

	No Dose Adjustment	Lower Dose Recommended	Use Caution	Avoid
Antipsychotics	• Aripiprazole • Asenapine* • Clozapine* • Iloperidone* • Loxapine (inhalation form) • Lurasidone* • Olanzapine* • Paliperidone* • Perphenazine* • Quetiapine* • Risperidone* • Ziprasidone	• Lurasidone (max 40 mg**) • Loxapine (oral form) • Olanzapine** • Quetiapine** • Risperidone (1 mg bid**)	• Chlorpromazine • Clozapine** • Haloperidol • Iloperidone • Molindone • Paliperidone** • Perphenazine** • Thiothixene	• Asenapine** • Fluphenazine • Iloperidone** • Trifluopera-zine
Anxiolytics and Hypnotics	• Alprazolam* • Eszopiclone* • Hydroxyzine* • Lorazepam* • Oxazepam • Pregabalin • Ramelteon*	• Buspirone* • Chlordiazepox-ide (5 mg qid) • Clonazepam* • Diazepam (reduce by 50%) • Diphenhydr-amine • Eszopiclone (1 mg**) • Lorazepam** Prazosin • Propranolol • Sodium oxybate (2.25 g/night divided) • Tiagabine • Zaleplon (5 mg max*) • Zolpidem (reduce by 50%) • Zopiclone (3.75 mg/day*)	• Alprazolam** • Clonazepam* • Clorazepate • Diazepam • Estazolam • Flurazepam • Hydroxyzine** • Midazolam • Quazepam • Temazepam • Triazolam	• Buspirone** • Clonazepam** • Zaleplon** • Zopiclone** • Ramelteon**

	No Dose Adjustment	Lower Dose Recommended	Use Caution	Avoid
Other	• Atomoxetine* • Methadone*	• Atomoxetine** • Methadone**	• Dextramphet-amine • Disulfiram • Methylphenidate	

* In mild to moderate impairment
** In severe impairment

Renal Disorder

Lithium, pregabalin, and gabapentin are almost entirely cleared by the kidneys. Lithium is contraindicated in acute renal failure but not in chronic renal failure.[7] Many clinicians prescribe two-thirds of the usual drug dose in renal dysfunction except for venlafaxine,[7] whose clearance is reduced by over 50% in patients undergoing dialysis.[8]

Table 15.2: Psychiatric Medication Recommendations
in Renal Disorders[3,4,6,7,8,9,12,13,14,16,17,18]

	No Dose Adjustment	Lower Dose Recommended	Use Caution	Avoid
Antidepressants	• Bupropion • Citalopram* • Desvenlafaxine* • Duloxetine* • Fluoxetine • Fluvoxamine • MAOIs* • Milnacipran* • Nefazodone • Paroxetine* • Sertraline • Trazodone • Vilazodone • Vortioxetine	• Desvenlafaxine (50 mg/day**) • Escitalopram (10 mg/day max) • Levomilnacipran (80 mg/day*, 40 mg/day**) • Mirtazapine • Milnacipran** • Paroxetine (reduce by 50%**) • Reboxetine • TCAs • Venlafaxine (reduce by 25%*/50%**)	• Citalopram** • Escitalopram** • Agomelatine* • Venlafaxine	• Duloxetine** • MAOIs** • Agomelatine**
Mood Stabilizers	• Carbamazepine • Valproate	• Gabapentin (200–300 mg/day *, 100–150 mg/day**) • Lamotrigine • Lithium* • Oxcarbazepine (lower dose*, reduce 50%**) • Topiramate (50–100 mg/day max)		• Lithium** • Oxcarbazepine XR**

	• No Dose Adjustment	• Lower Dose Recommended	Use Caution	Avoid
Antipsychotics	• Aripiprazole • Asenapine • Chlorpromazine • Clozapine* • Haloperidol • Iloperidone • Loxapine • Lurasidone* • Molindone • Olanzapine • Perphenazine • Quetiapine • Trifluoperazine • Ziprasidone*	• Clozapine** • Lurasidone (40 mg/day**) • Risperidone (0.5–1.5 mg) • Paliperidone (6 mg/day*, 3 mg/day**) • Ziprasidone (20–80 mg/day**)	• Fluphenazine • Thiothixene • Ziprasidone (IM)	
Anxiolytics & Hypnotics	• Buspirone* • Diazepam • Diphenhydramine • Eszopiclone • Hydroxyzine* • Lorazepam* • Oxazepam • Ramelteon • Prazosin • Propranolol • Tiagabine • Zaleplon*	• Alprazolam (0.25–0.5 mg tid) • Chlordiazepoxide (reduce by 50%) • Hydroxyzine (reduce by 50%**) • Midazolam (reduce by 50%**) • Pregabalin (divide dose) • Zaleplon** • Zolpidem (reduce by 50%) • Zopiclone (3.75 mg/day*)	• Clonazepam • Clorazepate • Estazolam • Flurazepam • Midazolam • Quazepam • Sodium oxybate • Temazepam • Triazolam	• Buspirone** • Lorazepam** • Zopiclone**
Others	• Atomoxetine • Disulfiram • Methadone*	• Methadone** • Lisdexamfet-amine	• Dextroamphet-amine • Methylphenidate	

*In mild to moderate impairment
**In severe impairment

HIV

The effective management of psychiatric conditions in patients with HIV can improve their quality of life and increase compliance with antiretroviral medications.[11] Clinicians should be familiar with the indications, adverse effects, and drug interactions of various psychiatric and antiretroviral agents. It is especially important to be aware of the interactions with cytochrome P450 metabolism, a common enzymatic pathway of many psychotropic and antiretroviral medications.[1,14,15]

Table 15.3: Psychotropic and Anti-retroviral Medication Interactions[5,6,7,9,11,12,13,14,15,16,17,18]

HIV Medications	Psychotropic Levels Affected	Antiretroviral Levels Affected	Lower Psychotropic Doses Recommended	Avoid
All Antiretrovirals			Alprazolam Clonazepam Diazepam	Chlorpromazine Clozapine Fluvoxamine Lithium Nefazodone Pimozide Thioridazine
Non-Nucleoside Reverse Transcriptase Inhibitors (NNRTIs)				
All NNRTIs	Trazodone ↑	↓ w/ Carbamazepine	Trazodone	
Efavirenz (EFV)	Bupropion ↓ 55% Sertraline ↓ 39% Vilazodone ↓			Alprazolam Clonazepam
Nevirapine (NVP)	Vilazodone ↓			
Protease Inhibitors (PIs)				
All PIs	Aripiprazole ↑ Desvenlafaxine ↑ Quetiapine ↑ Risperidone ↑ TCAs ↑ Trazodone ↑ Venlafaxine ↑ Vilazodone ↑ Ziprasidone ↑	↑ w/ Fluoxetine ↓ w/ Carbamazepine	Iloperidone *(50%)* Risperidone Trazodone Valproic Acid	Midazolam Triazolam
Darunavir[1] (DRV)	Paroxetine ↓ Sertraline ↓ 50%			
Fosamprenavir[1] (FPV)	Paroxetine ↓ 50%			
Indinavir (IDV)		↓ w/ Venlafaxine		Alprazolam
Nelfinavir (NFV)				

HIV Medications	Psychotropic Levels Affected	Antiretroviral Levels Affected	Lower Psychotropic Doses Recommended	Avoid
Ritonavir (RTV)	Lamotrigine ↓ 50%		Haloperidol	Alprazolam Clonazepam Bupropion
Tipranavir[1] (TPV)	Bupropion ↓ 46%			

[1]In combination with Ritonavir
↓ Levels Decreased
↑ Levels Increased

Important Notes Regarding Use of Psychotropic Drugs in HIV
Antidepressants[5,6,11,13,14,15]
- Citalopram, escitalopram, and sertraline have the fewest drug interactions.
- Fluoxetine is the most effective but may cause toxicity by increasing the levels of protease inhibitors.
- No interaction when efavirenz or etravirine are used with paroxetine.
- Nefazadone may cause significant problems with the HIV regimen; associated with hepatic failure.
- Mirtazapine can be used to promote appetite and sleep; however, it can adversely interact with CYP450 inhibitors such as ritonavir.
- Duloxetine is well-tolerated without dosage adjustment.
- Protease inhibitors increase TCA levels; should be closely monitored.

Anxiolytics[5,6,11,14,15]
- Benzos are generally contraindicated in patients taking protease inhibitors due to drug interactions, but they can be used on a short-term basis when necessary.[11]
- The safest benzos are lorazepam, oxazepam, and temazepam.

Antipsychotics[5,6,11,14,15]
- Atypicals are preferred antipsychotics for this population.
- Iloperidone: decrease the dose by 50% if used with strong CYP3A4 or CYP2D6 inhibitor, especially protease inhibitors.
- Lurasidone levels are increased by CYP3A4 inhibitors and decreased by CYP3A4 inducers.

Others[5,6,11,14,15]

- Psychostimulants such as amphetamines are one of the mainstays of treatment for HIV-induced fatigue.[5]
- Methylphenidate and dextroamphetamine may improve depression, energy level, and mood.
- Z drugs can interact with HIV medications; must be used with caution to prevent CNS depression.

References:

1. AIDS Info. 2013. "Guidelines for the Use of Antiretroviral Agents in HIV-1-Infected Adults and Adolescents: Tables 17 & 18." *Clinical Guidelines Portal.* Accessed February 3, 2015. http://aidsinfo. nih.gov/guidelines/html/1/adult-and-adolescent-treatment-guidelines/0.

2. Droroudgar, Shadi, Tony I. Chou, and Vicki I. Ellingrod. 2014. "How to modify psychotropic therapy for patients who have liver dysfunction." *Current Psychiatry* 13(12):46–49. Accessed February 3, 2015. http://www.currentpsychiatry.com/articles/savvy-psychopharmacology/article/how-to-modify-psychotropic-therapy-for-patients-who-have-liver-dysfunction/9d9e9690a4a8e30e5ec38b-cebd86b7db.html.

3. Elsevier Gold Standard, Inc. 2015. "Clinical Pharmacology." Accessed March 12, 2015. https://www.clinicalpharmacology.com.

4. Epocrates. 2015. Accessed March 25, 2015. https://online.epocrates.com.

5. Forstein, M., F. Cournos, A. Douaihy, K. Goodkin, M.L. Wainberg, and K.H. Wapenyi. 2006. "Guideline watch: practice guideline for the treatment of patients with HIV/AIDS." American Psychiatric Association Practice Guidelines. Accessed April 1, 2015. http://psychiatryonline.org/pb/assets/raw/sitewide/practice_guidelines/guidelines/hivaids-watch.pdf.

6. Hales, Robert. E., S. Yudofsky, and L. Roberts, eds. 2014. *The American Psychiatric Publishing Textbook of Psychiatry.* 6th ed. 1189–1352. Washington, DC: American Psychiatric Publishing.

7. Levenson, James. 2005, "Psychopharmacology in the Medically Ill." Accessed January 14, 2015. http://primarypsychiatry.com/psychopharmacology-in-the-medically-ill.

8. McIntyre, R., Baghdady, N., Banik, S., and Swartz, S. 2008. "The use of psychotropic drugs in patients with impaired renal function." *Primary Psychiatry* 15(1): 73–88. Accessed March 20, 2015. http://primarypsychiatry.com/the-use-of-psychotropic-drugs-in-patients-with-impaired-renal-function/.

9. Medscape. 2015. "Psychiatry and Mental Health." Accessed March 12, 2015. http://www.medscape.com/psychiatry.

10. National Institute of Diabetes and Digestive and Kidney Diseases. 2014. "Livertox Database." *US National Library of Medicine.* Accessed February 3, 2015. http://livertox.nih.gov/index.html.

11. Reid, Eloise, Kevin Stoloff, and John Joska. 2011. "Psychotropic Prescribing in HIV." Department of Psychiatry and Mental Health, UCT. 1–45. Accessed February 3, 2015. http://hivmentalhealth.co.za/wp-content/uploads/2011/11/Psychotropic-Drug-Booklet-PRESS-READY-Lo-Res.pdf.

12. RxList. 2015. "Drugs A-Z List." Accessed March 25, 2015. http://www.rxlist.com/drugs/alpha_a. htm.

13. Schatzberg, A.F., and C.B. Nemeroff, eds. 2009. *The American Psychiatric Publishing Textbook of Psychopharmacology*. 4th ed. 1309–1440. Washington, DC: American Psychiatric Publishing.

14. Schatzberg, A.F., Jonathan O. Cole, and Charles DeBattista. 2010. *Manual of Clinical Psychopharmacology*. 7th ed. 634–640. Washington, DC: American Psychiatric Publishing.

15. Thompson, A., B. Silverman, L. Dzeng, and G. Treisman. 2006. "Psychotropic medications and HIV." *Clin Infect Dis* 42(9):1305–1310. Accessed January 14, 2015. http://www.ncbi.nlm.nih.gov/pubmed/16586391.

16. Truven Health Analytics. 2015. *Micromedex 2.0*. Accessed March 20, 2015. http://www.micromedexsolutions.com/home/dispatch.

17. UpToDate. 2015. Accessed March 12, 2015. http://www.uptodate.com/home.

18. US National Library of Medicine. 2015. "Toxicology Data Network." Accessed March 17, 2015. http://toxnet.nlm.nih.gov.

19. University of Washington: Psychiatry Clerkship. 2007. "Lectures." Accessed February 3, 2015. http://depts.washington.edu/psyclerk/lectures.html.

Chapter 16
Psychiatric Emergencies And Their Management

Mental health clinicians may face many emergency psychiatric situations that require rapid intervention. These may involve acute disturbances of a patient's behavior, thought, or mood, which if untreated, may result in harm to self or others.[2,3] Careful diagnostic evaluation should follow crisis stabilization as well as ensuring the safety of the patient and his or her surroundings.[15]

Common psychiatric emergencies include[2,3,5]:
- Suicide
- Agitation and violent behavior
- Psychiatric medication-related emergencies (NMS, serotonin syndrome)

Suicide

Suicide is the eighth leading cause of death in the US.[15] More than 38,000 Americans and more than 800,000 people worldwide die from suicide every year.[14] People with major psychiatric illnesses commit 90% of all successful suicides, and up to 60% of psychiatric inpatients who kill themselves do so within six months of discharge from hospitals.[2,3] Males have higher incidences of committing suicide, but females make 2–3 times more attempts.[15] Higher suicide rates are seen in adolescents and the elderly, especially in elderly white males.[8] Among the elderly, the highest suicide rates are found among the divorced or widowed.[14] In the US, the highest suicide rates according to race are among Caucasians, American Indians, and Alaska Natives. Firearms are the most common means of completed suicide in both males and females. Methods commonly used by males in order of decreasing prevalence are firearms, hanging, and poisoning, while females commonly use poisoning, firearms, and hanging.[8,19]

Antisocial and borderline personality disorders are associated with increased suicide rates, and conduct disorder and borderline traits are associated with adolescent suicides.[8,17] Superimposition of substance abuse and depression to any of these conditions creates a lethal combination.

The etiology of suicidal behavior is multifactorial. Substantial factors include[3,10,19]:
- Biochemical alterations
- Genetic predispositions
- Life stressors
- Environmental factors
- Psychiatric disorders
- Personality disorders
- Chronic illness
- Substance abuse

Different psychiatric disorders have varied rates of suicide, with depression and bipolar disorder being of highest risk. The rates of suicide across different psychiatric disorders are[8,10]:

- MDD: 15%
- Bipolar Disorder: 10–15%
- Schizophrenia: 10%

- Antisocial PD: 5%
- Borderline PD: 4–9%
- Alcohol Dependence: 2%

Risk Factors

Acute risk factors are more predictive of emergent suicidality than chronic risk factors.[8] Acute risk factors include[8,15,19]:

- Psychic anxiety and panic attack
- Profound hopelessness
- Global insomnia
- Current suicidal ideations
- Previous suicidal attempt

- Acute loss/guilt/shame
- Mood congruent nihilistic delusions
- Recent discharge from psychiatric ward
- Active substance intoxication

Significant risk factors can be quickly analyzed with the mnemonic "SADPERSONS" scale[8,10]:

- **S**ex (male)
- **A**ge (very young or very old)
- **D**epression
- **P**revious attempt
- **E**thanol abuse
- **R**ational thinking loss (psychosis)
- **S**ocial supports lacking
- **O**rganized plan
- **N**o spouse
- **S**ickness (chronic illness)

Management

Safety of the patient [2,3,8,10,15]

- The safety of the patient is the foremost duty of the clinician. When deciding whether to hospitalize a potentially suicidal patient, due consideration must be given to all current and past risk factors.[15]
- The classical criteria for inpatient psychiatric hospitalization includes any patient with mental illness who has active suicidal/homicidal ideations, who is psychotic, who cannot attend to daily needs, and/or who is intoxicated.
- Ensuring safety requires inpatient hospital admission, close observation, reduced access to any means of suicide, and a redefined treatment plan once safety is established. Patients who are not hospitalized also need close follow-up with a multidisciplinary treatment plan and a detailed discharge plan.[15]

- Signed safety contracts are usually ineffective as a risk management strategy, despite their common use.

Assessment[3,4,8,10]

- Information may be obtained through direct questioning and observation. Specifics of any suicide plan must be inquired about, including but not limited to the nature, frequency, timing, and severity.
- Inquire about past suicidal ideations and attempts, as the highest predictor of suicide is past suicidal attempts.
- Determine the presence of acute crisis or stressors, such as loss of a loved one, job loss, acute financial or legal difficulties, acute shame or guilt, internal conflicts, and educational or family crisis.[4]
- Inquire about suicide in any family member, as it is a significant risk factor.

Medication[2,3,8,13,17]

- Newer medications with accelerated action (e.g., NMDA glutamic-acid antagonists like ketamine) may be available soon for the treatment of suicide; studies show a drastic, rapid reduction in suicidal ideation with these drugs.
- Benzos such as lorazepam promptly relieve risk factors including severe insomnia and psychic anxiety and can therefore be effective in emergency situations.[17]
- The rapid onset of action of antidepressants can be achieved by TCA-SSRI combo or by lithium augmentation of various antidepressants.[17]
- Clozapine and lithium have both demonstrated anti-suicidal effects.
- ECT may be lifesaving for profoundly depressed and acutely suicidal patients.[17]

Psychotherapy[15]

- Psychotherapy can be used to deal with contributing issues such as denial of symptoms and lack of insight.
- It may also help to manage high-risk symptoms such as hopelessness and anxiety.

Prevention

After resolving acute suicidality, clinicians must seek to prevent further attempts. The best forms of prevention include identification of clinically significant risk factors and warning signs, and prompt intervention.[2,3]

Practice guidelines for prevention[2,3,4,8,10,13,15]

- Formulate a structured plan at discharge.
- Ensure that an acutely suicidal patient is accompanied at all times.
- Restrict patient's access to any means of suicide.
- Develop a contingency plan to inform patient of contacts and resources if suicidal ideations return.
- Treat risk factors such as anxiety and insomnia, which can precipitate suicidality.
- Prepare plan to manage substance/alcohol use.

- Many depressed patients may attempt suicide by an overdose of medications, especially TCAs, MAOIs, or lithium[2,3,13]; prescribe drugs in small dosages to decrease the risk of overdose.
- After immediate risk of suicide subsides, monitor patient closely through outpatient management; reassess mood, suicidal ideation, and safety at each visit.
- The highest risk of suicide is during the first year after hospital discharge for MDD.

Agitation and Violence

The risk of violence in mental health patients is relatively low in contrast to general public opinion. However, highly publicized acts of violence by people with mental illness affect public perception.[9] People with psychiatric disorders are far more likely to be the victim of violence rather than the cause.[10] Studies show that people receiving treatment for mental illness are no more violent or dangerous than anyone else.[7,16] Although certain people with psychiatric disorders do commit assault and violent crime, research does not substantiate whether mental illness alone contributes to this behavior.[9]

The lifetime calculated risk of any person with schizophrenia seriously harming or killing someone is only 0.005%.[18] However, this risk increases 17 times in males and 80 times in females with the presence of comorbid alcoholism.[3,18] Antisocial personality disorder is associated with many instances of violence and vandalism, and impulse control disorder may also leads to the violation of many criminal laws.[16,20]

Symptoms of violence include demeaning or hostile verbal behavior, loud and abusive language, physical agitation, purposeless movements, aggression, irritability, intimidating behavior, refusal to cooperate, intense staring, and affective liability.[9,16] Acts of violence include homicide, rape, paraphilia, vandalism, domestic abuse, pyromania, and torture, among others.[9,10,20]

Causes and Risk Factors

Studies suggest that violence committed by people with mental illness is prompted by various overlapping factors including mental health diagnosis, family history, personal stressors, socioeconomic factors, substance abuse, and others.[9]

Mental disorders responsible for violent acts[2,3,9,20]

- Severe anxiety disorders
- Mood disorders
- Delusional disorders
- Substance abuse disorders
- Pervasive developmental disorder
- Dementia and delirium
- Malingering

- Traumatic brain injury
- Psychotic disorders, including schizophrenia, schizophreniform disorders, schizoaffective disorders
- Impulse control disorde
- Personality disorders: Antisocial, paranoid and borderline

Assessment of risk factors[2,3,9,10,15,20]

Predicting specific acts of violence is impossible given that they usually occur in highly emotional states. However, clinicians can make a general assessment of relative risks based on the following criteria[9,20]:

- *History of violence:* The best predictor for future violence. Victims of violent crime are also more likely to perpetrate it.[9]
- *Substance abuse:* The likelihood of committing violent crimes is 30 times greater in alcohol/substance abusers than in general population due to impaired judgment and disinhibition.[9]
- *Personality disorders:* Borderline personality disorders, antisocial personality disorders, and conduct disorders often manifest aggression and violence.[9] Patients with antisocial personality disorder with associated substance abuse have 100 times greater risk of being violent than the general population.
- *Psychosocial factors:* Young age, male gender, low socioeconomic status, unemployment, and divorce or separation, have all been implicated as predispositions to violent behavior.
- *Early exposure*: The risk of violence increases with childhood exposure to aggressive family fights, physical abuse, or having a parent with a criminal record.[9]
- *Nature of symptoms:* Patients with command hallucinations, paranoid delusions, or florid psychotic thoughts are more likely to act violently.[9]

Management

Violent patients can compromise the safety of themselves and others; immediate intervention must focus on ensuring safety.[3,10] With an imminently violent patient, attempt the least aggressive approaches first before resorting to more intrusive strategies.

Non-pharmacological management[2,3,9,10]

- Assess environment for potential dangers.
- Assess patient's physical demeanor.
- Take verbal threats seriously and stay away from patient.
- Don't hesitate to call security, as even a mere suggestion of resistance can be helpful.
- Always de-escalate crisis through supportive listening, reassurance, and a calm, empathetic approach towards the patient.
- *Physical restraint/seclusion:* No intervention is more effective for potentially violent patients than restraint.[17] If verbal interventions do not suffice, make sure there is a trained team of 5 or more people to help the patient into restraints.

Emergency medication[3,10,13,15,16,17,20]

- IM formulations and SL tabs have a faster onset than oral medications.
- IM atypicals are expensive and inferior in efficacy compared to IM typicals in managing agitated patients, but they have a faster onset and fewer EPS.

- For less severe agitation, benzos (lorazepam) can suffice at 1–2 mg/hour, max 10 mg/day.
- For agitated behavior, a benzo (e.g., lorazepam) and an antipsychotic (e.g., haloperidol) is a good combination.
- For severely agitated patients, a combination of different medications may be needed until hostility, agitation, and assaultiveness is reduced.
- Common combination includes 5 mg IM dose of haloperidol mixed with 2 mg Ativan (lorazepam) and 50 mg of Benadryl (diphenhydramine).
- IM formulations of ziprasidone, olanzapine, and aripiprazole are FDA approved for agitation associated with schizophrenia or bipolar mania.

Prevention
- Long-term intervention includes a range of psychosocial approaches such as DBT, conflict management, and substance abuse treatment.[9]
- Other methods include social-skills training, relapse prevention, problem-solving, etc.
- Researchers suggest that effectively treating mental illness and substance abuse may reduce the incidence of violence.[9]
- Practitoners should be aware that some psychiatric patients do pose a risk of violence, although most people who commit violence are not mentally ill.[9,20]

Psychiatric Medication-Related Emergencies

Neuroleptic Malignant Syndrome (NMS)[1,10,11,15]
NMS is a rare but serious complication of antipsychotic use that generally occurs with high doses of typical antipsychotics but may occur with atypical agents as well. It can be life-threatening and occurs shortly after the initiation of neuroleptic treatment or after dose increases.[11]
Symptoms: Involve the following triad—altered consciousness, muscular rigidity, and autonomic instability (hyperthermia, tachycardia, labile blood pressure, and diaphoresis).[1,15] Other symptoms include dyspnea, incontinence, pallor, psychomotor agitation, shuffling gait, tremor, and delirium.
Treatment[11,15,17]:
- Discontinue offending drugs
- Begin symptomatic treatment (e.g., cooling blanket, ice packs, intensive nursing)
- Begin hydration and alkalization of urine to prevent kidney failure
- Medications: Benzos (especially diazepam and lorazepam), bromocriptine (2.5–5 mg bid–tid), dantrolene (2.5mg/kg IV), and amantadine (100–200 mg/day)
- ECT may also be useful[1,10,11,15]

Serotonin Syndrome[6,7,12]

SSRIs used alone or in combination with other serotonergic agents can lead to a life-threatening condition known as serotonin syndrome. This syndrome is caused by the increased availability of serotonin in the CNS.[7] Life-threatening symptoms including rigidity and hyperthermia result only from stimulation of 5-HT$_2$ receptors. Only drugs that generally increase serotonergic effects are expected to cause serotonin toxicity.[12] The medications used with SSRIs that can lead to serotonin syndrome include[7]:

- TCAs
- MAOIs
- Lithium
- Trazodone
- Mirtazapine
- SNRIs: venlafaxine, duloxetine

- Opiates: meperidine, tramadol, pentazocine, dextromethorphan
- CNS stimulants: amphetamine, cocaine, methylphenidate
  Herbal medications: St. John's wort, ginseng, S-adenosyl-methionine (SAMe)

Symptoms: Abdominal cramps, agitation, altered mental status, confusion, diarrhea, dilated pupils, excessive sweating, fever, flushing, hypertension, hyperthermia, muscle rigidity, myoclonus, nausea, tachycardia, tremors.[6,12]

Age/sex ratio[6,7,10,12]:
- Women demonstrate a higher incidence of death related to toxicity.
- SSRI toxicity is highest among ages 19–39; in most cases, ingestion was intentional.
- Side-effect profile manifests more aggressively among the elderly.

Diagnosis[5,6,7,12]:
- Three or more of the following symptoms must be present: agitation, ataxia, diaphoresis, hyperreflexia, myoclonus, altered mental status, diarrhea, shivering, hyperthermia, tremor.[12]
- Rule out other causes, such as infection or substance abuse.
- Physical examination reveals increased HR, new onset hypertension, tremors, myoclonic jerks.
- EKG may indicate QT prolongation.
- Focus lab studies on obtaining drug levels from urine and serum samples.

Management: Serotonin syndrome is a medical emergency.[12,15]
- *Emergency department care:*
  - Stabilize airway, breathing, circulation
  - Begin supportive treatment
  - Manage cardiac arrhythmia
  - May administer naloxone if opioid medications have been used simultaneously
  - Administer benzos for agitated patients

- Administer serotonin antagonists (e.g., cyproheptadine) for severe cases
        - Use cooling blankets/ice packs for signs of hyperthermia
        - Ensure proper hydration in rhabdomyolysis to protect kidneys
    - *Medications:*
        - Adsorbent antidotes: activated charcoal
        - Serotonin antagonist: cyproheptadine
        - Sedatives: diazepam, lorazepam
        - Anti-hypertensive: nitoprusside
        - Neuromuscular-blocking agents: rocuronium, vecuronium

Complications: Aspiration pneumonia, seizure, acute renal failure, respiratory failure[12]

Important notes[6,12]:

- This syndrome has good prognosis with prompt medical attention.
- Patient follow-ups required after alleviation of symptoms, as rhabdomyolysis can cause acute kidney failure.
- Use available pharmacological agents judiciously; only alarming signs should warrant use.
- Counsel patients with multi-drug prescriptions about adverse interactions between medications.

References:

1. Adnet, P., P. Lestavel, and R. Krivosic-Horber. 2000. "Neuroleptic malignant syndrome." *British Journal of Anaesthesia* 85(1):129–135. doi: 10.1093/bja/85.1.129.

2. Allen, M.H., G.W. Currier, D.H. Hughes, M. Reyes-Harde, and John P. Docherty. 2001. "Treatment of Behavioral Emergencies." The Expert Consensus Guideline Series. 4–88. Accessed February 10, 2015.

3. Allen, M.H., G.W. Currier, D. Carpenter, R.W. Ross, and J.P. Docherty. 2005. "The expert consensus guideline series: Treatment of behavioral emergencies 2005." *J Psychiatr Pract* 11(suppl 1):5–108.

4. American Psychiatric Association (APA). 2010. "Practice guideline for the assessment and treatment of patients with suicidal behaviors." Accessed February 10, 2015. http://psychiatryonline.org/pb/assets/raw/sitewide/practice_guidelines/guidelines/suicide.pdf.

5. American Psychiatric Association (APA). 2013. *Diagnostic and Statistical Manual of Mental Disorders.* 5th ed. (DSM-5®). Washington, DC: American Psychiatric Publishing.

6. Boyer, E. W., and M. Shannon. 2005. "The serotonin syndrome." *N Engl J Med* 352(11):1112–1120. doi: 10.1056/NEJMra041867.

7. Buckley, Nicholas A, Andrew H Dawson, and Geoffrey K Isbister. 2014. "Serotonin Syndrome." *BMJ* 348:g1626. doi: 10.1136/bmj.g1626.

8. Fawcett, J., W.A. Scheftner, and D.C. Clark. 1990. "Time related predictors of suicide." *Am J Psychiatry* 147:1189–1194.

9.   Harvard Health Publications. 2011. "Mental illness and violence." Harvard Medical School. Accessed April 20, 2015. http://www.health.harvard.edu/newsletter_article/mental-illness-and-violence.

10. Hillard, J.R., ed. 1990. *Manual of Clinical Emergency Psychiatry.* 109–124. Washington, DC: American Psychiatric Publishing.

11. Medscape: Drugs & Diseases. 2015. "Neuroleptic Malignant Syndrome." Accessed February 10, 2015. http://emedicine.medscape.com/article/816018-overview.

12. Medscape: Drugs & Diseases. 2015. "Selective Serotonin Reuptake Inhibitor Toxicity." Accessed February 10, 2015. http://emedicine.medscape.com/article/821737-overview.

13. Preston, John D., and James Johnson. 2011. *Clinical Psychopharmacology Made Ridiculously Simple.* 7th ed. 54. Miami: MedMaster Inc.

14. Suicide Awareness Voices of Education (SAVE). 2015. "Suicide Facts." Accessed June 20, 2015. https://www.save.org/index.cfm?fuseaction=home.viewPage&page_id=705D5DF4-055B-F1EC-3F66462866FCB4E6&r=1&CFID=1216161&CFTOKEN=72273ece53938f 1c-9343DB65-5056-8A47-CE55B51C9A42B086

15. Schatzberg, A.F., and C.B. Nemeroff, eds. 2009. *The American Psychiatric Publishing Textbook of Psychopharmacology.* 4th ed. 1202–1212, 1287–1308. Washington, DC: American Psychiatric Publishing.

16. Schatzberg, A.F., and C. DeBattista. 1999. "Phenomenology and treatment of agitation." *J Clin Psychiatry* 60(suppl 15):17–20.

17. Schatzberg, A.F., Jonathan O. Cole, and Charles DeBattista. 2010. *Manual of Clinical Psychopharmacology.* 7th ed. 545–562. Washington, DC: American Psychiatric Publishing.

18. Swanson, Jeffery W., Marvin S. Swartz, Richard A. Van Dorn, Eric B. Elbogen, H. Ryan Wagner, Robert A. Rosenheck, T. Scott Stroup, Joseph P. McEvoy, and Jeffrey A. Lieberman. 2006. "A national study of violent behavior in persons with schizophrenia." *Archives of General Psychiatry* 63(5):490–499. doi: 10.1001/archpsyc.63.5.490.

19. Tsirigotis, Konstantinos, Wojciech Gruszczynski, and Marta Tsirigotis. 2011. "Gender differentiation in methods of suicide attempts." *Medical Science Monitor* 17(8):PH65-PH70. doi: 10.12659/MSM.881887.

20. Tupin, J. 1975. "Management of violent patients." In *Manual of Psychiatric Therapeutics.* Edited by R.I. Shader. 125–133. Boston: Little, Brown.

21. University of Washington: Psychiatry Clerkship. 2007. "Lectures." Accessed February 3, 2015. http://depts.washington.edu/psyclerk/lectures.html.

Chapter 17
Posttraumatic Stress Disorder And Its Treatment

Posttraumatic stress disorder (PTSD) is a psychiatric condition which can develop after a person is exposed to traumatic events such as sexual assault, life-threatening situations, abuse, injury, serious accidents, natural disasters, violent attacks, or any event that severely compromises physical or emotional wellbeing.[1] Once referred to as "shell shock" or battle fatigue, veterans of the Vietnam War first brought this post-war syndrome to public attention.[11] PTSD has only been recognized as a formal diagnosis since 1980.[3] Women are twice as likely to develop PTSD as men[11]; children are less likely to experience PTSD.[5] At least 5 million people currently suffer from PTSD in the US, and approximately 7–10% of people will develop it in their lifetime.[5,7] The incidence and prevalence of PTSD in combat/war veterans and rape victims is exorbitantly high.[5,7] Diagnosis is based on eight criteria from the DSM-5.

Symptoms include[3,4,5,7,11]:

- Recurring flashbacks/reliving traumatic event
- Numbing and avoidance of memories of event
- Hyperarousal
- Nightmares
- Emotional disturbance when reminded of event
- Avoiding places/activities connected with event
- Loss of memory, especially regarding important aspects of event
- Hypervigilant
- Feelings of guilt
- Hopelessness
- Self-destructive behavior
- Difficulty concentrating
- Insomnia
- Fearfulness

The five main types of PTSD are[8]:

1. Normal stress response
2. Acute stress disorder
3. Uncomplicated PTSD
4. Comorbid PTSD
5. Complex PTSD

Changes in DSM-5[1,7,9]

- PTSD has been moved from anxiety disorders into the new "Trauma and Stressor-related Disorders."
- Diagnosis now requires exposure to actual or threatened death, serious injury, or sexual violation.

- Symptoms are now divided into four clusters: intrusion, avoidance, negative alterations in cognitions and mood, and alterations in arousal and reactivity.
- Diagnosis now requires at least one avoidance symptom.
- Two new symptoms have been added:
  - *Criteria D:* persistent and distorted blame of self or others, persistent negative emotional state
  - *Criteria E:* reckless or destructive behavior
- Additional clinical subtype of "with dissociative symptoms" has been added.
- Separate diagnostic criteria are included for children ages six or younger.
- Distinction between acute and chronic phases of PTSD is eliminated; now requires disturbance to persist only for more than a month.

Management[2,3,4,5,6,7,10,11]

PTSD can usually be managed with a combination of psychotherapy and pharmacological approaches.

Psychotherapeutic Approaches

Psychological debriefing: Initial preventive treatment consists of interviews that allow an individual to share his or her feelings with a therapist immediately after the traumatic event.

Psychological therapies: Trauma-focused CBT, group therapy, individual and family therapy, play therapy, art therapy, hypnosis, relaxation techniques, anxiety management, eye movement desensitization and reprocessing (EDMR). Two interventions gaining popularity are MDMA-enhanced (ecstasy) psychotherapy and Virtual Reality (VR) exposure.

Pharmacological Treatment

Symptoms such as re-experiencing the event, hypervigilance, and increased arousal respond better to medication than symptoms of avoidance and withdrawal. It is recommended to give any medications use a full trial of 6–8 weeks to gauge efficacy.

Antidepressants[3,4,6,7,10]

- SSRIs are first-line medications, although they are required in higher doses for PTSD.
- Sertraline, paroxetine, and venlafaxine are FDA-approved for the treatment of PTSD.
- These medications may relieve all four symptom clusters.
- Improvement is usually seen within 4–6 weeks of initiation, and treatment should be maintained in responders for up to 1 year.
- Amitriptyline is helpful for hypervigilance, increased arousal, and avoidance; imipramine can be useful for intrusive symptoms.

Mood Stabilizers[3,4,6,7,10]

- These drugs reduce limbic-system sensitization that accompanies the weeks or months following a traumatic event.
- Carbamazepine decreases re-experiencing, insomnia, hyperarousal, impulsivity, and violent behavior.[3]
- Valproate is associated with improvement in avoidance/arousal but not re-experiencing symptoms.
- Topiramate may reduce PTSD symptoms unresponsive to other medication and may be effective in reducing flashbacks and nightmares.[3]
- Gabapentin can be helpful for sleep disturbance and nightmares.
- Lithium may improve hyperarousal symptoms.
- Lamotrigine may be useful for core symptoms of PTSD.

Adrenergic-inhibiting agents[3,4,6,7,10]

- Individuals with PTSD have elevated plasma levels of norepinephrine at rest and increased incidence of remembering trauma.[3]
- The beta-blocker propranolol decreases symptoms such as multiple nighttime awakenings, intrusive recollections, and physiological instability.
- Clonidine reduces impulsivity, hyperarousal, nightmares, and intrusive symptoms; does not reduce avoidance and numbness.[3]
- Prazosin can improve overall sleep quality and nightmares; may also improve re-experiencing symptoms, numbing, avoidance, and hyperarousal.[3]

Benzodiazepines[3,4,6,7,10]

- Recent studies suggest that benzos may actually cause symptoms to linger and may reduce the effectiveness of psychotherapeutic treatment.
- Benzos may also interfere with fear extinction; have limited utility for PTSD.[3]
- Studies on alprazolam and clonazepam suggest low efficacy in treating PTSD.
- Based on the above, it is recommended to avoid benzos to manage PTSD due to low efficacy, dissassociation, and risk of potential harm.

Antipsychotics[3,4,6,7,10]

- Atypical antipsychotics can help with dissociative symptoms and explosive, aggressive, or violent behavior.
- Risperidone may ameliorate intrusive thinking, irritability, and core PTSD symptoms.
- Olanzapine is effective as an adjunctive treatment for PTSD with associated depression and sleep problems unresponsive to SSRIs.
- Quetiapine improves insomnia and psychotic symptoms.

Other Medications[2,3,4,6,7,10]

- Buspirone may reduce hyperarousal symptoms.[11]
- Cyproheptadine can relieve associated sleep disorders and nightmares.[11]

- Eszopiclone improves overall PTSD severity and helps with sleep.[7]
- The use of methylenedioxymethamphetamine (MDMA, "ecstasy") with psycho-therapy is experimental but appears controversial.[11]
- ECT may help in severe depression with melancholic features plus PTSD.

References:

1. American Psychiatric Association (APA). 2013. "Posttraumatic Stress Disorder." Updated DSM-5. Accessed January 13, 2015. http://www.dsm5.org/Documents/PTSD%20Fact%20 Sheet.pdf.

2. Cukor, J., J. Spitalnick, J. Difede, A. Rizzo, and B.O. Rothbaum. 2009. "Emerging treatments for PTSD." *Clin Psychol Rev* 29(8):715–726. doi: 10.1016/j.cpr.2009.09.001.

3. Gabbard, Glen O., ed. 2007. *Gabbard's Treatments of Psychiatric Disorders*. 4th ed. 517–536. Washington, DC: American Psychiatric Publishing.

4. Hales, Robert. E., S. Yudofsky, and L. Roberts, eds. 2014. *The American Psychiatric Publishing Textbook of Psychiatry*. 6th ed. 455–498, 929–1004. Washington, DC: American Psychiatric Publishing.

5. Hembree, E.A., and E.B. Foa. 2000. "Posttraumatic stress disorder: psychological factors and psychosocial interventions." *J Clin Psychiatry* 61(7 suppl):33–39.

6. Ipser, J.C., and D.J. Stein. 2012. "Evidence-based pharmacotherapy of post-traumatic stress disorder (PTSD)." *Int J Neuropsychopharmacol.* 15(6):825–840. Accessed February 3, 2015. http://www.ncbi. nlm.nih.gov/pubmed/21798109.

7. Medscape: Drugs & Diseases. 2015. "Posttraumatic Stress Disorder." Accessed January 14, 2015. http://emedicine.medscape.com/article/288154-overview.

8. National Center for PTSD. 2013. "Types of PTSD," *Psych Central.* Accessed January 14, 2015. http://psychcentral.com/lib/types-of-ptsd/.

9. National Center for PTSD. 2014. "DSM-5 Diagnostic Criteria for PTSD Released." *US Department of Veteran Affairs.* Accessed January 14, 2015. http://www.ptsd.va.gov/professional/PTSD-overview/ diagnostic_criteria_dsm-5.asp.

10. Schatzberg, A.F., and C.B. Nemeroff, eds. 2009. *The American Psychiatric Publishing Textbook of Psychopharmacology*. 4th ed. 1171–1200. Washington, DC: American Psychiatric Publishing.

11. Wikipedia Contributors. 2015. "Posttraumatic Stress Disorder." *Wikipedia, the Free Encyclopedia.* Accessed January 14, 2015. http://en.wikipedia.org/wiki/Posttraumatic_stress_disorder.

Chapter 18
Eating Disorders And Their Treatment

Eating disorders are debilitating psychiatric conditions characterized by severely disturbed and aberrant eating habits, involving either extremely insufficient food intake or excessive binge eating.[1] Some eating disorders can have severe physical and emotional effects, often leading to death. Early detection and prompt intervention are imperative for combatting these types of diseases.[5,6]

The mortality rate of anorexia is the highest among psychiatric disorders at around 20% without treatment.[5] Mortalities from anorexia nervosa are primarily due to cardiac arrest or suicide.[5] The lifetime prevalence of anorexia nervosa in the US is estimated at 0.3–1%, with disordered eating behavior occurring in 13% of US adolescent girls.[5] Anorexia is significantly more frequent in Caucasian populations but has been reported within all races.[5] The female-to-male ratio is 10–20:1, with 85% of patients experiencing the onset of the symptoms between the ages of 13 and 18 years.[5] Bulimia nervosa is more prevalent than anorexia and has a better prognosis.[6]

The exact cause of anorexia is unknown, but genetic factors and social stresses are thought to play a major role. Since Western society often cultivates and reinforces the desire for thinness, eating disorders are more common in industrialized societies with an abundance of food where slimness is considered attractive, especially for women.[5] Although the etiology of bulimia is unclear, the disorder likely results from a combination of family history, social values, and certain personality traits. The prognosis of eating disorders is variable: one-third of those afflicted recover, one-third fluctuate between recovery to relapse, and one-third suffer chronically.[9]

DSM-5 Types[1,2,5,6,8]
The types of eating disorders classified in DSM-5 include:
- Bulimia Nervosa
- Anorexia Nervosa
- Binge Eating Disorder
- Feeding or Eating Disorders Not Elsewhere Classified
- Other Eating Disorders (orthorexia, body dysmorphic disorder, night eating disorder, pica)

Testing[3,5,6]
Psychological tests: Eating-disorder-specific psychometric tests, eating-attitude tests, body-attitude questionnaire, eating disorder inventory, SCOFF questionnaire.

Lab tests: Comprehensive blood chemistry panel, CBC, urinalysis, urine toxicology screen, pregnancy test, amylase level, ECG, DEXA.

Management

Anorexia Nervosa[3,4,5,7,8,9]

Treatment: Multimodal—nutritional/feeding programs, psychosocial interventions, medications, therapy, and other modalities

Medications:

- SSRIs, TCAs, topiramate, valproic acid, and methylphenidate
- TCAs such as amitriptyline and imipramine can promote weight gain
- SGAs—particularly olanzapine, risperidone, and quetiapine—are useful in patients with delusions, obsessions, and severe resistance to weight gain
- Chlorpromazine may help very disturbed patients if given before meals in small doses
- Other medications include zinc supplements and cortisol

Relapse prevention: Fluoxetine (max 60 mg/day)

Non-pharmacological treatment:

- *Therapy:* Group therapy, CBT, acceptance and commitment therapy, dialectical behavioral therapy, EMDR, guided imagery, interpersonal psychotherapy, psychodynamic psychotherapy, stress management, ego-oriented individual therapy, motivational enhancement therapy
- *Other modalities:* Self-help groups, nutritional management, supportive family therapy, family-based treatment

Binge Eating Disorder[3,4,9]

Treatment: Combination of dietary and psychosocial treatments, nutritional rehabilitation, behavioral weight control, CBT

Medications:

- Vyvanse is the only drug approved by the FDA for this disorder
- SSRIs (fluoxetine, sertraline, fluvoxamine) are preferred choice due to likelihood of co-morbid depression in patients with binge eating disorder
- Appetite suppressants (orlistat, pramilintide)
- Antiepileptic agents topiramate and zonisamide appear to reduce binge eating frequency and promote weight loss better than other agents

Bulimia Nervosa[3,4,6,9]

Treatment: Multimodal—nutritional rehabilitation and counseling, psychosocial interventions, psychotherapy, medications, coordinating care and collaborating with other clinicians

Medications:

- SSRIs, TCAs, topiramate, valproic acid, and methylphenidate

- Fluoxetine is FDA-approved for treatment of bulimia nervosa
- Sertraline reduces symptoms by causing progressive muscle relaxation
- After treatment, continue antidepressants for up to 1 year in the maintenance phase
- Methylphenidate can be helpful in patients with both bulimia nervosa and ADHD

Non-pharmacological treatment: CBT, interpersonal psychotherapy, nutritional rehabilitation and counseling, family therapy

Prevention[3,5,6]

Prevention strategies include:

- Educating patients about nutrition and health
- Promoting positive body image
- Noticing changes in body weight and appearance and providing early counseling

References:

1. American Psychiatric Association (APA). 2013a. *Diagnostic and Statistical Manual of Mental Disorders.* 5th ed. (DSM-5®). Washington, DC: American Psychiatric Publishing.

2. American Psychiatric Association (APA). 2013b. "Highlights of Changes from DSM-IV-TR to DSM-5." Last accessed January 13, 2015. http://www.dsm5.org/Documents/changes%20from%20 dsm-iv-tr%20to%20dsm-5.pdf.

3. Gabbard, Glen O., ed. 2007. *Gabbard's Treatments of Psychiatric Disorders.* 4th ed. 703–732. Washington, DC: American Psychiatric Publishing.

4. Hales, Robert. E., S. Yudofsky, and L. Roberts, eds. 2014. *The American Psychiatric Publishing Textbook of Psychiatry.* 6th ed. 557–586, 929–1004. Washington, DC: American Psychiatric Publishing.

5. Medscape: Drugs & Diseases. 2015a. "Anorexia Nervosa." Accessed February 3, 2015. http://emedicine.medscape.com/article/912187-overview.

6. Medscape: Drugs & Diseases. 2015b. "Bulimia Nervosa." Accessed February 3, 2015. http://emedicine.medscape.com/article/286485-overview.

7. Menaster, M. 2005. "Use of olanzapine in anorexia nervosa." *J Clin Psychiatry* 66:654–655, author reply 655–656.

8. National Association of Anorexia Nervosa and Associated Disorders (ANAD). 2015. "Important Changes in Eating Disorder Diagnoses in DSM-V." Accessed February 3, 2015. http://www.anad. org/news/important-changes-in-eating-disorder-diagnoses-in-dsm-v.

9. Schatzberg, A.F., and C.B. Nemeroff, eds. 2009. *The American Psychiatric Publishing Textbook of Psychopharmacology.* 4th ed. 1027–1044, 1231–1240. Washington, DC: American Psychiatric Publishing.

Chapter 19
Personality Disorders And Their Treatment

All individuals possess various personality traits, but personality disorders are often characterized by deviant behavioral tendencies that are associated with dysfunction in personal, social, and occupational performance.[1,5,9] They are characterized by enduring maladaptive patterns of behavior, cognition, and inner experience, exhibited across many contexts and markedly deviating from those accepted by the individual's culture, leading to distress or impairment.[1,6] They cannot be diagnosed in children or adolescents because personality development is incomplete at these ages, as traits present during childhood or adolescence may not persevere into adulthood.[5,6] Personality disorders have a complex etiology and are created by an innate disposition that manifests as a result of subsequent evolvement from environmental cues.[9]

Categorization
There are 10 types of personality disorders categorized into three clusters:

Table 19.1 Personality Disorder Clusters[1,3,4,6]

Cluster	**A** (Odd personality)	**B** (Dramatic, erratic, or emotional personality)	**C** (Fearful or anxious personality)
Disorder	Paranoid Schizoid Schizotypal	Antisocial Borderline Histrionic Narcissistic	Avoidant Dependent Obsessive-compulsive

Management
Personality disorders are often disabling and can disrupt an individual's personal and social life. Management is challenging, as most patients lack insight to their own condition.[3,6] As a result, effective management of these disorders requires individualized approaches and an understanding of their multidimensional effects and coexisting morbidities.[6,9]

Therapy
Psychotherapy is the mainstay of treatment.[3,4,7] The most frequently used techniques include:[7]

- Psychodynamic psychotherapy
- CBT
- Interpersonal therapy
- Therapeutic community approach
- Mentalization-based treatment
- Group psychotherapy
- Dialectic behavior therapy

Medication

Medications are seldom used, as they are not very helpful for any personality disorders.[2,3] Medications are only useful as adjuncts to psychotherapy and in comorbid disorders.[2,9]

Cluster A

Limited trials suggest that the medications of choice are conventional antipsychotics.[2] Atypicals should be tried first because of their better safety profile.[9]

Cluster B

Medications may help control impulsivity, affective instability, and self-injurious behavior.[3,8,9] The use of medication in BPD patients has increased by up to 40% in the past six years.[2]

Antipsychotics[2,3,4,8,9]
- Haloperidol has a broad-spectrum effect in symptom domains, including schizotypal, affective, and impulsive-behavioral.
- Reduction of acute-distress symptoms can be achieved with aripiprazole, olanzapine, risperidone, or quetiapine.

Antidepressants[2,3,4,9]
- Sertraline, paroxetine, escitalopram, and mirtazapine abate impulsive and aggressive symptoms.
- Fluvoxamine at 20–60 mg/day may relieve depression and impulsive aggression rapidly.
- Venlafaxine (SNRI) significantly reduces global symptomatology.
- TCAs and MOAIs have limited efficacy for BPD.

Anxiolytics[2,3,4,9]
- SSRIs or antipsychotics can relieve somatic anxiety.
- Psychic anxiety may respond to long-acting benzos or gabapentin.
- Benzos, although conducive for anxiety symptoms, increase risk of impulsivity and dependence.[6]

Mood Stabilizers[2,3,4,9]
- Lithium may ameliorate anger and suicidal tendencies in BPD patients.[9]
- Carbamazepine provides significant behavioral control but has only modest effects on mood.[9]
- Divalproex may be efficacious in tempering impulsive aggression.[9]
- Lamotrigine 75–300 mg/day improves overall functioning.[9]

Antisocial Personality Disorder

- Milieu approaches such as token economies, therapeutic-residential communities, and mentalization-based treatments can be effective preventive and therapeutic modes.[3]
- Four medications have been demonstrated to diminish symptoms: benzos, lithium, fluoxetine, and propranolol.[4]
- Lithium and propranolol enhance affective aggression but may inhibit predatory aggression via the noradrenergic system.
- Phenytoin and carbamazepine enhance affective and predatory aggression via electrical "kindling."[3]

Cluster C

Numerous studies have shown the efficacy of MAOIs and SSRIs in social phobia, including its generalized subtype.[3,9] SSRIs may be useful in treating obsessive-compulsive and dependent personality traits.[9]

Important notes[3,4,5,6]

- Schizotypal personality disorder is associated with a risk of developing brief psychotic disorder, schizophreniform disorder, and delusional disorder.
- Paranoid personality disorder may be a prodrome to delusional disorder or frank schizophrenia.[6]
- Homicide may be a potential complication of paranoid/antisocial personality disorder.
- Histrionic personality disorder may exhibit somatoform disorders.[6]
- Narcissistic personality disorder may be associated with anorexia nervosa, substance abuse, and depression.[6]
- Avoidant personality disorder may be associated with anxiety disorders and phobias.[6]
- Dependent personality disorder may be associated with anxiety and adjustment disorder.[6]
- Hospitalization is often necessary in BPD patients for suicidal/self-injurious behavior.[5]
- Prescribe medications in BPD at minimum dosage with great caution because of risk of overdose.
- Antisocial personality disorder is associated with anxiety disorders, substance abuse, somatization disorder, and pathologic gambling.[6]

References:

1. American Psychiatric Association (APA). 2013. *Diagnostic and Statistical Manual of Mental Disorders.* 5th ed. (DSM-5®). Washington, DC: American Psychiatric Publishing.

2. Bellino, S., E. Paradiso, and F. Bogetto. 2008. "Efficacy and tolerability of pharmacotherapies for borderline personality disorder." *CNS Drugs* 22:671–692.

3. Gabbard, Glen O., ed. 2007. *Gabbard's Treatments of Psychiatric Disorders.* 4th ed. 757–844. Washington, DC: American Psychiatric Publishing.

4. Hales, Robert. E., S. Yudofsky, and L. Roberts, eds. 2014. *The American Psychiatric Publishing Textbook of Psychiatry.* 6th ed. 854–894, 929–1004. Washington, DC: American Psychiatric Publishing.

5. Medscape: Drugs & Diseases. 2015a. "Borderline Personality Disorder." Accessed February 3, 2015. http://emedicine.medscape.com/article/913575-overview.

6. Medscape: Drugs & Diseases. 2015b. "Personality Disorders." Accessed February 3, 2015. http://emedicine.medscape.com/article/294307-overview.

7. National Alliance on Mental Illness (NAMI). 2015. "Psychotherapy." Accessed April 2, 2015. https://www.nami.org/Learn-More/Treatment/Psychotherapy.

8. Rocca, P., L. Marchiaro, E. Cocuzza, and F. Bogetto. 2002. "Treatment of borderline personality disorder with risperidone." *J Clin Psychiatry* 63:241–244.

9. Schatzberg, A.F., and C.B. Nemeroff, eds. 2009. *The American Psychiatric Publishing Textbook of Psychopharmacology.* 4th ed. 1045–1060, 1267–1286. Washington, DC: American Psychiatric Publishing.

Chapter 20
ECT, VNS, And Other Brain Stimulation Therapies

These modalities are non-pharmacological, often invasive methods used to treat depression and other disorders through direct activation of the brain by a variety of stimulation including electricity and magnets.[9] Among these modalities, electroconvulsive therapy (ECT) is the most researched stimulation therapy.[9] The most commonly used brain stimulation therapies include[4]:

- Electroconvulsive therapy (ECT)
- Vagus nerve stimulation (VNS)
- Repetitive transcranial magnetic stimulation (rTMS)
- Magnetic seizure therapy (MST)
- Deep brain stimulation (DBS)
- Fisher Wallace stimulator
- Transcranial direct current stimulation (TDCS)
- Focal electrical alternating current therapy (FEAT)

Electroconvulsive Therapy (ECT)[2,4,9,10]

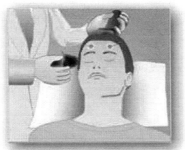

Figure 20.1: ECT (NIMH 2015)

ECT is a non-pharmacological treatment in which seizures are electrically induced in patients for therapeutic purposes. ECT is reserved for treatment-resistant cases of various disorders: MDD, schizophrenia, mania, and catatonia.[4,9] First developed in 1938, ECT did not gain popularity initially because of associated complications and controversies; however, the procedure has improved significantly and is now considered safe and effective.[9] ECT is considered the gold standard of treatment for treatment-resistant depression.[4]

FDA approved for: Treatment-resistant depression

Other potential uses (off-label): Bipolar disorder, post-partum depression, schizophrenia (acute and catatonia), severe depression, suicidal patients

MOA: No definite MOA; may alter brain's neurochemistry[9]

Prerequisites:
- Informed consent must be obtained from patient or designate
- Sedation with general anesthesia is needed before procedure[9]
- Muscle relaxant to decrease movement is required during procedure[9]

Procedure:
- Electrodes are placed at precise locations on head[9]
- Electric current passes through the brain, inducing a seizure that lasts for about 1 min[9]

Stimulation sites: Bifrontal, bitemporal, left anterior, right unilateral

Types: Unilateral ECT, bilateral ECT

Dosage: Use approximately 3x/week until symptoms are reduced (6–12 sessions), followed by maintenance treatment in cases of recurrence (one session/week to one session/1–2 months)

Side effects: Amnesia, GI disturbance, headache, muscle aches

Contraindications:
- No absolute contraindications[4]
- *Relative contraindications:* intracranial space-occupying lesion, recent MI, unstable angina, severe CHF, severe valvular heart disease, bleeding vascular aneurism or malformation, recent cerebral infarction, severe pulmonary dysfunction[4]

Lab tests recommend: CBC, serum potassium, sodium levels, EKG, pregnancy test, anesthesia-eligibility tests

Special populations:
Pregnancy: Safe during all trimesters
Lactation: Considered safe
Elderly: Considered safe but closely monitor mental status
Hepatic impairment: Use caution
Renal impairment: Use caution, monitor electrolytes closely

Important notes:
- Monitor vitals like BP, HR, and respiratory rate throughout the procedure[9]
- Profound short-term efficacy demonstrated in major depression
- Increases the efficacy of antidepressants/mood stabilizers
- Studies reveal that a "brief pulse" of electricity at frequent intervals is less likely to cause memory loss[9]
- Patients wake after several minutes with some dizziness, become alert after several hours, and then can resume normal activities
- Cognitive side effects seem to be troublesome but usually resolve within six months[4]

Vagus Nerve Stimulation (VNS)[2,4,5,9]

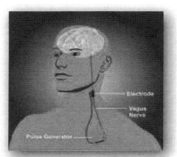

Figure 20.2: VNS (NIMH 2015)

VNS is used as an adjunct for treatment-resistant depression. Despite receiving FDA approval in 2005, VNS remains a controversial treatment for depression because studies have not shown promising outcomes.[9]

FDA approved for: Chronic or recurrent medication-resistant depression with four failed treatments, refractory partial seizures

Other potential uses (off-label): Epilepsy (intractable)

MOA: Alters mood-associated neurotransmitters (e.g., GABA, glutamate, serotonin, norepinephrine)

Procedure:

- Pulse generator is implanted into the upper left subclavicular region
- Lead wire is attached to left vagus nerve and connected to pulse generator[9]
- Typically, electrical pulses lasting 30 sec are sent every 5 min from generator to the vagus nerve; duration/frequency of pulses vary with generator programming[9]
- Vagus nerve transmits signals to brain following stimulation[9]

Stimulation site: Cervical cranial nerve

Dosage: Up to 1 mA initially, clinical benefits assessed over several months **Side effects:** Breathing problems, cough, additional surgery, dysphagia, headache, implantation site discomfort, infection from implant surgery, pain in the neck, sore throat

Contraindications: Patients with bilateral or left cervical vagotomy

Important notes:

- The FDA has approved a humanitarian device exemption for VNS in treatment-resistant depression
- Surgical implantation of device may cause infection, vocal cord paralysis, and bradycardia

- Symptoms like cough and hoarseness of voice may occur during nerve-stimulation process, but in general, the patient does not feel any sensation while the device works[9]
- Device can be monitored by a personal computer or PDA[5]
- Device may be deactivated for certain periods of time by placing a magnet over the chest where the pulse generator is implanted; device reactivates when magnet is removed[9]
- No cognitive side effects; improves neurocognitive performance by improving depression

Repetitive Transcranial Magnetic Stimulation (rTMS)[2,4,9]

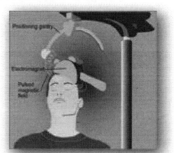

Figure 20.3 rTMS (NIMH 2015)

This procedure uses a magnet instead of an electrical current to activate the brain. Studies have shown some efficacy in management of treatment-resistant major depression, psychosis, and other disorders. [9]

FDA approved for: Class II (special controls) medical device; approved for depression not responding to medication, and migraine headache

Other potential uses (off-label): Psychosis

MOA: Similar to ECT but is used to target specific group of neurons (very localized action); the magnetic field enters the cortex and activates the resting nerve cells[4]

Procedure:

- Electromagnetic coil is held against the forehead near a specific brain area, followed by short electromagnetic pulses to the nerve cells[9]
- Magnetic field has the same strength as an MRI scan[9]

Stimulation site: Cortical

Dosage: Repeated pulses delivered at 1–20 Hz for 30–60 min, repeated 5 days/week for 4–6 weeks

Side effects: Discomfort at magnet site, mild headache or lightheadedness, seizure, twitching, or contracture of muscles of scalp, jaw, or face

Contraindications:
- Increased ICP, epilepsy, severe CV disease
- Cranial implants, brain stimulators, or electrodes

Important notes:
- No requirement of anesthesia during procedure, unlike ECT
- Hearing loss may occur due to large clicking sounds produced by the machine; the use of earplugs advised
- Minor side effects; patients can return to work after each treatment session
- Usually not covered by insurance, as it is expensive[4]

Magnetic Seizure Therapy (MST)[4,9,10]

MST is another non-pharmacological approach for depression using the principles of ECT and rTMS.

FDA approved for: None

Other potential uses (off-label): Treatment-resistant depression

MOA: Same as ECT but allows enhanced control over stimulation site and seizure initiation

Procedure:
- Patient must be anesthetized and adminstred muscle relaxant to prevent any movement
- Magnetic pulse used instead of electricity to stimulate specific brain target
- Induces a seizure similar to ECT but pulse given at higher frequency than in rTMS

Common side effects: Amnesia

Contraindications: Pacemakers, implanted devices

Important notes:
- Goal of therapy is ECT-like efficacy with reduction in cognitive side effects[9]
- Extensively studied as a treatment for patients unresponsive to antidepressant medication and those who cannot tolerate ECT

Deep Brain Stimulation (DBS)[2,4,7,8,9]

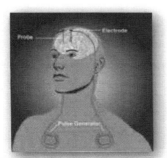

Figure 20.4 DBS (NIMH 2015)

DBS utilizes invasive electrode implanation to send electrical impulses to a targeted area in the brain.

FDA approved for: Parkinson's disease, treatment-resistant depression (humanitarian device exemption)

Other potential uses (off-label): Dystonia, chronic pain, essential tremor, OCD

MOA: Impulses "reset" the malfunctioning area of brain, allowing it to resume working normally again[9]

Prerequisites:
- Brain MRI; used by surgeon as a guide during surgery[9]
- Catheter inserted into brain through two drilled holes in head; electrodes placed on specific brain areas[9]
- After electrode implantation, patient receives general anesthesia; electrodes are then attached to wires inside the body where a pair of battery-operated generators are implanted[9]

Procedure: A pair of electrodes implanted in the brain is controlled by a generator implanted in the chest providing continuous stimulation, although electrical frequency and level are adjusted according to the requirement[9]

Stimulation Site: Subcortical

Side effects: Confusion, disorientation, infection, intracranial hemorrhage, mood changes, movement disorders, seizures

Contraindications: Medical conditions requiring multiple MRI exposures, diathermy

Important notes:
- Invasive procedure; electrodes must be implanted surgically
- Reaches deeper brain structures than ECT or TMS
- DBS is currently being investigated for schizophrenia, substance abuse, and obesity[4]

Fisher Wallace Stimulator[3,10,13]

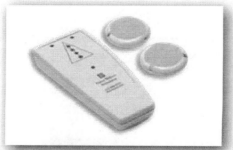

Figure 20.5 Fisher Wallace Stimulator (2015)

The Fisher Wallace Stimulator is a portable, battery-powered cranial electrotherapy stimulation (CES) device that has been cleared by the FDA for the symptomatic relief of depression, anxiety, and insomnia. The device is a handheld pulse generator that delivers very low electric outputs to the brain. It does not interfere with medication and does not cause serious side effects.

FDA approved for: None (approval pending)

Indications: FDA cleared to treat depression, insomnia, and anxiety

MOA: Delivers mild electrical stimulation to brain to stimulate production of neuro-chemicals such as serotonin, GABA, and endorphins

Dosage:
- Depression and anxiety: Use device for 20 min 1–2x/day for 6 weeks, then less frequently as needed
- Insomnia: Use device for 20 min before sleeping

Side effects: Dizziness, headache, skin irritation

Contraindications: Demand or sensing-type cardiac pacemakers

Important notes:
- If approved, device will become only FDA-approved medical device for insomnia and anxiety and only home-use device approved for depression
- Comparatively cheaper than other invasive devises (cost approx $600–$800)
- Can be used at home by patient without a doctor's supervision

Transcranial Direct Current Stimulation (TDCS)[4,6,9,12]

TDCS is a noninvasive means of electrically polarizing neurons in the brain.[4]

FDA approved for: None

Other potential uses (off-label): Depression, stroke, substance abuse

MOA/Procedure: Current stimulation of brain cortex via electrodes causes depolarization and hyperpolarization of cortical neuron; anodal stimulation facilitates cortical function while cathodal stimulation inhibits cortical function

Side effects: Dizziness, headache, nausea, skin irritation

Contraindications: Pacemaker, implanted medication pump, metal plate in skull, craniotomy

Important notes:
- Noninvasive, portable, inexpensive, relatively few side effects
- More extensive studies needed to establish safety/efficacy

Focal Electrical Alternating Current Therapy (FEAT)[1]

FEAT is an investigational treatment for depression.

MOA/Procedure: Uses alternating current to produce transcranial stimulation for focal modulation of brain activity

Stimulation site: Cortical
Important notes:
- Fewer cognitive side effects than ECT

References

1. BehaveNet. 2015. "Focal electrical alternating current seizure therapy." Accessed March 12, 2015. http://behavenet.com/focal-electrical-alternating-current-seizure-therapy.

2. Cusin, C., and D.D. Dougherty. 2012. "Somatic therapies for treatment-resistant depression: ECT, TMS, VNS, DBS." *Biol Mood Anxiety Disord* 2(1):14. doi: 10.1186/2045-5380-2-14.

3. Fisher Wallace Stimulator. 2015. "How It Works." Accessed February 3, 2015. http://www.fisher-wallace.com.

4. Gabbard, Glen O., ed. 2007. *Gabbard's Treatments of Psychiatric Disorders.* 4th ed. 449–466. Washington, DC: American Psychiatric Publishing.

5. George, Mark S., Ziad Nahas, Daryl E. Bohning, Qiwen Mu, F. Andrew Kozel, Jeffrey Borckhardt, and Stewart Denslow. 2004. "Mechanisms of action of vagus nerve stimulation (VNS)." *Clinical Neuroscience Research* 4(1–2):71–79. doi: http://dx.doi.org/10.1016/j.cnr.2004.06.006.

6. Johns Hopkins Medicine. 2015. "Transcranial Direct Current Stimulation." Accessed March 12, 2015. http://www.hopkinsmedicine.org/psychiatry/specialty_areas/brain_stimulation/tdcs.html.

7. Lyons, Mark K. 2011. "Deep Brain Stimulation: Current and Future Clinical Applications." *Mayo Clinic Proceedings* 86(7):662–672. doi: 10.4065/mcp.2011.0045.

8. Mayo Clinic. 2015. "Deep Brain Stimulation." Accessed March 12, 2015. http://www.mayoclinic.org/tests-procedures/deep-brain-stimulation/basics/how-you-prepare/prc-20019122.

9. National Institutes of Mental Health (NIMH). 2015. "Brain Stimulation Therapies." Accessed January 14, 2015. http://www.nimh.nih.gov/health/topics/brain-stimulation-therapies/brain-stimulation-therapies.shtml.

10. Psychiatric Times. 2015. "The Rise of Cranial Electrotherapy." Accessed January 14, 2015. http://www.psychiatrictimes.com/electroconvulsive-therapy/rise-cranial-electrotherapy?cid=dlvr.it.

11. Schatzberg, A.F., and Charles B. Nemeroff, eds. 2009. *The American Psychiatric Publishing Textbook of Psychopharmacology.* 4th ed. 1097–1098. Washington, DC: American Psychiatric Publishing.

12. Schlaug, Gottfried, and Vijay Renga. 2008. "Transcranial direct current stimulation: a non-invasive tool to facilitate stroke recovery." *Expert review of medical devices* 5(6):759–768. doi: 10.1586/17434440.5.6.759.

13. YouTube. 2012. "Dr. Xenakis at FDA Hearing for CES." Accessed June 18, 2014. https://www.youtube.com/watch?v=dYjq_-HLVz4.

*Figures 20.1, 20.2, 20.3, and 20.4 are available via public domain from the NIMH at http://www.nimh.nih.gov/health/topics/brain-stimulation-therapies/brain-stimulation-therapies.shtml. Image 20.5 courtesy of Fisher Wallace Laboratories, www.FisherWallace.com.

Chapter 21
Dietary, Herbal, And OTC Medications In Psychiatry

Over the past two decades in the US, patients have increasingly sought complementary and alternative medicine (CAM) for various reasons, including the high cost of prescriptions, desire to use natural medications, and stigma associated with seeing a psychiatrist.[6,10] Recent surveys show that up to 40% of the US population uses alternative medication, with 9.8% doing so for psychiatric reasons.[3,6] In some countries, such as France and Germany, herbal medicine continues to coexist with modern pharmacology.[6] However, many herbal medications lack scientific evidence of efficacy, as they are considered dietary food supplements and are not subject to the same FDA standards as all prescription drugs.[9] Therefore, unless standardized, it is impossible to determine whether herbal supplements possess the actual quality, quantity, efficacy, or safety advertised by producers. Nevertheless, psychiatrists must be fairly knowledgeable about these alternatives and should propagate proper information to interested patient groups. Additionally, recommending a healthy diet may be more useful to patients than recommending vitamins and dietary and herbal supplements.[9]

Psychiatric disorders treated with alternative medication[2,3,5,6,7,8,9,10]

- *Cognitive disorders:* Ginkgo biloba, vitamin E
- *Anxiety, sleep problems:* Valerian, lavender, kava, melatonin
- *Depression, bipolar disorder:* St. John's wort, s-adenosylmethionine (SAMe), vitamin B, inositol, DHEA, omega-3 fatty acids
- *Psychosis:* Choices limited; rauwolfia, omega-3 fatty acids
- *Movement disorders:* Vitamin E, melatonin, ginkgo biloba
- *Addictions:* Valerian, passion flower, St. John's wort, kudzu, iboga

Clinical guidelines

- Remind patients that CAMs may not always be safe; some have dangerous side effects
- Educate patients about potential risks and interactions
- Seek specialist advice before using CAM in cases where the patient is a child, elderly, pregnant, or breastfeeding

Common CAMs

DHEA (Dehydroepiandrosterone)[4,7,8,9]
Generic name: DHEA
Brand name: DHEA generics only
FDA approved for: None

Other potential uses (off-label): Aging, Alzheimer's disease, erectile dysfunction, MDD, menopause

Dosage forms: *Cap* (25, 50 mg); *tab* (25, 50 mg); *chewing gum, SL drops* (5 mg/drop [600-drop bottle])

Dosage:

- Alzheimer's disease: 25–400 mg po qd
- Depression: 50–200 mg po qd
- Erectile dysfunction: 20–75 mg po qd
- Menopausal hot flashes: 10–50 mg po qd

MOA: Increases sex-hormones androgen and estrogen, which prompts an anti-aging effect

Warnings: Can decrease effectiveness of medications treating estrogen-sensitive cancers

Drug interactions:

- Can interfere with estrogen-lowering agents
- Increases toxicity of Halcion (triazolam)

Common side effects: Acne, hair loss, hirsutism, hypertension, liver dysfunction, palpitation, voice deepening (women)

Contraindications: Patients with hormone-sensitive conditions (e.g., endometriosis, fibroids, or breast, uterine, or ovarian cancer)

Recommended lab tests: LFTs

Tapering/withdrawal: Gradual taper recommended

Important notes:

- Moderately effective for osteoporosis and lupus

Folate and Vitamin B12[4,6,8,9]

Generic name: Folic acid (folate), cyanocobalamin (B12)

Brand name: Folate, FA-8, vitamin B12 generics, Folgard, Folgard RX, Folvite, others

FDA approved for: Various anemias

Other potential uses (off-label): Depression

Dosage forms:

- **Folic acid:** *Tab* (0.4, 0.8, 1 mg); *tab* (800 mcg);cap (5mg, 2000 mcg); *injection* (5 mg/ml)
- **B12:** *Tab* (25, 50, 100, 250, 500, 1000 mcg); *SL tab* (1000, 2500, 5000 mcg); *IM* (100, 1000 mcg/ml); *nasal spray:* (500 mcg/0.1 ml); *oral lozenge* (50, 250, 500, 1000 mcg)

Dosage:

- Folate: 800 mcg/day
- Oral B12: 500–1000 mcg bid

MOA: Major determinants of one-carbon metabolisms, playing a major role in mood regulation

Warnings: Severe allergy and angioedema reported with B12 injections

Drug interactions: Estrogen, barbiturates, anticonvulsants, cancer and antibiotic medications

Common side effects: Arthralgia, bad taste in mouth (folate), B12-injection-site pain, dizziness, headache; in large doses: confusion, irritability, loss of appetite, nausea

Contraindications: Hypersensitivity

Lab tests recommend: CBC

Overdose:

- Folate: skin rash, nausea, seizures
- B12: extremely uncommon; may cause pruritus, burning sensation, other tactile responses

Important notes:

- L-Methylfolate is a cofactor in the synthesis of monoamines
- Beneficial in people with deficiency (e.g., geriatrics, alcoholics, patients who have undergone gastric resection)
- Could be useful during pregnancy to reduce the risk of neural tube defects in offspring

Gingko[3,8,9,10]

Generic name: *Ginkgo biloba*

Brand name: Ginkgo biloba generics only

FDA approved for: None

Other potential uses (off-label): Age-related memory impairment, dementia, PMS,[9] SSRI-induced sexual dysfunction

Dosage forms: After refining/processing, gingko leaves are made into tablets, capsules and liquid solutions[9]

Dosage:

- Cognitive function: 120–600 mg po divided bid
- Dementia: 120–240 mg po divided bid–tid
- PMS: 80–320 mg po divided bid
- SSRI-induced sexual dysfunction: 60–240 mg po daily

MOA: Antioxidant which may increase 5-HT_{1A} receptors, α_2- and β-adrenergic receptors; increases acetylcholine, norepinephrine, serotonin, and endogenous nitric oxide[2]

Warnings:

- Avoid in patients with hypertension or clotting disorders
- Can prolong bleeding; avoid use before surgery

Drug interactions:
- May stimulate mania with antidepressants
- Avoid with anticoagulants due to inhibition of platelet-activating factors
- Can reduce effectiveness of anticonvulsants

Common side effects: Allergic reaction, bleeding, confusion, dizziness, GI issues, headache

Contraindications: Recent hemorrhage, blood clotting and platelet disorder

Recommended lab tests: Coagulation profile

Tapering/withdrawal: Gradual taper recommended

Important notes:
- Currently under investigation for prophylaxis of Alzheimer's dementia
- Top-selling herbal supplement in the US
- Likely helpful for mild-to-moderate cerebrovascular disease and peripheral vascular disease
- Possibly helpful for movement disorders, specifically in reducing TD

Inositol [4,8,9]

Generic name: Inositol, Myo-inositol

Brand name: Inositol, inositol nicotinate generics only

FDA approved for: Not approved

Other potential uses (off-label): Depression, OCD, panic disorder, PCOS

Dosage forms: *Tab* (650 mg); *cap* (500 mg); *powder* (454 g bottle)

Dosage:
- Varies—500 mg/day initially, can go up to 6–12 g/day based on tolerability/efficacy

MOA: Plays a role in how neurotransmitters work; possibly reverses desensitization of serotonin receptors and mediates effects of lithium and various antidepressants

Drug interactions: Fishy odor with inositol-lecithin combination

Common side effects: GI distress

Lab tests recommend: None

Tapering/withdrawal: Gradual taper recommended

Important notes:
- Inositol, is also known as vitamin B8, a natural isomer of glucose

Kava [3,5,8,9]

Generic name: Piper methysticum

Brand name: Kava generics only

FDA approved for: None

Other potential uses (off-label): Agitation, anxiety, sleep problems

Dosage forms: Available as fresh root, liquid, extract, capsule

Dosage:
- Anxiety disorders:
  - *Kava-lactones:* 75–150 mg/day po
  - *Root tea:* 1 cup po qd–tid, 2–4 g root/150 ml water
- Benzo withdrawal/prevention: 50 mg po qd initially, increase to max 300 mg/day over 1 week while tapering benzo over 2 weeks
- Insomnia: *Kava-lactones*—180–210 mg po qhs

MOA: Kava lactone acts as GABA agonist; may down-regulate β-adrenergic activity and act on limbic structures, promoting relaxation without sedation

Warnings: Can cause severe liver damage and toxicity

Drug interactions: Inhibits CYP2E1

Common side effects: Ataxia, euphoria, GI distress, headache, liver toxicity, sedation

Contraindications: Patients with preexisting liver disease

Recommended lab tests: LFTs

Overdose: Liver failure

Tapering/withdrawal: Gradual taper recommended; extended use may cause dependence

Important notes:
- Can cause severe hepatic toxicity; banned in several countries

Melatonin[6,8,9,10]

Generic name: Melatonin

Brand name: Melatonin generics

FDA approved for: Not approved

Other potential uses (off-label): Cancer, insomnia, jet lag, migraine

Dosage forms: *Cap, tab, SL tab, ER tab* (0.2, 0.3, 1, 3, 5, 10, 20 mg)

Dosage:
- Insomnia: 2.5–5mg hs, max 10 mg
- Jet Lag: 0.5–5 mg hs for 4 days

MOA: Hormone made by pineal gland at dark hours; aids resetting of circadian rhythm in sleep

Warnings: Severe sedation with alcohol

Drug interactions: Prednisone, CNS depressants, warfarin

Common side effects: Fatigue, GI distress, sedation, somnolence

Contraindications: None

Lab tests recommend: None

Overdose: Lethargy, drowsiness, agitation; OD rare

Important notes:
- Common hypnotic for children, especially those with ADHD

- Should be taken at early evening, not at bedtime

Omega-3 Fatty Acids[4,6,8,9,10]
Generic name: Omega-3 fatty acid
Brand name: Omega-3 fatty acid generics, Lovaza, Vascazen
FDA approved for: Lovaza approved for reducing very high triglycerides
Other potential uses (off-label): ADHD, bipolar disorder, dementia, depression
Dosage forms: *Cap* (1 g)
Dosage:
- Hypertriglyceridemia (Lovaza): 2–4 g daily
- Dietary supplement: 1–2 g tid with meals
- Depression: 1 g/day or 2 g/day divided bid
- Bipolar disorder: 9.6 g/day

MOA: May have similar signal-transduction impact to lithium, deficiency of some omega acids may be associated with bipolar disorder
Warnings:
- Use caution with preexisting liver disease, coagulation disorder, heart disease
- Can increase blood sugar levels

Drug interactions: Use caution with warfarin and other blood thinners
Common side effects: Belching, bloating, diarrhea, gas
Contraindications: Hypersensitivity, allergy to fish or soy
Recommended lab tests: LFTs, lipid panel, coagulation profile
Overdose: Increased risk of bleeding, high LDL level, blood-sugar control problem, increased HR
Tapering/withdrawal: No withdrawal symptoms
Important notes:
- The efficacy in treatment of depression is still debated
- Fish, plant, and nut oils are the primary dietary source of omega-3 fatty acids
- Found in cold water fish such as salmon, mackerel, halibut, sardines, tuna, and herring
- Recommended in conjunction with standard mood stabilizers
- May reduce negative side effects of antipsychotics (e.g., weight gain)

SAMe (S-Adenosylmethionine)[4,6,8,9,10]
Generic name: S-Adenosylmethionine
Brand name*:* S-Adenosylmethionine (SAMe) generics, AdoMet, Natrol
FDA approved for: None
Other potential uses (off-label): Depression, fibromyalgia, liver disease, osteoarthritis
Dosage forms: *Tab* (200, 400 mg)

Dosage:
- Depression: 400–1600 mg/day

MOA: Inhibits monoamine uptake, increases serotonin levels

Warnings: Can precipitate mania in susceptible patients

Drug interactions: Risk of serotonin syndrome with antidepressants, dextromethorphan, meperidine, pentazocine, tramadol

Common side effects: Anxiety, insomnia, nausea, tremors, vomiting

Contraindications: Bipolar disorder

Recommended lab tests: None

Tapering/withdrawal: Gradual taper recommended

Important notes:
- Good natural antidepressant for mild-to-moderate depression
- Augments effect of standard antidepressants
- Used mainly as nutrition supplement
- Considered safer option in nursing, especially for mothers with infants >2 months old
- Popular among patients with HIV due to relatively few side effects

St. John's Wort[1,3,6,8,9,10]

Generic name: Hypericum perforatum

Brand name: St. John's wort generics only

FDA approved for: None

Other potential uses (off-label): Mild-to-moderate depression, OCD, PMS

Dosage forms: Extracted from Hypericum perforatum; crude (1g/1ml); standardized (0.3% hypericin, 2–4.5% hyperforin)

Dosage:
- Depression (mild-to-moderate):
  - *Hypericin 0.3% standardized extract:* 300 mg po tid or 1800 mg po qd
  - *Crude:* 2–4 ml/day po, may be divided tid
- OCD:
  - *Hypericin 0.3% standardized extract (XR):* 450 mg po bid
- PMS:
  - *Hypericin 0.3% standardized extract:* 300 mg/day po

MOA: Resembles SSRIs (called "natural Prozac") but more complicated, contains multiple substances that may act on dopamine, norepinephrine, and GABA receptors

Warnings:
- May cause serotonin syndrome with other SSRIs
- May cause photosensitivity and rash in fair-skinned people
- Risk of organ rejection in patients who undergo organ transplant
- Can precipitate mania in bipolar patients

Drug interactions:
- Can increase sedative effect of drugs like benzos, barbiturates, alcohol
- Can decrease effects of some anticonvulsants, anticoagulants, oral contraceptives, HIV and cancer medications
- Increases expression of P-glycoprotein

Common side effects: Anxiety, fatigue, GI upset, photosensitivity, rash, restlessness
Contraindications: Pregnancy, lactation, schizophrenia, bipolar disorder
Recommended lab tests: None
Overdose: Rare
Tapering/withdrawal: Gradual taper recommended; sudden cessation can cause withdrawal symptoms
Important notes[9]:
- Popular first-line agent in Germany for treating mild anxiety and depression
- Discontinue at least 3 days before starting an SSRI

Valerian[3,6,8,9]
Generic name: Valeriana officinalis
Brand name: Valerian generics only
FDA approved for: None; food supplement classified GRAS (generally recognized as safe)
Other potential uses (off-label): Anxiety, insomnia
Dosage forms: Extracted from root of Valeriana officinalis, available in mixtures
Dosage:
- Insomnia: use for max 28 days
  - *Aqueous extract:* 400–900 mg po hs
  - *Ethanolic extract:* 600 mg po hs
  - *Root (fresh/dried):* 2–3 g po qd
  - *Combinations with hops/lemon balm:* 320–500 mg po hs

MOA: 5-HT and GABA receptor agonist, blocks reuptake of GABA and MAO
Warnings: Avoid in patients with liver disease or seizure disorders
Drug interactions:
- Potentiates effect of CNS depressants, such as benzos, alcohol, etc.
- Can interact with some anticoagulants, anticonvulsants, antifungals, OCP, HIV or cancer treatments

Common side effects: Confusion, dizziness, drowsiness, sedation, fatigue
Recommended lab tests: None
Overdose: Confusion, CNS depression
Tapering/withdrawal: Gradual taper recommended
Important notes:
- Improves insomnia by reducing sleep latency and increasing REM sleep[9]

References:

1. American Botanical Council (ABC). 2002. "St. John's Wort." *The ABC Clinical Guide to Herbs.* Accessed March 20, 2015. http://abc.herbalgram.org/site/DocServer/SJW.pdf?docID=168.

2. De La Barrera, Jaime. 2015. "Herbal Information." *Info Herb.* Accessed February 3, 2015. http://www.infoherb.com/sample-page.

3. Hicks, K. "Herbal Medicines." Ohio State University. Accessed February 3, 2015. https://osuwmc-digital.osu.edu/sitetool/sites/psychiatry2public/documents/psychiatry_documents/hicks.pdf.

4. Life Extension Vitamins. 2015. "Depression, Part 4 - Vitamins and Minerals to Fight Depression." Accessed March 20, 2015. http://www.lifeextensionvitamins.com/depa4viandmi.html.

5. Medscape: Drugs & Diseases. 2015. "Kava (Herbs/Suppl)." Accessed January 14 2015. http://reference.medscape.com/drug/ava-pepper-awa-kava-344543.

6. Preston, John D., and James Johnson. 2011. *Clinical Psychopharmacology Made Ridiculously Simple.* 7th ed. 57–60. Miami: MedMaster Inc.

7. Psychiatric Times. 2004. "DHEA Lessens Depressive Symptoms, NIMH Study Shows." Accessed March 20, 2015. http://www.psychiatrictimes.com/articles/dhea-lessens-depressive-symptoms-nimh-study-shows.

8. Royal College of Psychiatrists (RCPSYCH). 2015. "Complementary and Alternative Medicines 1." Accessed February 3, 2015. http://www.rcpsych.ac.uk/mentalhealthinfoforall/treatments/complementarytherapy.aspx#germ.

9. Schatzberg, A.F., Jonathan O. Cole, and Charles DeBattista. 2007. *Manual of Clinical Psychopharmacology.* 6th ed. 595–612. Washington, DC: American Psychiatric Publishing.

10. Wegmann, J. 2008. *Psychopharmacology: Straight Talk on Mental Health Medications.* 135–144. Eau Claire: Pesi, LLC.

Chapter 22
Future Advances In Mental Health

Mental health conditions exact a heavy human and economic toll. The NIMH estimates that 1 in 4 American adults—about 61.5 million people—have been diagnosed with a mental health disorder, costing the US more than $317 billion annually in lost wages, healthcare expenditures, and disability benefits.[9]

Given that one in five American adults now take at least one psychiatric drug, it is surprising that the global pharmaceutical industry has significantly decreased its investment in new treatments for psychiatric disorders—almost all industry research dollars are currently invested in cancer, metabolism, autoimmunity, or other diseases.[5] While mental-disorder research can be difficult, many new and promising medications and mechanisms are being explored to treat a variety of disorders. Although the development of new and effective treatments has been decelerating, but the emerging field of pharmacogenetics appears promising.[4] Pharmacogenetics involves the use of genetic testing to guide the delivery and administration of drugs. These tests can be utilized to predict an individual's treatment response, guiding medication choice, dosing, and assessing safety. Presumably, pharmacogenetics will lead to the development of personalized treatment plans through gene scanning, RNA fingerprinting, brain mapping, and brain imaging.[11,15] Genetic tests are available on the market today for many genotypes including: CYP2D6, CYP2C19, CYP3A4, ADRA2A, CYP1A2, CYP2B6, COMT, GRIK4, HTR2A, HTR2C, MTHFR, and SLC6A4/5-HTT.[4]

Identification of clinical biomarkers can be a useful strategy for finding newer medications to treat various psychiatric conditions. However, much work remains to be done: greater understanding of gene-environment interactions is needed, as is innovation in developing novel psychosocial therapies and preventative measures for people at high risk for psychiatric disorders.[9,10] Advancements in psychiatry, psychopharmacology, and neuroscience may eventually clarify the underlying pathology of mental disorders, eliminating much of the conjecture involved in choosing medications.[15]

Studies, Trials, and Newer Modalities

The process of developing and distributing new drugs is long and expensive process. According to a report by the Pharmaceutical Research and Manufacturers of America (PhRMA), it takes an average of $1.2 billion and 10–15 years for an experimental drug to advance from the lab to patients.[9] Only 5 in 5,000 compounds progress to human testing, and only one of those five will be approved for sale.[9,10]

Drug Trials

Drug trials proceed through a series of distinct phases established by the FDA.[10,13] These phases are as follows[12]:

- **Phase 0:** A compound is administered in an initial exploratory study carefully involving limited human exposure. No therapeutic or diagnostic goals are involved yet.
- **Phase 1:** Low doses of a compound are administered to a small group of healthy volunteers who are closely supervised to determine any frequent or serious adverse events and monitor how the drug is metabolized and excreted.
- **Phase 2:** This phase involves a larger number of trial participants (up to several hundred) who usually have the medical condition that the experimental therapy is intended to treat. The goal is to determine the efficacy of the proposed drug in the target population.
- **Phase 3:** The drug's safety and efficacy are examined in thousands of patients across multiple locations and populations before submitting it for approval to the FDA.
- **Phase 4:** This final step, post marketing studies, takes place after FDA approval of the drug. Post-marketing studies gather information about a drug's effect in various populations and any side effects associated with long-term use. Adverse drug effects in the US are usually obtained from voluntary reporting to the pharmaceutical company or to the FDA.

Future Medications

In 2014, a slight reduction in the amount of pharmaceutical company research on new psychotropic drugs entering the pipeline began. Nevertheless, US drug companies are currently developing 119 products for use in psychiatry.[9,10] Many of these potential treatments are listed in Table 22.1 below.

Table 22.1: Future Medications[2,8,9,10]

Drug name	Molecule/Mechanism	Use
Alzheimer's Disease (AD)		
AVP-923	Dextromethorphan hydrobromide and quinidine sulfate	Agitation in AD
Brexpiprazole	D_2 receptor partial agonist	Agitation in AD, ADHD, PTSD
ELND005	Inositol stereoisomer	Agitation and aggression in AD
Anxiety Disorders		
Aloradine nasal spray	Sensory receptor cell modulator	Social anxiety disorder (works within 15 min)
AVN-101	$5\text{-}HT_6$ receptor antagonist	Anxiety in AD
Bitopertin	Glycine transporter type 1 inhibitor	OCD
Ganaxolone	Modulates GABA through activation of $GABA_A$ receptors	Drug-resistant epilepsy, PTSD, other CNS disorders
Guanfacine ER	Selective α_{2A}-receptor agonist	Anxiety disorders
Nepicastat	Dopamine β-hydroxylase inhibitor	PTSD, substance abuse
ADHD		
SEP-225289 and EB-1020	Triple reuptake inhibitors	Once-daily treatment of ADHD
SPN-810	ER formulation of molindone	Impulsive aggression in ADHD
Brexpiprazole	D_2 receptor partial agonist	Adult ADHD, PTSD
Eltoprazine	$5\text{-}HT_{1A}$ and $5\text{-}HT_{1B}$ receptor agonist, $5\text{-}HT_{2C}$ receptor antagonist	Adult ADHD
SPN-812	Selective norepinephrine reuptake inhibitor	Adult ADHD
AR08	Adrenergic receptor agonist	ADHD
d-ATS	Dexamphetamine transdermal	ADHD
Edivoxetine	Selective norepinephrine reuptake inhibitor	ADHD

Drug name	Molecule/Mechanism	Use
NT0102	Methylphenidate XR-ODT	ADHD
Autism Spectrum Disorder (ASD)		
AT001	Fluoxetine rapid dissolve	ASD (fast track), depression
CNDO-201	Oral trichuris suis ova	ASD
RG7314	Vasopressin-1 receptor antagonist	ASD
Syntocinon nasal spray	Oxytocin	ASD, schizophrenia
Bipolar Disorder		
Cariprazine	D_2 and D_3 receptor partial agonist	Bipolar I disorder, MDD
Depression		
Esketamine intranasal	S-enantiomer of ketamine	Treatment-resistant depression (works within 10 min)
ALKS-5461	Buprenorphine and samidorphan	MDD augmentation
AZD6423	NMDA antagonist	Suicidal ideation
CERC-301	NR2B (GluN2B) antagonist	MDD adjunctive, suicidal ideation
Amitifadine	Triple reuptake inhibitor	MDD
Ademetionine (prescription)	S-adenosylmethionine (SAMe)	MDD
Armodafinil	Modafinil	Major depression in bipolar disorder, binge eating disorder
Botox	Onabotulinum toxin A	MDD
Brexpiprazole	D_2 receptor partial agonist	MDD, ADHD, schizophrenia
Cariprazine	D_2 and D_3 receptor partial agonist; atypical antipsychotic	MDD, bipolar depression
GLYX-13	Selective weak partial agonist of glycine site of NMDA receptor	MDD
HT-2157	Glutamate receptor antagonist	MDD

Drug name	Molecule/Mechanism	Use
Mifepristone	Progesterone and glucocorticoid receptor antagonist	MDD with psychosis
MIN-117	$5\text{-}HT_{1A}$/5-HTT receptor antagonist	MDD
RG1578	mGluR2 antagonist	MDD adjunctive
RG7090	mGluR5 antagonist	Treatment-resistant depression
R04995819	K_{ATP} channel opener	MDD
Tedatioxetine	Triple reuptake inhibitor, also antagonizes $5\text{-}HT_{2A}$, $5\text{-}HT_{2C}$, $5\text{-}HT_3$ and α_{1A}-adrenergic receptors	MDD
Viibryd	Vilazodone	MDD (children, adolescents), GAD
Schizophrenia		
ITI-214	PDE1 inhibitor	Cognitive impairment associated with schizophrenia
OMS824	PDE10 inhibitor	Schizophrenia
PF-02545920	PDE10 inhibitor	Schizophrenia, Huntington's disease
ABT-126	Alpha-7 NNR antagonist	Cognitive impairment associated with schizophrenia
AQW051	Alpha-7 nicotinic acetylcholine receptor agonist	Cognitive impairment associated with schizophrenia
Encenicline	Alpha-7 nicotinic acetylcholine receptor partial agonist	Cognitive impairment associated with schizophrenia
AVN-211	$5\text{-}HT_6$ receptor antagonist	Schizophrenia
ALKS 9072	Aripiprazole lauroxil	Schizophrenia
Bitopertin	GlyT1 inhibitor	Schizophrenia
Brexpiprazole	D_2 receptor partial agonist	Schizophrenia, MDD, ADHD
ADX71149/JNJ-40411813	mGluR2 PAM modulator	Schizophrenia

Drug name	Molecule/Mechanism	Use
ALKS 3831	Olanzapine/samidorphan fixed-dose combination	Schizophrenia
ITI-007	5-HT_{2A} receptor antagonist	Schizophrenia
MIN-101	5-HT_{2A}, 1 and sigma-2 receptor antagonist	Schizophrenia
Pimavanserin	Inverse agonist of serotonin	Parkinson's disease/AD psychosis
RBP-7000	Long-acting formulation of risperidone via SC injection, D_2, 5-HT_2 antagonist	Schizophrenia
RP5063	Partial agonist of D_2, D_3 and D_4 receptors and 5-HT_{1A} and 5-HT_{2A} receptors, antagonist of 5-HT_6 and 5-HT_7 receptors	Schizophrenia
Syntocinon nasal spray	Oxytocin based	Schizophrenia, ASD
Zicronapine	Antagonist at D_1, D_2, and 5-HT_{2A} receptors	Schizophrenia, psychosis
Substance abuse		
TA-CD	Cocaine vaccine	Cocaine
SYN117	DOPAMINE β-HYDROXYLASE INHIBITOR	Cocaine dependence
RBP-8000	Cocaine esterase	Cocaine intoxication
TV-1380	Form of human plasma butyrylcholinesterase	Cocaine dependence
MN-166	PD-4 inhibitor	Methamphetamine dependence
AD01	Ondansetron/topiramate	Alcohol use disorder
AD04	Low-dose ondansetron	Alcohol use disorder
LY2940094	Nocioceptin-1 antagonist	Alcohol dependence
Naloxone nasal spray	Opioid antagonist	Opioid overdose
Lofexidine	α_{2A}-adrenergic receptor agonist	Opioid withdrawal
RBP-6000	Buprenorphine depot	Opioid dependence
OMS405	PPAR gamma agonist	Opioid use disorder, nicotine withdrawal

Drug name	Molecule/Mechanism	Use
Others		
AZD5213	H$_3$ receptor antagonist	Tourette syndrome
Ecopipam	Selective D$_1$/D$_5$ receptor antagonist	Tourette syndrome
Armodafinil	Modafinil	Binge eating disorder, depression
LDX	Lisdexamfetamine	Binge eating disorder
PH80-PMD	Synthetic peptide	PMDD, PMS

The Future of Mental Health

Advancements in technology, an inexhaustible agglomeration of information available on the internet, the unprecedented opportunity of social networking, and commendable legislation conjointly provide the impetus for psychiatry to embark upon its voyage into the future.

Recent advancements in legislation such as the Affordable Care Act (2010) and the Mental Health Parity and Addiction Equity Act (2008) provide an opportunity to increase general access to mental health care. The implementation of these laws is an important step towards exterminating the stigma associated with many forms of psychiatric illness, as mental health conditions are now lawfully treated on par with medical conditions.[3]

The Internet has revolutionized in the way in which patients select their physicians, as word-of-mouth recommendations have been steadily replaced by online search engines and web reviews as trusted resources for researching physicians. Optimizing the accessibility and efficiency of a practice's website is vital to the success of clinicians and other healthcare professionals. Physicians can also take advantage of social-networking websites to communicate with their patients, peers, and community. For example, *doximity.com* allows healthcare professionals to connect with each other by providing physician-only forums for discussion. *Zocdoc.com* offers prospective patients access to nearby healthcare providers, screens physicians based on their availability and accepted forms of insurance, and even allows patients to book an appointment immediately. Patients are also asked to rate aspects of their experience such as the physician's knowledge, office wait time, and bedside manner, as well as provide any additional comments. Patients are also able to rate their providers on websites such as *healthgrades.com, rateMDs.com, vitals.com*, and others.

Smartphone apps have brought in an unparalleled opportunity for their usage in cognitive training or "brain training," which has grown steadily in popularity and gained substantial attention in mental health research.[6] By taking advantage of the brain's natural plasticity, cognitive training exercises can enhance intelligence via the global domains of cognitive function, such as memory, attention, processing speed, etc.[6] Popular cognitive training programs include *Lumosity*, *Cognitive Fit*, *Posit Science*, and *Train Your Brain*.

Telepsychiatry is another great example of the consortium of technology with psychiatry. This advancement involves the delivery of psychiatric assessment and care through telecommunications technology, usually videoconferencing.[14] This method is transforming the way that clinicians see clients, as it allows patients in remote or under-served areas to receive psychiatric services.[1] By treating patients at home, telepsychiatry may be a practical, inexpensive, and user-friendly modality.[1]

All of the aforementioned advancements are reassuring to the future of mental health. Due to this plethora of newer enterprises, the highlight of which is the BRAIN Initiative (a gallant step by the NIH), the day when clinicians will be able to utilize personalized medicine, identify genetic risk factors for psychiatric disorders, and develop better objective diagnostic tests, genetic markers, and novel medications is not too far off.[7] Politicians, academics, corporations, and the public working in unison can help to eradicate the stigma surrounding psychiatric treatment and improve care for all individuals suffering from mental health disorders.

References:

1.   American Psychiatric Association (APA). 2015. "Telepsychiatry." Accessed March 20, 2015. http://www.psychiatry.org/practice/professional-interests/underserved-communities/telepsychiatry.

2.   Center Watch. 2015. "FDA Approved Drugs by Therapeutic Area." Accessed February 3, 2015. http://www.centerwatch.com/drug-information/fda-approved-drugs/therapeutic-area/17/psychiatry-psychology.

3.   Community Preventive Services Task Force. 2015. "Recommendation for Mental Health Benefits Legislation." *American Journal of Preventive Medicine.* 48(6):767–770.

4.   Genelex. 2014. "Clinically Actionable Pharmacogenetic Tests." Accessed January 15, 2015. http://genelex.com/pharmacogenetic-tests/.

5.   Hyman, S. 2013. "Psychiatric Drug Development: Diagnosing a Crisis." Accessed April 10, 2015. http://www.dana.org/Cerebrum/Default.aspx?id=39489.

6.   Kueider, Alexandra M., Jeanine M. Parisi, Alden L. Gross, and George W. Rebok. 2012. "Computerized Cognitive Training with Older Adults: A Systematic Review." *PLoS ONE* 7(7):e40588. doi: http://journals.plos.org/plosone/article?id=10.1371/journal.pone.0040588.

7. National Institutes of Health (NIH). 2014. "The Brain Initiative." Accessed February 10, 2015. http://www.braininitiative.nih.gov/nih-brain-awards.htm.

8. National Institute of Mental Health (NIMH). 2015. "Statistics." Accessed April 10, 2015. http://www.nimh.nih.gov/health/statistics/index.shtml.

9. Pharmaceutical Research and Manufacturers of America (PhRMA). 2014. "Mental Health Medicines in Development Report, 2014." Accessed January 12, 2014. http://www.phrma.org/mental-health-medicines-in-development-report-2014.

10. Pharmaceutical Research and Manufacturers of America (PhRMA). 2015. "Selected Medicines in Development for Mental Illness." Accessed February 3, 2015. http://www.phrma.org/research/selected-medicines-development-mental-illness.

11. Sinclair, L. 2014. "Med Check." *Psychiatric News*. Accessed February 3, 2015. http://psychnews.psychiatryonline.org/doi/full/10.1176/pn.47.7.psychnews_47_7_26-a.

12. Stahl, S.M. 2008. *Essential Psychopharmacology: Neuroscientific Basis and Practical Applications*. 3rd ed. 223–246. New York: Cambridge Press.

13. US National Institutes of Health (NIH). 2015. "Glossary Definition: Phase." Accessed March 20, 2015. https://clinicaltrials.gov/ct2/help/glossary/phase.

14. Wang, Lidong, and Cheryl Ann Alexander. 2014. "Telepsychiatry: Technology Progress, Challenges, and Language and Transcultural Issues." *Journal of Translational Medicine and Developmental Disorders* 1(1):1–11.

15. Wegmann, J. 2008. *Psychopharmacology: Straight Talk on Mental Health Medications*. 145–148. Eau Claire: Pesi, LLC.

Appendix A
Helpful Resources

Books/Guides:
- *Handbook of Psychiatric Drugs,* 2011 Edition
  Lawrence J. Albers, Rhoda K. Hahn, and Christopher Reist
- *Diagnostic and Statistical Manual of Mental Disorders*, Fifth Edition (DSM-5®)
  American Psychiatric Association (APA)
- *Gabbard's Treatments of Psychiatric Disorders,* Fourth Edition
  Glen O. Gabbard, ed.
- *The American Psychiatric Publishing Textbook of Psychiatry,* Sixth Edition
  Robert. E. Hales, S. Yudofsky, and L. Roberts, eds.
- *Clinical Psychopharmacology Made Ridiculously Simple,* Seventh Edition
  John D. Preston and James Johnson
- *Condensed Psychopharmacology 2013: A Pocket Reference for Psychiatry and Psychotropic Medications*
  Leonard Rappa and James Viola
- *The American Psychiatric Publishing Textbook of Psychopharmacology,* Fourth Edition
  Alan F. Schatzberg and Charles B. Nemeroff, eds.
- *Manual of Clinical Psychopharmacology,* Seventh Edition
  Alan F. Schatzberg, Jonathan O. Cole, and Charles DeBattista
- *Essential Psychopharmacology: Neuroscientific Basis and Practical Applications,* Third Edition
  Stephen M. Stahl
- *Essential Psychopharmacology: the Prescriber's Guide,* Fourth Edition
  Stephen M. Stahl
- *Psychopharmacology: Straight Talk on Mental Health Medications*
  Joseph Wegmann

Databases/Websites
- Centers for Disease Control and Prevention (CDC): http://www.cdc.gov.
- Center Watch, FDA Approved Drugs by Therapeutic Area: http://www.centerwatch.com/drug-information/fda-approved-drugs/therapeutic-area/17/psychiatry-psychology.
- Elsevier Gold Standard, Inc, Clinical Pharmacology: https://www.clinicalpharmacology.com.
- Epocrates: https://online.epocrates.com.

- Medscape, Psychiatry and Mental Health: http://www.medscape.com/psychiatry.
- Medscape Drugs & Diseases, Psychiatrics: http://reference.medscape.com/drugs/psychiatrics.
- National Alliance on Mental Illness (NAMI): https://www.nami.org.
- National Institute of Diabetes and Digestive and Kidney Diseases, Livertox Database: http://livertox.nih.gov/index.html.
- National Institute of Mental Health (NIMH): http://www.nimh.nih.gov.
- RxList, Drugs A-Z List: http://www.rxlist.com/drugs/alpha_a.htm.
- Substance Abuse and Mental Health Services Administration (SAMHSA): http://www.samhsa.gov.
- Truven Health Analytics, Micromedex 2.0: http://www.micromedexsolutions.com/home/dispatch.
- UpToDate: http://www.uptodate.com/home.
- US Food and Drug Administration (FDA): http://www.fda.gov.
- US National Library of Medicine, Daily Med: http://dailymed.nlm.nih.gov.
- US National Library of Medicine, Drugs and Lactation Database (LactMed): http://toxnet.nlm.nih.gov/newtoxnet/lactmed.htm.
- US National Library of Medicine, Toxicology Data Network: http://toxnet.nlm.nih.gov.

Appendix B
Medical/Psychiatric Abbreviations

AA	Alcoholics Anonymous	CAM	Complimentary and Alternative Medicine
AC	Before Meals		
ACH	Acetylcholine	CAP	Capsule
ACHE	Acetylcholinesterase	CBC	Complete Blood Count
AD	Alzheimer's Disease	CBT	Cognitive Behavior Therapy
ADD	Attention Deficit Disorder		
ADHD	Attention Deficit Hyperactivity Disorder	CD	Controlled Dose
		CDC	Centers for Disease Control and Prevention
AIDS	Acquired Immune Deficiency Syndrome		
		CES	Cranial Electrotherapy Stimulation
AIMS	Abnormal Involuntary Movement Scale		
		CHF	Congestive Heart Failure
AM	Before Noon	CMP	Comprehensive Metabolic Panel
ANC	Absolute Neutrophil Count		
		CNS	Central Nervous System
APA	American Psychiatric Association	CONC	Concentrate
		COPD	Chronic Obstructive Pulmonary Disease
APA	American Psychological Association		
		CPAP	Continuous Positive Airway Pressure
APPROX	Approximately		
AS	Autism Spectrum	CPT	(Physician's) Current Procedural Terminology
ASD	Autism Spectrum Disorder		
AV	Atrioventricular	CR	Controlled Release
AZT	Azidothymidine	CYP	Cytochrome P450
BARB	Barbiturate	D/C, DISC	Discontinue or Discharge
BDNF	Brain-Derived Neurotrophic Factor	DA, D	Dopamine
		DAWN	Drug Abuse Warning Network
BENZO(S)	Benzodiazepine(s)		
BID	Twice Daily	DBS	Deep Brain Stimulation
BMI	Body Mass Index	DBT	Dialectical Behavioral Therapy
BP	Blood Pressure		
BP-1	Bipolar Type 1	DHEA	Dehydroepiandrosterone
BPD	Borderline Personality Disorder	DKA	Diabetic Ketoacidosis
		DM	Diabetes Mellitus
BUN	Blood Urea Nitrogen	DMT	Dimethyltryptamine

DNA	Deoxyribonucleic Acid	FGA	First Generation
DOM	2,5-Dimethoxy-4-		Antipsychotic
	Methylamphetamine	G	Gram
DR	Delayed Release	GABA	Gamma Amino Butyric
DRESS	Drug Reaction with		Acid
	Eosinophilia and Systemic	GAD	Generalized Anxiety
	Symptoms		Disorder
DSM	Diagnostic and Statistical	GAF	Global Assessment of
	Manual of Mental		Functioning
	Disorders	GERD	Gastroesophageal Reflux
DSM-IV(-TR)	Diagnostic and Statistical		Disease
	Manual of Mental	GI	Gastrointestinal
	Disorders, 4th Edition (-	GRAS	Generally Recognized As
	Text Revision)		Safe
DSM-5	Diagnostic and Statistical	GU	Genitourinary
	Manual of Mental	HDL	High-density lipoprotein
	Disorders, 5th Edition	HS	At Bedtime
DT	Delirium Tremens	HG	Mercury
DX	Diagnosis	HIV	Human
ECA	Epidemiological		Immunodeficiency Virus
	Catchment Area	HR	Heart Rate, Hour
ECT	Electroconvulsive Therapy	HRS	Hours
EEG	Electroencephalogram	HSR	Hypersensitivity Reaction
EKG	Electrocardiogram	HTN	Hypertension
EMDR	Eye Movement	IBD	Inflammatory Bowel
	Desensitization and		Disease
	Reprocessing	IBS	Irritable Bowel Syndrome
EPS	Extra Pyramidal Symptom	ICD	International
ER	Emergency Room,		Classification of Diseases
	Extended Release	ICP	Intracranial Pressure
ET	And	ICU	Intensive Care Unit
ETO	Emergency Treatment	IM	Intramuscular
	Order	INR	International Normalized
ETOH	Ethanol		Ratio
FDA	(US) Food and Drug	IOP	Intraocular Pressure
	Administration	IPT	Interpersonal Therapy
FEAT	Focal Electrical	IR	Immediate Release
	Alternating Current	IV	Intravenous
	Therapy	KG	Kilogram
		L	Liter

LA	Long Acting	NIH	National Institutes of Health
LDH	Lactate Dehydrogenase		
LDL	Low-Density Lipoprotein	NIMH	National Institute of Mental Health
LIQ	Liquid		
LFT	Liver Function Test	NMDA	N-Methyl-D-Aspartate
LSD	Lysergic Acid Diethylamide	NMS	Neuroleptic Malignant Syndrome
MAO	Monoamine Oxidase	NRT	Nicotine Replacement Therapy
MAOI	Monoamine Oxidase Inhibitor	NSAID	Non-Steroidal Anti-Inflammatory Drug
MAX	Maximum		
MCG	Microgram	NRI	Norepinephrine Reuptake Inhibitors
MDA	3,4-Methylene-dioxyamphetamine	OCD	Obsessive-Compulsive Disorder
MDD	Major Depressive Disorder		
MDMA	Methylene Dioxymethamphetamine	OCP	Oral Contraceptive Pill
		OD	Overdose
MEQ	Milliequivalent	ODT	Orally Disintegrating Tablet
MET	Motivational Enhancement Therapy	OSA	Obstructive Sleep Apnea
MG	Milligram	OTC	Over the Counter
MI	Myocardial Infarction	OZ	Ounce
ML	Milliliter	PCOS	Polycystic Ovary Syndrome
MMSE	Mini Mental State Examination	PCP	Phencyclidine
MOA	Mechanism of Action	PDD	Pervasive Developmental Disorder
MRI	Magnetic Resonance Imaging	PDE	Phosphodiesterase
MS	Metabolic Syndrome	PDMP	Prescription Drug Monitoring Program
MSE	Mental Status Exam		
MST	Magnetic Seizure Therapy	PET	Positron Emission Tomography
MT	Melatonin		
NAMI	National Alliance for Mental Illness	PFT	Pulmonary Function Test
		PM	Afternoon
NAS	Neonatal Abstinence Syndrome	PMDD	Premenstrual Dysphoric Disorder
NCD	Neurocognitive disorder/disease	PPHN	Persistent Pulmonary Hypertension
NG	Nanogram	PO	By Mouth, Orally

PRN	As Needed	SJS	Stevens-Johnson Syndrome
PT	Prothrombin Time	SL	Sublingually, Under the
PTSD	Posttraumatic Stress		Tongue
	Disorder	SNP	Single Nucleotide
PVD	Peripheral Vascular		Polymorphism
	Disease	SNRI	Serotonin Norepinephrine
Q	Every, Per		Reuptake Inhibitor
QAM	Every Day before Noon	SOL	Solution
QD	Every Day	SQ, SUBQ	Subcutaneous
QHS	Every Night at Bedtime	SR	Sustained Release
QID	Four Times a Day	SSRI	Selective Serotonin
QPM	Every Day after Noon or		Reuptake Inhibitor
	Every Evening	STAT	Immediately
QTC	Corrected QT interval	SX	Symptoms
QWK	Every Week	T, TAB	Tablet
REM	Rapid Eye Movement	TBI	Traumatic Brain Injury
REMS	Risk Evaluation and	TCA	Tricyclic Antidepressant
	Mitigation Strategy	TD	Tardive Dyskinesia
RFT	Renal Function Test	TDCS	Trans-Cranial Direct
RIS	Risperidone		Current Stimulation
RLS	Restless Leg Syndrome	TEN	Toxic Epidermal
RTMS	Repetitive Transcranial		Necrolysis
	Magnetic Stimulation	TF-CBT	Trauma-Focused
RX	Prescription		Cognitive Behavioral
SA	Sinoatrial		Therapy
SAD	Seasonal Affective	TIA	Transient Ischemic Attack
	Disorder	TID	Three Times Daily
SAMHSA	Substance Abuse and	TMAX	Time to Maximum Plasma
	Mental Health Services		Concentration
	Administration	TMS	Transcranial Magnetic
SARI	Serotonin Antagonist and		Stimulation
	Reuptake Inhibitor	TSF	12-Step Facilitation
SC, SUBC	Subcutaneous	TSH	Thyroid Stimulating
S/E	Side Effects		Hormone
SEC	Seconds	TRH	Thyroid Releasing
SGA	Second Generation		Hormone
	Antipsychotic	T1/2	Half-Life
SIADH	Syndrome of Inappropriate	T3	Triiodothyronine
	Antidiuretic Hormone	URTI	Upper Respiratory Tract
	Secretion		Infection

VNS	Vagus Nerve Stimulator	X	Times
VPA	Valproic Acid	XR	Extended Release
W/O	Without	YRS	Years
WBC	White Blood Cell	α	Alpha
WHO	World Health Organization	β	Beta
		5-HT	Serotonin

References:

1. Illinois Department of Human Services. 2014. "Review of Psychotropic Drugs, 2014 Key." Accessed February 3, 2015. https://www.dhs.state.il.us/OneNetLibrary/27896/documents/By_Division/Division%20of%20DD/HumanRights/PsychotropicDrugsList.pdf.

2. Rappa, Leonard, and James Viola. 2012. "Condensed Psychopharmacology 2013: A Pocket Reference for Psychiatry and Psychotropic Medications. 1–5. RXPSYCH, LLC.

3. Texas Education Agency. 2012. "Psychiatric Terminology." Accessed February 13, 2015. http://cte.unt.edu/content/files/_HS/documents/curriculum/med_terminology/psychiatric.pdf.

4. Vermont Department of Mental Health. 2015. "Acronyms & Abbreviations." Accessed January 13, 2015. http://mentalhealth.vermont.gov/acronym.

Index

About the Author

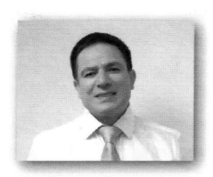

Tanveer A. Padder, MD is an award-winning psychiatrist certified by the American Board of Psychiatry and Neurology, American Board of Addiction Medicine and holds additional certification from the American Board of Clinical Psychopharmacology. He is a preeminent expert in psychopharmacology and has been awarded a Master Psychopharmacologist certification by Dr. Stahl's Neuroscience Education Institute.

A highly sought-after psychiatrist, Dr. Padder is a leading expert in mood, anxiety, substance abuse, and psychotic disorders. He is currently the medical director of two mental health clinics in Maryland, where he is actively involved in treating complex patient populations. He authored *Organized Wisdom Bipolar 101 & 102* and has published extensively in national and international medical and psychiatric journals.

Dr. Padder has distinguished himself as a very talented psychiatrist, as evidenced by his impressive academic and clinical track record. He graduated medical school with honors and was the best outgoing graduate. His compassionate approach to serving mental health patients has garnered him numerous local and national awards, including 2010 and 2011 directory of America's Top Psychiatrists, provided by the Consumer Federation of America.

In his own words, he believes his greatest achievements are, "the smiles I have been able to bring, the difference I have been able to make, and the comfort I have been able to provide to the lives of people who have little or no voice and are suffering silently."

Dr. Padder lives in Maryland with his wife and three children.

Made in the USA
San Bernardino, CA
05 December 2016